Comprehensive Pharmacy Review for NAPLEX

Practice Exams, Cases, and Test Prep

Eighth Edition

Comprehensive Pharmacy Review for NAPLEX

Practice Exams, Cases, and Test Prep

Eighth Edition

EDITORS

Alan H. Mutnick, PharmD, FASHP, RPh

Corporate Director, Clinical Services
Catholic Health Partners
Cincinnati, Ohio

Paul F. Souney, MS, RPh

Vice President
Medical Affairs and Pharmacotherapy Management
Medical Outcomes Management, Inc.
Sharon, Massachusetts

Larry N. Swanson, PharmD, FASHP, RPh

Professor and Chairman
Department of Pharmacy Practice
Campbell University College of Pharmacy and Health Sciences
Buies Creek, North Carolina

Leon Shargel, PhD, RPh

President
Applied Biopharmaceutics
Raleigh, North Carolina

Affiliate Associate Professor
Department of Pharmaceutics
School of Pharmacy
Virginia Commonwealth University
Richmond, Virginia

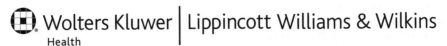

Wolters Kluwer | Lippincott Williams & Wilkins
Health

Philadelphia • Baltimore • New York • London
Buenos Aires • Hong Kong • Sydney • Tokyo

Acquisitions Editor: Sirkka Howes
Product Manager: Michael Marino
Marketing Manager: Joy Fisher Williams
Design Coordinator: Teresa Mallon
Production Services: Absolute Service, Inc.

Eighth Edition
Copyright © 2013, 2010, 2007, 2004, 2001 by Lippincott Williams & Wilkins, a Wolters Kluwer business.

351 West Camden Street   Two Commerce Square
Baltimore, MD 21201   2001 Market Street
                            Philadelphia, PA 19103

Printed in China

9 8 7 6 5 4 3 2 1

Library of Congress Cataloging-in-Publication Data

Comprehensive pharmacy review for NAPLEX : practice exams, case studies and test prep / editors, Alan H. Mutnick ... [et al.]. — 8th ed.
   p. ; cm.
 Rev. ed. of: Comprehensive pharmacy review practice exams / editors, Alan H. Mutnick ... [et al.]. 7th ed. c2010.
 Companion to Comprehensive pharmacy review for NAPLEX / editors, Leon Shargel ... [et al.]. 8th ed. c2013.
  ISBN 978-1-4511-1987-9 (pbk.)
 I. Mutnick, Alan H. II. Comprehensive pharmacy review practice exams. III. Comprehensive pharmacy review for NAPLEX.
 [DNLM: 1. Pharmacy—Examination Questions. QV 18.2]

 615.1076—dc23

                                                                2012023402

DISCLAIMER
        Care has been taken to confirm the accuracy of the information present and to describe generally accepted practices. However, the authors, editors, and publisher are not responsible for errors or omissions or for any consequences from application of the information in this book and make no warranty, expressed or implied, with respect to the currency, completeness, or accuracy of the contents of the publication. Application of this information in a particular situation remains the professional responsibility of the practitioner; the clinical treatments described and recommended may not be considered absolute and universal recommendations.
        The authors, editors, and publisher have exerted every effort to ensure that drug selection and dosage set forth in this text are in accordance with the current recommendations and practice at the time of publication. However, in view of ongoing research, changes in government regulations, and the constant flow of information relating to drug therapy and drug reactions, the reader is urged to check the package insert for each drug for any change in indications and dosage and for added warnings and precautions. This is particularly important when the recommended agent is a new or infrequently employed drug.
        Some drugs and medical devices presented in this publication have Food and Drug Administration (FDA) clearance for limited use in restricted research settings. It is the responsibility of the health care provider to ascertain the FDA status of each drug or device planned for use in their clinical practice.
        To purchase additional copies of this book, call our customer service department at **(800) 638-3030** or fax orders to **(301) 223-2320**. International customers should call **(301) 223-2300**.
        Visit Lippincott Williams & Wilkins on the Internet: http://www.lww.com. Lippincott Williams & Wilkins customer service representatives are available from 8:30 a.m. to 6:00 p.m., EST.

Contents

Preface

This practice exam book is a companion to *Comprehensive Pharmacy Review*. Whereas *Comprehensive Pharmacy Review* presents most of the subjects in the pharmacy curriculum in outline form with review questions interspersed, this booklet offers two examinations that are similar in format and coverage to those in the licensing examination required of all pharmacists.

Both patient profile–based and free-standing test items are included in the examinations. The questions are of two general types. In the first type (Example 1), the correct response most accurately completes a statement or answers a question. In the second type (Example 2), three statements are given. The correct answer may include one, two, or all three of these statements; these questions are to be answered according to the direction block that accompanies them.

EXAMPLE 1 (MULTIPLE-CHOICE)

Drugs that demonstrate nonlinear pharmacokinetics show which of the following properties?

A. A constant ratio of drug metabolites is formed as the administered dose increases.
B. The elimination half-life increases as the administered dose is increased.
C. The area under the curve (AUC) increases in direct proportion to an increase in the administered dose.
D. Both low and high doses follow first-order elimination kinetics.
E. The steady-state drug concentration increases in direct proportion to the dosing rate.

EXAMPLE 2 (MULTIPLE TRUE–FALSE)

Antimuscarinic agents are used in the treatment of Parkinson disease and in the control of some neuroleptic-induced extrapyramidal disorders. These agents include which of the following?

I. ipratropium
II. benztropine
III. trihexyphenidyl

I only
III only
I and II
II and III
I, II, and III

Allow a maximum of 4 hours for each examination. Answers, with explanations, are given at the end of each test. Additional cases, questions, and calculations exercises are included following the two practice tests. Also, several appendices are included at the back of the book for reference.

Contributors

Connie Lee Barnes, PharmD
Professor
Director, Drug Information Center
Department of Pharmacy Practice
Campbell University College of Pharmacy and Health Sciences
Buies Creek, North Carolina

Brooke Bernhardt, PharmD, BCOP
Clinical Pharmacy Specialist, Hematology/Oncology
Texas Children's Hospital
Houston, Texas

K. Paige D. Brown, PharmD
Assistant Director of Experiential Education
Assistant Professor of Pharmacy Practice
Campbell University College of Pharmacy and Health Sciences
Buies Creek, North Carolina

Todd A. Brown, MHP, RPh
Clinical Instructor and Vice Chair
Department of Pharmacy Practice
Bouve College of Health Sciences School of Pharmacy
Northeastern University
Boston, Massachusetts

Marcia L. Buck, PharmD, FCCP, FPPAG
Clinical Pharmacy Coordinator, Children's Hospital
Associate Professor, Pediatrics
School of Medicine
Clinical Associate Professor
School of Nursing
University of Virginia Health System, Department of Pharmacy
    Services
Charlottesville, Virginia

Dean S. Collier, PharmD, BCPS
Assistant Professor
Department of Pharmacy Practice
University of Nebraska Medical Center
Clinical Pharmacist
Department of Pharmacy Practice
The Nebraska Medical Center
Omaha, Nebraska

Robert B. Greenwood, RPh, PhD
Associate Dean of Academic Affairs
Professor of Pharmaceutical Sciences
Campbell University College of Pharmacy and Health Sciences
Buies Creek, North Carolina

James B. Groce III, PharmD, CACP
Professor, Department of Pharmacy Practice
Campbell University College of Pharmacy and Health Sciences
Clinical Assistant Professor of Medicine, Department of Medicine
University of North Carolina School of Medicine
Clinical Pharmacy Specialist—Anticoagulation
Department of Pharmacy
Cone Health
Greensboro, North Carolina

Terri S. Hamrick, PhD
Associate Professor
Department of Pharmaceutical Sciences
College of Pharmacy and Health Sciences
Campbell University
Buies Creek, North Carolina

Julie J. Kelsey, PharmD
Clinical Pharmacy Specialist
Women's Health and Family Medicine
Department of Pharmacy Services
University of Virginia Health System
Charlottesville, Virginia

D. Byron May, PharmD, BCPS
Professor
Department of Pharmacy Practice
Campbell University College of Pharmacy and Health Sciences
Buies Creek, North Carolina
Clinical Specialist in Adult Internal Medicine
Department of Pharmacy
Duke University Hospital
Durham, North Carolina

Alan H. Mutnick, PharmD, FASHP, RPh
Corporate Director/Clinical Services
Catholic Health Partners
Cincinnati, Ohio

Andrew J. Muzyk, PharmD
Assistant Professor
Department of Pharmacy Practice
Campbell University College of Pharmacy and Health Sciences
Buies Creek, North Carolina
Clinical Pharmacy Specialist
Department of Pharmacy
Duke University Hospital
Durham, North Carolina

Roy A. Pleasants II, PharmD
Associate Professor
Department of Pharmacy Practice
Campbell University College of Pharmacy and Health Sciences
Buies Creek, North Carolina
Clinical Assistant Professor
Division of Pulmonary Medicine
Duke University School of Medicine
Durham, North Carolina

Robert A. Quercia, MS, RPh
Editor and Co-Coordinator of Focus Column Formulary Journal
Medical Editor, University of Connecticut/Hartford Hospital
Evidenced-based Practice Center
Hartford, Connecticut
Adjunct Associate Clinical Professor
University of Connecticut School of Pharmacy
Storrs, Connecticut

Gerald E. Schumacher, PharmD, MS, PhD
Professor of Pharmacy, Emeritus
Bouve College of Health Sciences School of Pharmacy
Northeastern University
Boston, Massachusetts

Jennifer D. Smith, PharmD, CPP, BC-ADM, CDE, C-TTS
Associate Professor
Department of Pharmacy Practice
Campbell University College of Pharmacy and Health Sciences
Buies Creek, North Carolina
Clinical Pharmacist Practitioner
Wilson Community Health Center
Wilson, North Carolina

Paul F. Souney, RPh, MS
Vice President
Medical Affairs and Pharmacotherapy Management
Medical Outcomes Management, Inc.
Sharon, Massachusetts

Linda M. Spooner, PharmD, BCPS with Added Qualifications in Infectious Diseases
Associate Professor of Pharmacy Practice
Department of Pharmacy Practice
Massachusetts College of Pharmacy and Health Sciences
School of Pharmacy-Worcester/Manchester
Worcester, Massachusetts
Clinical Pharmacy Specialist in Infectious Diseases
Department of Pharmacy
Saint Vincent Hospital
Worcester, Massachusetts

Gilbert A. Steiner, PharmD
Associate Professor
Department of Pharmacy Practice
Campbell University College of Pharmacy and Health Sciences
Buies Creek, North Carolina

Larry N. Swanson, PharmD, FASHP, RPh
Professor and Chairman
Department of Pharmacy Practice
Campbell University College of Pharmacy & Health Sciences
Buies Creek, North Carolina

Ryan S. Swanson, PharmD, RPh
Clinical Pharmacist
Kerr Drug
Fuquay-Varina, North Carolina

Heather A. Sweeney, PharmD, RPh
Clinical Manager
Pharmaceutical Distribution
Cardinal Health
Cincinnati, Ohio

Tina Harrison Thornhill, PharmD, FASCP, CGP
Associate Professor
Department of Pharmacy Practice
Campbell University College of Pharmacy and Health Sciences
Buies Creek, North Carolina
Clinical Specialist, Geriatrics and Acute Rehabilitation
Wake Forest Baptist Health
The Sticht Center on Aging and Rehabilitation
Winston-Salem, North Carolina

Jenny A. Van Amburgh, BS Pharm, PharmD, FAPhA, BCACP, CDE
Associate Clinical Professor & Assistant Dean of Academic Affairs
School of Pharmacy
Northeastern University
Boston, Massachusetts
Director of Clinical Pharmacy Services & Residency Program
    Director
Harbor Health Services, Inc.
Dorchester, Massachusetts

Anthony E. Zimmermann, BS, PharmD
Professor and Chair
Department of Pharmacy Practice
College of Pharmacy
Western New England University
Springfield, Massachusetts

Taking a Test

One of the least attractive aspects of pursuing an education is the necessity of being examined on the material that has been presented. Instructors do not like to prepare tests, and students do not like to take them.

However, students are required to take many examinations during their learning careers, and little if any time is spent acquainting them with the positive aspects of tests and with systematic and successful methods for approaching them. Students perceive tests as punitive and sometimes feel as if they were merely opportunities for the instructor to discover what the student has forgotten or has never learned. Students need to view tests as opportunities to display their knowledge and to use them as tools for developing prescriptions for further study and learning.

While preparing for any exam, class and board exams as well as practice exams, it is important that students learn as much as they can about the subject they will be tested and are prepared to discover just how much they may not know. Students should study to acquire knowledge, not just to prepare for tests. For the well-prepared student, the chances of passing far exceed the chances of failing.

MATERIALS NEEDED FOR TEST PREPARATION

In preparing for a test, most students collect far too much study material, only to find that they simply do not have time to go through all of it. They are defeated before they begin because either they cannot get through all the material, leaving areas unstudied, or they race through the material so quickly that they cannot benefit from the activity.

It is generally more efficient for the student to use materials already at hand—that is, class notes, one good outline to cover and strengthen all areas and to quickly review the whole topic, and one good text as a reference for complex material that requires further explanation.

Also, many students attempt to memorize far too much information, rather than learning and understanding less material and then relying on that learned information to determine the answers to questions at the time of the examination. Relying too heavily on memorized material causes anxiety, and the more anxious students become during a test, the less learned knowledge they are likely to use.

ATTITUDE AND APPROACH

A positive attitude and a realistic approach are essential to successful test taking. If the student concentrates on the negative aspects of tests or on the potential for failure, anxiety increases and performance decreases. A negative attitude generally develops if the student concentrates on "I must pass" rather than on "I can pass." "What if I fail?" becomes the major factor motivating the student to run from failure rather than toward success. This results from placing too much emphasis on scores. The score received is only one aspect of test performance. Test performance also indicates the student's ability to use differential reasoning.

In each question with five alternatives, of which one is correct, there are four alternatives that are incorrect. If deductive reasoning is used, the choices can be viewed as having possibilities of being correct. The elimination of wrong choices increases the odds that a student will be able to recognize the correct choice. Even if the correct choice does not become evident, the probability of guessing correctly increases. Eliminating incorrect choices on a test can result in choosing the correct answer.

Answering questions based on what is incorrect is difficult for many students because they have had nearly 20 years of experience taking tests with the implied assertion that knowledge can be displayed only by knowing what is correct. It must be remembered, however, that students can display knowledge by knowing something is wrong, just as they can display it by knowing something is right.

PREPARING FOR THE EXAMINATION

1. **Study for yourself.** Although some of the material may seem irrelevant, the more you learn now, the less you will have to learn later. Also, do not let the fear of the test rob you of an important part of your education. If you study

to learn, the task is less distasteful than studying solely to pass a test.

2. **Review all areas.** You should not be selective by studying perceived weak areas and ignoring perceived strong areas. Cover all of the material, putting added emphasis on weak areas.

3. **Attempt to understand, not just to memorize, the material.** Ask yourself: To whom does the material apply? When does it apply? Where does it apply? How does it apply? Understanding the connections among these points allows for longer retention and aids in those situations when guessing strategies may be needed.

4. **Try to anticipate questions that might appear on the test.** Ask yourself how you might construct a question on a specific topic.

5. **Give yourself a couple days of rest before the test.** Studying up to the last moment will increase your anxiety and cause potential confusion.

TAKING THE EXAMINATION

1. Be sure to pace yourself to use the test time optimally. You should use all of your allotted time; if you finish too early, you probably did so by moving too quickly through the test.

2. Read each question and all the alternatives carefully before you begin to make decisions. Remember, the questions contain clues, as do the answer choices.

3. Read the directions for each question set carefully. You would be amazed at how many students make mistakes in tests simply because they have not paid close attention to the directions.

4. It is not advisable to leave blanks with the intention of coming back to answer questions later. If you feel that you must come back to a question, mark the best choice and place a note in the margin. Generally speaking, it is best not to change answers once you have made a decision. Your considered reaction and first response are correct more often than are changes made out of frustration or anxiety.

5. Do not let anxiety destroy your confidence. If you have prepared conscientiously, you know enough to pass. Use all that you have learned.

6. Do not try to determine how well you are doing as you proceed. You will not be able to make an objective assessment, and your anxiety will increase.

7. Do not become frustrated or angry about what appear to be bad or difficult questions. You simply do not know the answers; you cannot know everything.

SPECIFIC TEST-TAKING STRATEGIES

Read the entire question carefully, regardless of format. Test questions have multiple parts. Concentrate on picking out the pertinent key words that will help you problem-solve. Words such as *always, all, never, mostly, primarily,* and so forth play significant roles. In all types of questions, distractors with terms such as *always* or *never* most often are incorrect. Adjectives and adverbs can completely change the meaning of questions—pay close attention to them. The knowledge and application of grammar often are key to dissecting questions.

Multiple-Choice Questions

Read the question and the choices carefully to become familiar with the data provided. Remember, in multiple-choice questions there is one correct answer and there are four distractors, or incorrect answers. (Distractors are plausible and possibly correct, or they would not be called distractors.) They are generally correct for part of the question but not for the entire question. Dissecting the question into parts helps eliminate distractors.

Many students think that they must always start at option A and make a decision before they move to B, thus forcing decisions they are not ready to make. Your first decisions should be made on those choices you feel the most confident about.

Compare the choices with each part of the question. To be wrong, a choice needs to be incorrect for only part of the question. To be correct, it must be totally correct. If you believe a choice is partially incorrect, tentatively eliminate that choice. Make notes next to the choices regarding tentative decisions. One method is to place a minus sign next to the choices you are certain are incorrect and a plus sign next to those that potentially are correct. Finally, place a zero next to any choice you do not understand or need to come back to for further inspection. Do not feel that you must make final decisions until you have examined all choices carefully.

When you have eliminated as many choices as you can, decide which of those that remain has the highest probability of being correct. Above all, be honest with yourself. If you do not know the answer, eliminate as many choices as possible and choose reasonably.

Multiple-Choice True-False Questions

Multiple-choice questions are not as difficult as some students make them. There are two general types of multiple-choice questions including (1) the more traditional single answer type question in which the candidate must decide one of five choices (a, b, c, d, or e) and (2) the combined response ("K" type) multiple-choice question which is shown below. In this case, these are the questions for which you must select from the following choices:

A if **only I** is correct
B if **only III** is correct
C if **I and II** are correct
D if **II and III** are correct
E if **I, II, and III** are correct

Remember that the name for this type of question is *multiple true–false,* and then use this concept. Become familiar with each choice, and make notes. Then concentrate on the one choice you feel is definitely incorrect. If you can find one incorrect alternative, you can eliminate three choices immediately and be down to a 50/50 probability of guessing the correct answer. If choice A is incorrect, so are C and E; if choice B is incorrect, so are choices D and E. Therefore, you are down to a 50/50 probability of guessing the correct answer.

After eliminating the choices you are sure are incorrect, concentrate on the choice that will make your final decision. For instance, if you discard choice I, you have eliminated alternatives A, C, and E. This leaves B (III) and D (II and III). Concentrate on choice II, and decide if it is true or false. (Take the path of least resistance and concentrate on the smallest possible number of items while making a decision.) Obviously, if none of the choices is found to be incorrect, the answer is E (I, II, III).

Guessing

Nothing takes the place of a firm knowledge base, but having little information to work with, you may find it necessary to guess at the correct answer. A few simple rules can help increase your guessing accuracy. Always guess consistently if you have no idea what is correct—that is, after eliminating all that you can, make the choice that agrees with your intuition or choose the option closest to the top of the list that has not been eliminated as a potential answer.

When guessing at questions that present with choices in numeric form, you will often find the choices listed in an ascending or descending order. It is generally not wise to guess the first or last alternative because these are usually extreme values and are most likely incorrect.

USING A PRACTICE EXAM TO LEARN

All too often, students do not take full advantage of practice exams. There is a tendency to complete the exam, score it, look up the correct answer to those questions missed, and then forget the entire thing.

In fact, great educational benefits could be derived if students would spend more time using practice tests as learning tools. As mentioned previously, incorrect choices in test questions are plausible and partially correct, or they would not fulfill their purpose as distractors. This means that it is just as beneficial to look up the incorrect choices as the correct choices to discover specifically why they are incorrect. In this way, it is possible to learn better test-taking skills as the subtlety of question construction is uncovered.

In addition, it is advisable to go back and attempt to restructure each question to see if all the choices can be made correct by modifying the question. By doing this, you will learn four times as much. By all means, look up the right answer and explanation. Then, focus on each of the other choices, and ask yourself under what conditions, if any, they might be correct.

SUMMARY

Ideally, examinations are designed to determine how much material students have learned and how that material is used in the successful completion of the examination. Students will be successful if these suggestions are followed:

- Develop a positive attitude, and maintain that attitude.
- Be realistic in determining the amount of material you attempt to master and in the score you hope to attain.
- Read the directions for each type of question and the questions themselves closely, and follow the directions carefully.
- Bring differential reasoning to each question in the examination.
- Guess intelligently and consistently when guessing strategies must be used.
- Use the test as an opportunity to display your knowledge and as a tool for developing prescriptions for further study and learning.

Board examinations are not easy. They may be almost impossible for those who have unrealistic expectations or for those who allow misinformation concerning the exams to produce anxiety out of proportion to the task at hand. Examinations are manageable if they are approached with a positive attitude and with consistent use of all of the information the student has learned.

Michael J. O'Donnell

Introduction to the NAPLEX

After graduation from an accredited pharmacy program, the prospective pharmacist must demonstrate the competency to practice pharmacy. The standards of competence for the practice of pharmacy are set by each state board of pharmacy. NAPLEX—The North American Pharmacist Licensure Examination—is the principal instrument used by the state board of pharmacy to assess the knowledge and proficiency necessary for a candidate to practice pharmacy. The National Association of Boards of Pharmacy (NABP) is an independent, international, and impartial association that assists member boards and jurisdictions in developing, implementing, and enforcing uniform standards for the purpose of protecting the public health. NABP develops examinations that enable boards of pharmacy to assess the competence of candidates seeking licensure to practice pharmacy. Each state board of pharmacy may impose additional examinations. The two major examinations developed by NABP are

- The North American Pharmacist Licensure Examination (NAPLEX)
- Multistate Pharmacy Jurisprudence Examination (MPJE)

Foreign pharmacy graduates must pass the Foreign Pharmacy Graduate Equivalency Examination (FPGEE) as part of the Foreign Pharmacy Graduate Equivalency Certification process. Foreign-educated pharmacists awarded FPGEC Certification are considered to have partially fulfilled eligibility requirements for licensure in those states that accept the certification.

A description of these computerized examinations and registration information may be found on the NABP website online at www.nabp.net. Before submitting registration materials, the pharmacy candidate should contact the board of pharmacy for additional information regarding procedures, deadline dates, and required documentation.

The NAPLEX is a computer-adaptive test. These questions measure *the prospective pharmacist's ability to measure pharmacotherapy and therapeutic outcomes, prepare and dispense medications, and implement and evaluate information for optimal health care*. The computer adaptive exam tests a candidate's knowledge and ability by assessing the answers before presenting the next test question. If the answer is correct, the computer will select a more difficult question from the test item pool in an appropriate content area; if the answer is incorrect, an easier question will be selected by the computer. The NAPLEX score is based on the difficulty level of the questions answered correctly.

NAPLEX consists of 185 multiple-choice test questions. 150 questions are used to calculate the test score. The remaining 35 items served as pretest questions and do not affect the NAPLEX score. Pretest questions are administered to evaluate the item's difficulty level for possible inclusion as a scored question in future exams. These pretest questions are dispersed throughout the exam and cannot be identified by the candidate. A majority of the questions on the NAPLEX are asked in a scenario-based format (i.e., patient profiles with accompanying test questions). To properly analyze and answer the questions presented, the candidate must refer to the information provided in the patient profile. Some questions appear in a standalone format and should be answered solely from the information provided in the question.

NAPLEX Blueprint

THE NAPLEX COMPETENCY STATEMENTS

All NAPLEX questions are based on competency statements that are reviewed and revised periodically. The NAPLEX Competency Statements describe the knowledge, judgment, and skills that the candidate is expected to demonstrate as an entry-level pharmacist. A complete description of the NAPLEX Competency Statements is published on the NABP website and is reproduced, with permission of NABP. A strong understanding of the Competency Statements will aid in your preparation to take the examination.

Area 1: Assess Pharmacotherapy to Assure Safe and Effective Therapeutic Outcomes (Approximately 56% of Test)

1.1.0 Identify, interpret, and evaluate patient information to determine the presence of a disease or medical condition, assess the need for treatment and/or referral, and identify patient-specific factors that affect health, pharmacotherapy, and/or disease management.

1.1.1 Identify and assess patient information including medication, laboratory, and disease state histories.

1.1.2 Identify patient specific assessment and diagnostic methods, instruments, and techniques and interpret their results.

1.1.3 Identify and define the etiology, terminology, signs, and symptoms associated with diseases and medical conditions and their causes and determine if medical referral is necessary.

1.1.4 Identify and evaluate patient genetic, and biosocial factors, and concurrent drug therapy, relevant to the maintenance of wellness and the prevention or treatment of a disease or medical condition.

1.2.0 Evaluate information about pharmacoeconomic factors, dosing regimen, dosage forms, delivery systems and routes of administration to identify and select optimal pharmacotherapeutic agents, for patients

1.2.1 Identify specific uses and indications for drug products and recommend drugs of choice for specific diseases or medical conditions.

1.2.2 Identify the chemical/pharmacologic classes of therapeutic agents and describe their known or postulated sites and mechanisms of action.

1.2.3 Evaluate drug therapy for the presence of pharmacotherapeutic duplications and interactions with other drugs, food, and diagnostic tests.

1.2.4 Identify and evaluate potential contraindications and provide information about warnings and precautions associated with a drug product's active and inactive ingredients.

1.2.5 Identify physicochemical properties of drug substances that affect their solubility, pharmacodynamic and pharmacokinetic properties, pharmacologic actions, and stability.

1.2.6 Evaluate and interpret pharmacodynamic and pharmacokinetic principles to calculate and determine appropriate drug dosing regimens.

1.2.7 Identify appropriate routes of administration, dosage forms, and pharmaceutical characteristics of drug dosage forms and delivery systems, to assure bioavailability and enhance therapeutic efficacy.

1.3.0 Evaluate and manage drug regimens by monitoring and assessing the patient and/or patient information, collaborating with other health care professionals, and providing patient education to enhance safe, effective, and economic patient outcomes.

1.3.1 Identify pharmacotherapeutic outcomes and endpoints.

1.3.2 Evaluate patient signs and symptoms, and the findings of monitoring tests and procedures to determine the safety and effectiveness of pharmacotherapy. Recommend needed followup evaluations or tests when appropriate.

1.3.3 Identify, describe, and provide information regarding the mechanism of adverse reactions, allergies, side effects, iatrogenic, and drug-induced illness, including their management and prevention.

1.3.4 Identify, prevent, and address methods to remedy medication non-adherence, misuse, or abuse.

1.3.5 Evaluate current drug regimens and recommend pharmacotherapeutic alternatives or modifications.

Area 2: Assess Safe and Accurate Preparation and Dispensing of Medications (Approximately 33% of Test)

2.1.0 Demonstrate the ability to perform calculations required to compound, dispense, and administer medication.

2.1.1 Calculate the quantity of medication to be compounded or dispensed; reduce and enlarge formulation quantities and calculate the quantity or ingredients needed to compound the proper amount of the preparation.

2.1.2 Calculate nutritional needs and the caloric content of nutrient sources.

2.1.3 Calculate the rate of drug administration.

2.1.4 Calculate or convert drug concentrations, ratio strengths, and/or extent of ionization.

2.2.0 Demonstrate the ability to select and dispense medications in a manner that promotes safe and effective use.

2.2.1 Identify drug products by their generic, brand, and/or common names.

2.2.2 Identify whether a particular drug dosage strength or dosage form is commercially available and whether it is available on a nonprescription basis.

2.2.3 Identify commercially available drug products by their characteristic physical attributes.

2.2.4 Assess pharmacokinetic parameters and quality assurance data to determine equivalence among manufactured drug products, and identify products for which documented evidence of inequivalence exists.

2.2.5 Identify and provide information regarding appropriate packaging, storage, handling, administration, and disposal of medications.

2.2.6 Identify and provide information regarding the appropriate use of equipment and apparatus required to administer medications.

2.3.0 Demonstrate the knowledge to prepare and compound extemporaneous preparations and sterile products.

2.3.1 Identify techniques, procedures, and equipment related to drug preparation, compounding, and quality assurance.

2.3.2 Identify the important physicochemical properties of a preparation's active and inactive ingredients.

2.3.3 Identify the mechanism of and evidence for the incompatibility or degradation of a product or preparation and methods for achieving its stability.

Area 3: Assess, Recommend, and Provide Health care Information that Promotes Public Health (Approximately 11% of Test)

3.1.0 Identify, evaluate, and apply information to promote optimal health care.

3.1.1 Identify the typical content of specific sources of drug and health information for both health care providers and consumers, and recommend appropriate resources to address questions or needs.

3.1.2 Evaluate the suitability, accuracy, and reliability of clinical and pharmacoeconomic data by analyzing experimental design, statistical tests, interpreting results, and formulating conclusions.

3.2.0 Recommend and provide information to educate the public and healthcare professionals regarding medical conditions, wellness, dietary supplements, and medical devices.

3.2.1 Recommend and provide health care information regarding the prevention and treatment of diseases and medical conditions, including emergency patient care and vaccinations.

3.2.2 Recommend and provide health care information regarding nutrition, lifestyle, and other non-drug measures that promote health or prevent the progression of a disease or medical condition.

3.2.3 Recommend and provide information regarding the documented uses, adverse effects, and toxicities of dietary supplements.

3.2.4 Recommend and provide information regarding the selection, use, and care of medical/surgical appliances and devices, self-care products, and durable medical equipment, as well as products and techniques for self-monitoring of health status and medical conditions.

NABP offers candidates who are preparing for the NAPLEX the Pre-NAPLEX, which is similar to the actual NAPLEX, and allows candidates to gain experience in answering questions before examination day. The Pre-NAPLEX can be accessed via the Internet at the following website: www.nabp.net/prenaplex/. For foreign pharmacy graduates, the FPGEE Study Guide is available from NABP and includes information about the blueprint of the FPGEE, sample questions, and a list of textbooks commonly used in United States pharmacy schools.

Use the patient profile below to answer questions 1 to 10.

MEDICATION PROFILE (COMMUNITY)

Patient Name: Rachel Honors
Address: 5 Duke Dog Ln.
Age: 55   Height: 5′4″
Sex: F   Race: Caucasian   Weight: 140 lb   BP: 162/104 (9/22)
Allergies: No known drug allergies

DIAGNOSIS

Primary   (1)   Status post-STEMI, 9/15
Secondary   (1)   Hypertension
             (2)   Hypercholesterolemia
             (3)   GERD

MEDICATION RECORD (Prescription and OTC)

	Date	Rx No.	Physician	Drug and Strength	Quan	Sig	Refills
(1)	7/20	12233	Johnsie	Gemfibrozil 600 mg	60	i tab bid 30 min before breakfast and dinner	6
(2)	7/20	12234	Johnsie	Simvastatin 40 mg	30	i tab hs	6
(3)	7/20	12235	Johnsie	Hydrochlorothiazide 25 mg	30	i tab A.M.	6
(4)	7/20	12236	Johnsie	Aspirin 81 mg	100	i tab A.M.	3
(5)	8/21	14001	Johnsie	Doxazosin 2 mg	30	i tab A.M.	6
(6)	8/21	14002	Johnsie	Ramipril 5 mg	30	i tab A.M.	6
(7)	8/29	15005	Colon	Rabeprazole 20 mg	30	i tab A.M.	0
(8)	9/22	16500	Johnsie	Clopidogrel 75 mg	30	i tab A.M.	6
(9)	9/22	16501	Johnsie	Metoprolol 100 mg	60	i tab bid	6
(10)	9/22	16502	Johnsie	Nitroglycerin 0.4 mg	100	as directed	6

PHARMACIST NOTES AND OTHER PATIENT INFORMATION

	Date	Comments
(1)	7/20	New patient with new Rxs.
(2)	7/20	Contacted physician regarding potential problem with the current prescriptions.
(3)	7/20	Physician agreed with suggestion and acknowledged the oversight.
(4)	7/20	One medication was discontinued based on the recommendation to Dr. Johnsie.

(5)   8/21   Contacted physician regarding new prescriptions received, based on findings from the ALLHAT study; however, Dr. Johnsie disagreed with suggestion to delete either of the prescriptions.

(6)   8/21   Patient instructed on proper technique to take blood pressure daily at the same time, before taking morning medications, and to make sure prescriptions are refilled promptly each month.

(7)   9/22   Updated patient medication profile to reflect current medications.

(8)   9/22   Contacted Dr. Johnsie to reiterate findings from ALLHAT study, and this time he agreed to discontinue the medication.

1. Which medications prompted the pharmacist to call Dr. Johnsie on 7/20 owing to potential problems?

   I.   gemfibrozil
   II. simvastatin
   III. hydrochlorothiazide

   A. I only
   B. III only
   C. I and II
   D. II and III
   E. I, II, and III

2. Based on the ALLHAT study, which of the prescriptions written by Dr. Johnsie on 8/21 was the pharmacist hoping to have discontinued due to its potential negative effects in a hypertensive patient like Ms. Honors?

   I.   doxazosin
   II. ramipril
   III. hydrochlorothiazide

   A. I only
   B. III only
   C. I and II
   D. II and III
   E. I, II, and III

3. The seventh report of the Joint National Committee (JNC-7) guidelines for the treatment of hypertension include "compelling" indications that recommend the use of select drug therapies. Which of the following represent examples of compelling indications and their suggested therapy?

   I.   heart failure (diuretics, β-blockers, angiotensin-converting enzyme [ACE] inhibitors)
   II. chronic kidney disease (ACE inhibitors, angiotensin II receptor blockers [ARBs])
   III. recurrent stroke prevention (diuretics, ACE inhibitors)

   A. I only
   B. III only
   C. I and II
   D. II and III
   E. I, II, and III

4. Which of the following statements would justify the prescription written on 9/22 for metoprolol for Ms. Honors?

   I.   treatment of hypertension in a patient who is post–myocardial infarction (MI) as a compelling indication
   II. prevention of sudden death in a post-MI patient
   III. secondary prevention of stroke

   A. I only
   B. III only
   C. I and II
   D. II and III
   E. I, II, and III

5. Which of the following agents, assuming no contra-indications for use, was likely to have been given to Ms. Honors upon arrival to the hospital for the treatment of ST-segment elevated myocardial infarction (STEMI), assuming she arrived for treatment within 12 hours of her symptoms?

   I. alteplase (recombinant tissue-type plasminogen activator [rt-PA])
   II. reteplase (recombinant plasminogen activator [r-PA])
   III. tenecteplase (TNKase)

   A. I only
   B. III only
   C. I and II
   D. II and III
   E. I, II, and III

6. After her heart attack, Ms. Honors presents with a prescription for clopidogrel. What is the indication for clopidogrel in this patient?

   I. used in the prevention of arrhythmias
   II. used in hypertensive patients who have a compelling indication
   III. used in the prevention of acute coronary syndromes

   A. I only
   B. III only
   C. I and II
   D. II and III
   E. I, II, and III

7. Ms. Honors is receiving rabeprazole for which of the following indications?

   A. post-MI for prevention of sudden death
   B. gastroesophageal reflux disease (GERD)
   C. hypercholesterolemia
   D. hypertension
   E. none of the above

8. Which of the following patient information items should be addressed when Ms. Honors receives the nitroglycerin prescription?

   I. The tablet should be dissolved under the tongue only if the patient has difficulty swallowing.
   II. The tablets should be placed in an easy-to-open plastic container for future use.
   III. The tablets should be taken for an acute angina attack or before an activity that might induce an attack (i.e., strenuous exercise, anxiety).

   A. I only
   B. III only
   C. I and II
   D. II and III
   E. I, II, and III

9. Based on JNC-7 guidelines and the antihypertensive therapy being prescribed, which of the following best describes Ms. Honors' blood pressure classification?

   A. prehypertension
   B. stage I hypertension
   C. stage II hypertension
   D. stage III hypertension
   E. malignant hypertension

10. Based on Ms. Honors' patient profile, which of the following medications should be used cautiously, if at all?

   I. acetaminophen
   II. ibuprofen
   III. celecoxib

   A. I only
   B. III only
   C. I and II
   D. II and III
   E. I, II, and III

End of this patient profile; continue with the examination.

11. Untreated hypertension can result in which of the following types of target organ damage?

   I. renal
   II. cerebral
   III. retinal

   A. I only
   B. III only
   C. I and II
   D. II and III
   E. I, II, and III

12. Which of the following agents would *not* be considered a first-line antihypertensive agent in an otherwise healthy patient with stage I hypertension?

   A. amiloride
   B. chlorthalidone
   C. chlorothiazide
   D. indapamide
   E. hydrochlorothiazide

13. Parenteral products, such as half-normal saline solution, with an osmotic pressure less than that of blood are referred to as:

    A. isotonic solutions.
    B. hypotonic solutions.
    C. hypertonic solutions.
    D. isoosmotic solutions.
    E. neutral solutions.

14. Epoetin α (Epogen) is used in chronic kidney disease to treat:

    A. peripheral neuropathy.
    B. anemia.
    C. hyperphosphatemia.
    D. metabolic alkalosis.
    E. hyperuricemia.

15. Which of the following statements apply to insulin resistance?

    I. Insulin resistance occurs only in type 1 diabetes.
    II. Patients with insulin resistance may present with abdominal obesity, acanthosis nigricans, and polycystic ovarian syndrome.
    III. Insulin resistance can be treated successfully with appropriate drug therapy.

    A. I only
    B. III only
    C. I and II
    D. II and III
    E. I, II, and III

16. Lanolin

    I. is a natural product obtained from the wool of sheep.
    II. is used as an emollient thereby preventing water loss.
    III. is a water-soluble base containing propylene glycol or polyethylene glycol, which increases evaporation.

    A. I only
    B. III only
    C. I and II
    D. II and III
    E. I, II, and III

17. Which pair of OTC agents below has been shown to be safe and effective for the treatment of acute nonspecific diarrhea?

    A. bismuth subsalicylate and loperamide
    B. kaolin and pectin
    C. attapulgite and pectin
    D. loperamide and attapulgite
    E. attapulgite and bismuth subsalicylate

18. Which of the following statements about carbidopa/levodopa is/are true?

    I. Levodopa crosses the blood–brain barrier.
    II. Carbidopa does not cross the blood–brain barrier.
    III. Carbidopa inhibits the peripheral conversion of levodopa to dopamine.

    A. I only
    B. III only
    C. I and II
    D. II and III
    E. I, II, and III

19. Conditions that might predispose a patient to toxicity from a highly protein-bound drug include which of the following?

    I. hypoalbuminemia
    II. hepatic disease
    III. malnutrition

    A. I only
    B. III only
    C. I and II
    D. II and III
    E. I, II, and III

20. The mechanism of action of salmeterol is that of a:

    A. sympathomimetic agonist with high β_2 selectivity.
    B. sympathomimetic agonist with high β_1 selectivity.
    C. sympathomimetic antagonist with high β_2 selectivity.
    D. sympathomimetic antagonist with high β_1 selectivity.
    E. leukotriene receptor antagonist.

Use the patient profile below to answer questions 21 to 32.

MEDICATION PROFILE (COMMUNITY)

Patient Name: Alan Mutrick
Address: 5 Cinnamon Terrace
Age: 54   Height: 5′9″
Sex: M   Race: White   Weight: 175 lb
Allergies: No known allergies

DIAGNOSIS

Primary	(1)	Hypertension (9/10)
	(2)	Heart failure (8/10)
Secondary	(1)	Anemia (8/10)
	(2)	Chronic kidney disease (8/10)

MEDICATION RECORD (Prescription and OTC)

	Date	Rx No.	Physician	Drug and Strength	Quan	Sig	Refills
(1)	6/15	110555	Davis	Prednisone 10 mg	60	i bid	2
(2)	8/10	111002	Davis	Ferrous sulfate 325 mg	100	i tid	6
(3)	8/10	111003	Wonders	Lanoxin 0.25 mg	30	i q A.M.	6
(4)	8/10	111004	Wonders	Lasix 40 mg	30	i q A.M.	3
(5)	8/10	111005	Wonders	Slow-K 600 mg	90	i tid	3
(6)	9/10	113001	Wonders	Vasotec 5 mg	30	i qd	3
(7)	9/10	113002	Wonders	Hydrochlorothiazide 50 mg	30	i bid	3
(8)	9/10	113002	Wonders	Isordil 40 mg	120	i qid	3
(9)	9/10	113003	Wonders	Hydralazine 50 mg	60	i bid	3
(10)	12/1	200001	Wonders	Coreg 3.125 mg	30	i bid	0
(11)	12/1	200002	Wonders	Altace 2.5 mg	30	i q A.M.	0
(12)	12/15	200604	Wonders	Coreg 6.25 mg	30	i bid	0
(13)	1/2	201003	Wonders	Altace 5.0 mg	30	i q A.M.	3
(14)	1/2	201004	Wonders	Coreg 12.5 mg	60	i bid	0
(15)	1/16	203010	Wonders	Altace 10 mg	30	i q A.M.	6

PHARMACIST NOTES AND OTHER PATIENT INFORMATION

	Date	Comments
(1)	8/10	Pharmacist on duty contacted Dr. Wonders regarding the prescriptions just received with a question regarding one of the prescriptions; Slow-K is DC'd.
(2)	9/10	Patient presents with new prescriptions and tells pharmacist that Dr. Wonders wanted him to stop taking the Lanoxin.
(3)	9/10	Pharmacist contacted Dr. Wonders with questions about several of the prescriptions in patient profile as well as new prescriptions presented to pharmacy.
(4)	9/10	DC Lasix.
(5)	9/10	DC Lanoxin.
(6)	12/1	DC Isordil 40 mg, hydralazine 50 mg, and Vasotec 5 mg.
(7)	12/15	Pharmacist contacted Dr. Wonders regarding Coreg prescription initially filled on 12/1 and received requested verbal prescription.
(8)	1/2	Contacted Dr. Wonders regarding indication for increase in Altace prescription.

21. Based on the medication profile presented on 8/10, which of the following describe potential causes for Mr. Mutrick's heart failure?

    I. high-output failure caused by anemia
    II. low-output failure caused by prednisone
    III. high-output failure caused by myocardial infarction

    A. I only
    B. III only
    C. I and II
    D. II and III
    E. I, II, and III

22. Which of the following statements describe the interaction that should have taken place when Mr. Mutrick was having his prescriptions filled on 8/10?

    I. No significant interaction is needed with the new prescriptions.
    II. The pharmacist should advise Dr. Wonders of the potential problem of giving a potassium supplement in a patient with chronic kidney disease.
    III. The pharmacist should call Dr. Wonders regarding the potential use of a β-blocker in this newly diagnosed heart failure patient.

    A. I only
    B. III only
    C. I and II
    D. II and III
    E. I, II, and III

23. Why did the pharmacist contact Dr. Wonders on 12/15 regarding the Coreg prescription?

    I. Coreg is an ARB, which is currently not indicated in the treatment of heart failure.
    II. Coreg is a β-adrenergic blocker; in the treatment of heart failure, the dose must be closely titrated up to the optimal dose.
    III. β-Adrenergic blockers should not be abruptly discontinued in cardiac patients.

    A. I only
    B. III only
    C. I and II
    D. II and III
    E. I, II, and III

24. Which group of symptoms is most often associated with a patient who has signs of left-sided heart failure?

    A. shortness of breath, rales, paroxysmal nocturnal dyspnea
    B. jugular venous distention, hepatojugular reflux, pedal edema, shortness of breath
    C. hepatojugular reflux, jugular venous distention, pedal edema, abdominal distention
    D. paroxysmal nocturnal dyspnea, pedal edema, jugular venous distention, hepatojugular reflux
    E. fatigue, abdominal distention, hepatomegaly, rales

25. What is the therapeutic indication for ramipril (Altace) that might have prompted the pharmacist's call to Dr. Wonders on 1/2?

    I. hypertension
    II. renal dysfunction
    III. heart failure

    A. I only
    B. III only
    C. I and II
    D. II and III
    E. I, II, and III

26. How many milligrams of elemental iron does Mr. Mutrick receive with his daily dose of ferrous sulfate?

    A. 117 mg
    B. 195 mg
    C. 150 mg
    D. 322 mg
    E. 975 mg

27. Which action best describes how the drug Lasix would affect Mr. Mutrick?

    I. reduction of excess sodium and water in the patient
    II. direct pulmonary dilation
    III. increased preload through cytokine release

    A. I only
    B. III only
    C. I and II
    D. II and III
    E. I, II, and III

28. Which pharmacologic mechanisms relate primarily to the use of Vasotec in this patient?

    I. ACE inhibitors indirectly reduce preload by decreasing aldosterone secretion.
    II. ACE inhibitors reduce afterload by decreasing angiotensin II production.
    III. ACE inhibitors decrease levels of bradykinin.

    A. I only
    B. III only
    C. I and II
    D. II and III
    E. I, II, and III

29. Which of the following may potentially alter Lanoxin effects in Mr. Mutnick?

    I. renal dysfunction
    II. heart failure
    III. Lasix

    A. I only
    B. III only
    C. I and II
    D. II and III
    E. I, II, and III

30. Which drug used in the treatment of heart failure has been associated with systemic lupus erythematosus?

    A. Apresoline
    B. Lanoxin
    C. Vasotec
    D. Lasix
    E. Isordil

31. Which of the following drugs were recently given a Class III recommendation—"conditions for which there is evidence and/or general agreement that a procedure/therapy is not useful/effective and in some cases may be harmful"—in the treatment of heart failure?

    I. inamrinone
    II. dobutamine
    III. dopamine

    A. I only
    B. III only
    C. I and II
    D. II and III
    E. I, II, and III

32. Which statements best represent the actions that a pharmacist should take if presented with a prescription for a nonsteroidal anti-inflammatory drug (NSAID) for Mr. Mutrick?

    I. Contact the physician regarding the history of anemia in the patient and the current disease profile.
    II. Contact with the physician is not necessary.
    III. Fill the prescription and counsel the patient on the correct method for taking the NSAID with meals.

    A. I only
    B. III only
    C. I and II
    D. II and III
    E. I, II, and III

End of this patient profile; continue with the examination.

33. Which of the following statements does *not* accurately describe the current role that β-adrenergic blockers play in the treatment of heart failure?

    A. β-Adrenergic blockers have been shown to decrease the risk of death and hospitalization as well as to improve the clinical status of heart failure patients.
    B. Current guidelines recommend the use of β-adrenergic blockers in all patients with stable heart failure as a result of left ventricular dysfunction, unless they have a contraindication to their use or are unable to tolerate their effects owing to hypotension, bradycardia, bronchospasm, and the like.
    C. β-Adrenergic blockers are generally used in conjunction with diuretics and ACE inhibitors.
    D. Side effects to β-adrenergic blockers may occur during the early days of therapy but do not generally prevent their long-term use, and progression of the disease may be reduced.
    E. β-Adrenergic blockers are contraindicated in the treatment of heart failure because of their strong negative inotropic effects, which further reduce cardiac output.

34. The use of atropine sulfate in the treatment of sinus bradycardia centers around its anticholinergic activity. What hemodynamic response should be monitored for when the drug is administered?

    A. Initial doses may cause constipation.
    B. High doses will cause pupillary constriction.
    C. Initial doses may exacerbate the bradycardia.
    D. High doses will cause diarrhea.
    E. Initial doses will cause extreme sweating.

35. Which cardiac drugs are available in extended-release dosage forms?

    I. Quinaglute
    II. Coreg
    III. Plendil

    A. I only
    B. III only
    C. I and II
    D. II and III
    E. I, II, and III

36. Which agents would be an alternative therapy in an intensive care unit (ICU) patient nonresponsive to dopamine or dobutamine?

    A. timolol
    B. verapamil
    C. disopyramide
    D. inamrinone
    E. atenolol

37. Which agent works by irreversibly blocking the proton pump of parietal cells, thereby inhibiting basal gastric acid secretion?

    A. Tagamet
    B. Carafate
    C. Sandostatin
    D. Prevacid
    E. Pepcid

38. The serum creatinine level, along with the age, weight, and gender of the patient, may be used to estimate creatinine clearance. Creatinine clearance is a measurement of

    A. glomerular filtration rate (GFR).
    B. active tubular secretion.
    C. muscle metabolism.
    D. hepatic function.
    E. effective renal plasma flow.

39. Which of the following agents may induce an acute attack of gout?

    I. low-dose aspirin
    II. nicotinic acid
    III. cytotoxic drugs

    A. I only
    B. III only
    C. I and II
    D. II and III
    E. I, II, and III

40. When used as a topical decongestant, oxymetazoline

    I. is recommended for administration every 12 hours.
    II. has limited use, generally ≤ 3 days.
    III. acts as a direct-acting parasympathomimetic agent.

    A. I only
    B. III only
    C. I and II
    D. II and III
    E. I, II, and III

41. The elimination half-life for a newly released antimicrobial agent is approximately 2 hours. The drug has been shown to demonstrate first-order elimination characteristics. What percent of this drug would be eliminated from the body 6 hours after it is administered as an intravenous (IV) bolus dose?

   A. 12.5%
   B. 25.0%
   C. 50.0%
   D. 75.0%
   E. 87.5%

42. The culture and sensitivity report from a sputum specimen indicates the following minimum inhibitory concentrations (MICs) against a gram-negative bacterial isolate:

   ceftazidime 8 μg/mL
   gentamicin 4 μg/mL
   cefepime 1 μg/mL
   meropenem 2 μg/mL
   ciprofloxacin 32 μg/mL

   Based on the results of the report, which of the listed antimicrobials is the most potent single agent against this specific bacterial isolate?

   A. ceftazidime
   B. gentamicin
   C. cefepime
   D. meropenem
   E. ciprofloxacin

Use the patient profile below to answer questions 43 to 58.

MEDICATION PROFILE (COMMUNITY)

Patient Name: Kenneth Farmer
Address: 6152 Heavendale Ct.
Age: 70   Height: 5'9"
Sex: M   Race: Caucasian   Weight: 176 lb
Allergies: No known allergies

DIAGNOSIS

Primary   (1)   Diabetes mellitus
              (2)   Osteoarthritis
              (3)   Hypertension
              (4)   Hyperlipidemia
Secondary   (1)   Hx of peptic ulcer disease

MEDICATION RECORD (Prescription and OTC)

	Date	Rx No.	Physician	Drug and Strength	Quan	Sig	Refills
(1)	1/12			Tylenol 500 mg	100	Every 4h prn pain	OTC
(2)	1/12			Unisom sleep tabs	24	Tablet hs prn sleep	OTC
(3)	1/30	290311	Wilson	Celecoxib 200 mg	30	1 po qd	12
(4)	1/30	290313	Wilson	Ramipril 10 mg	30	1 po q A.M.	12
(5)	1/30	290314	Wilson	Simvastatin 20 mg	30	1 po q P.M.	6
(6)	1/30	290315	Wilson	Metformin 500 mg	60	1 po bid	3
(7)	2/15	297312	Wilson	Omeprazole 20 mg	30	1 po qd	2
(8)	4/27	301666	Drake	Pioglitazone 15 mg	30	1 po qd	3
(9)	7/25	325000	Drake	ACTOplus met 15/500	30	1 po qd	3
(10)	8/25	328111	Wilson	ACTOplus met 15/500	60	1 po bid	6
(11)	9/30			Alka-Seltzer Plus Day Cold			

PHARMACIST NOTES AND OTHER PATIENT INFORMATION

	Date	Comments
(1)	1/12	Patient complains of some pain in his right knee; he indicates that there is no redness or swelling; recommended Tylenol to treat.
(2)	1/12	Patient complains of insomnia; recommended Unisom sleep tablets when needed.
(3)	1/30	Annual check-up reveals the following for apparently untreated primary conditions:

a. Type 2 diabetes (A_{1C} greater than 7.3%, fasting blood sugar [FBS] of 140 mg/dL, postprandial glucose of 175 mg/dL)

b. Hypertension (blood pressure [BP] 150/110), hypercholesterolemia (total cholesterol 220 mg/dL, low-density lipoprotein [LDL] 160 mg/dL, high-density lipoprotein [HDL] 50 mg/dL)

c. Osteoarthritis with pain occurring off and on in right knee

d. Ongoing gastrointestinal (GI) complaints of indigestion and sour stomach

	Date	Comments
(4)	2/15	Contacted Dr. Drake as patient appeared concerned over increase in stomach pain since beginning celecoxib prescription who DC'd and added new prescription for omeprazole.
(5)	7/25	Contacted Dr. Drake to obtain permission to DC the previous single prescriptions for metformin and pioglitazone with the initiation of ACTOplus met.
(6)	9/30	Patient complained of symptoms of a common cold.

43. Which of the following *best* identifies the major clinical classifications for diabetes mellitus?

    A. type 1, type 2, hyperglycemia
    B. prediabetes, hyperosmolar hyperglycemic state (HHS), type 3
    C. type 1, type 2, and gestational diabetes mellitus
    D. Cushing syndrome, diabetic ketoacidosis, thiazide diuretic diabetes
    E. prediabetes, gestational diabetes mellitus, ketonemia

44. Diagnostic criteria used to make the diagnosis of diabetes mellitus in Mr. Farmer included

    I. a fasting plasma glucose level of 140 mg/dL.
    II. a hemoglobin A_{1C} level 7.3%
    III. a 2-hour plasma glucose level of 175 mg/dL during an oral glucose tolerance test using 75 g anhydrous glucose dissolved in water.

    A. I only
    B. III only
    C. I and II
    D. II and III
    E. I, II, and III

45. Mr. Farmer indicates to you that his physician said something about a "hemoglobin-type test to check how my blood sugar was doing." Which of the following applies to hemoglobin A_{1C} in diabetes?

    I. A value of $< 7\%$ (based on 6.5% as the upper limit of normal) would be a desired therapeutic endpoint.
    II. Another name for this is the glycosylated hemoglobin test.
    III. This reflects the average blood glucose level over the preceding 2 to 3 months.

    A. I only
    B. III only
    C. I and II
    D. II and III
    E. I, II, and III

46. Glyburide is an example of

    I. an oral insulin secretagogue.
    II. an oral hypoglycemic agent.
    III. a sulfonylurea.

    A. I only
    B. III only
    C. I and II
    D. II and III
    E. I, II, and III

47. Based on Mr. Farmer's profile, which of the following prescription(s) filled on 1/30 should have prompted a call to the physician?

    I. ramipril
    II. metformin
    III. celecoxib

    A. I only
    B. III only
    C. I and II
    D. II and III
    E. I, II, and III

48. Which of the following information applies to the prescription for metformin given to Mr. Farmer?

    I. It can be used in combination with several other classes of hypoglycemic agents.
    II. It is classified as an insulin sensitizer.
    III. It is contraindicated in situations that have the potential for increased risk of lactic acidosis.

    A. I only
    B. III only
    C. I and II
    D. II and III
    E. I, II, and III

49. When would the drug acarbose be a likely addition to Mr. Farmer's treatment regimen?

    I. If Mr. Farmer demonstrates significant postprandial hyperglycemia with current therapy.
    II. If Mr. Farmer is unable to lower his baseline blood glucose levels with current therapy.
    III. If Mr. Farmer develops an allergy to metformin, as it has a similar mechanism of action.

    A. I only
    B. III only
    C. I and II
    D. II and III
    E. I, II, and III

50. Mr. Farmer is interested in a blood glucose monitor that allows him to test at other sites besides the finger. The use of an alternate site for testing would *not* be appropriate

    I. in the fasting states, such as when he wakes in the morning.
    II. when he has an episode of hypoglycemia.
    III. immediately after a meal.

    A. I only
    B. III only
    C. I and II
    D. II and III
    E. I, II, and III

51. Mr. Farmer had been treated for osteoarthritis in his right knee. Which of the following are characteristic of osteoarthritis?

    I. It was formerly known as degenerative joint disease.
    II. It is the most common form of arthritis.
    III. It has a significant inflammatory component.

    A. I only
    B. III only
    C. I and II
    D. II and III
    E. I, II, and III

52. Mr. Farmer requested something to help him with his sleep problem. Which of the following applies to Mr. Farmer and his use of Unisom Sleep Tabs?

    I. This product contains doxylamine as the active ingredient.
    II. This product should be used cautiously in the elderly because of potential adverse central anticholinergic effects.
    III. As an elderly man, Mr. Farmer may have prostate enlargement, and this agent may produce polyuria, which could confuse the interpretation of his diabetes symptoms.

    A. I only
    B. III only
    C. I and II
    D. II and III
    E. I, II, and III

53. Which of the following statements regarding sulfonylureas (SUs) is *not* true?

    I. SUs are associated with weight loss.
    II. SUs may cause significant hypoglycemia.
    III. The SUs have been used since their introduction in the late 1950s.

    A. I only
    B. III only
    C. I and II
    D. II and III
    E. I, II, and III

54. Which of the following medications continues to be the subject of significant controversy regarding its possible link with cardiovascular disease and now has restricted distribution within the United States?

    A. insulin glargine
    B. rosiglitazone
    C. sitagliptin
    D. ramipril
    E. celecoxib

55. Which of the following represent properties associated with exenatide?

    I. It is resistant to deactivation by DPP-4.
    II. It needs to be administered within 60 minutes prior to meals.
    III. It is a synthetic version of a peptide secreted by the Gila monster.

    A. I only
    B. III only
    C. I and II
    D. II and III
    E. I, II, and III

56. Which of the following best represents the strategy applied by Dr. Drake for the prescriptions he provided for Mr. Farmer?

    I. Pioglitazone (Actos) was prescribed to provide an additive effect to metformin, in order to increase glucose control.
    II. Pioglitazone/metformin (ACTOplus met) was prescribed to replace the individual agents as combination therapy to simplify the patient's long-term regimen.
    III. Pioglitazone/metformin (ACTOplus met) was being titrated up to the ideal dose necessary for maximal glucose control.

    A. I only
    B. III only
    C. I and II
    D. II and III
    E. I, II, and III

57. Giving Alka-Seltzer Plus Day Cold Liquid-Gel Capsules to Mr. Farmer to treat his common cold symptoms would not be recommended because

   I. the oral decongestant phenylephrine in the product may increase his blood sugar.
   II. it is shotgun therapy with multiple active ingredients; one should usually treat specific symptoms with single-agent products.
   III. it contains acetaminophen, which may push Mr. Farmer into a toxic dose.

   A. I only
   B. III only
   C. I and II
   D. II and III
   E. I, II, and III

58. Which of the following hypoglycemic agents has been shown to be prone to primary and/or secondary failure when given to type 2 diabetes patients?

   A. glyburide (DiaBeta)
   B. exenatide (Byetta)
   C. acarbose (Precose)
   D. pioglitazone (Actos)
   E. sitagliptin (Januvia)

End of this patient profile; continue with the examination.

59. Jean, a regular customer in your pharmacy, shows you her newborn baby's head and asks you to recommend treatment. Upon examining the baby, you notice that he has an accumulation of skin scales on the scalp. You tell her that the baby has cradle cap and recommend that she treat the baby by

   A. washing the baby's head with coal tar solution daily for 2 weeks.
   B. washing his head with an antifungal shampoo (Nizoral AD).
   C. applying topical antibiotics such as Neosporin daily until resolved.
   D. massaging the scalp with baby oil followed by washing his head with a mild shampoo, such as Johnson & Johnson's baby shampoo.
   E. applying a moisturizer to the scalp daily until resolved.

60. Sunscreens should generally not be used in children < 6 months of age because

   A. the products commonly cause a severe rash in this age group.
   B. infants produce too much sweat, which can dilute the sunscreen.
   C. the metabolic and excretory systems of infants are not fully developed.
   D. overexposure to the sun can interfere with vitamin D production.
   E. infants have a lot of dermal melanin, which causes them to burn more easily.

61. Common warts are treated with which acid?

   A. glycolic acid
   B. salicylic acid
   C. lactic acid
   D. muriatic acid
   E. galactic acid

62. Which virus is responsible for common warts?

   A. herpes simplex virus (HSV)
   B. Epstein-Barr virus
   C. coronavirus
   D. HIV
   E. human papillomavirus

Use the patient profile below to answer questions 63 to 69.

PATIENT RECORD (INSTITUTION/NURSING HOME)

Patient Name: Salvatore Torres
Address: 369 Cherry St.
Age: 59   Height: 5'10"
Sex: M   Race: Hispanic   Weight: 170 lb
Allergies: Sulfonamide drug–induced Stevens–Johnson syndrome

DIAGNOSIS

Primary	(1)	Hypertension
Secondary	(1)	Drug-induced erythema multiforme
	(2)	Status post–acute coronary syndrome
	(3)	Asthma

LAB/DIAGNOSTIC TESTS

	Date	Test
(1)	11/3	WBC 5500/mm^3
(2)	11/3	BUN 15 mg/dL
(3)	11/3	SCr 1.0 mg/dL
(4)	11/3	BP 170/100 mm Hg
(5)	11/3	Electrolytes within normal limits
(6)	11/5	Total cholesterol 250 mg/dL; elevated LDL

MEDICATION ORDERS (Including Parenteral Solutions)

	Date	Drug and Strength	Route	Sig
(1)	11/3	Atenolol 50 mg	po	i bid
(2)	11/3	Hydrochlorothiazide (HCTZ) 25 mg	po	i q A.M.
(3)	11/3	Nitroglycerin 0.4 mg	sl	prn
(4)	11/3	Spironolactone 50 mg	po	i bid
(5)	11/3	Theo-24 400 mg	po	i q A.M.
(6)	11/5	Irbesartan 150 mg	po	i qd
(7)	11/5	Simvastatin 40 mg	po	i hs
(8)	11/5	Nitroprusside infusion	IV	1 μg/kg/min titrated to desired BP
(9)	11/5	Morphine sulfate 5 mg	IV	q4h prn chest pain

ADDITIONAL ORDERS

	Date	Comments
(1)		None

DIETARY CONSIDERATIONS (Enteral and Parenteral)

	Date	Comments
(1)	11/3	Low-fat diet.
(2)	11/3	Limit sodium intake to no additional salt with meals.

PHARMACIST NOTES AND OTHER PATIENT INFORMATION

	Date	Comments
(1)	11/3	Discontinue HCTZ and replace with spironolactone.
(2)	11/5	Blood pressure not responding to initial therapy; begin nitroprusside infusion.
(3)	11/5	Begin lipid-lowering therapy.
(4)	11/5	Schedule for coronary catheterization in the morning.

63. The decision to discontinue hydrochlorothiazide therapy in Mr. Torres and begin spironolactone therapy was based on which of the following?

   I. inappropriate therapeutic effect by thiazide diuretics in hypertensive patients
  II. lack of proven benefit in reducing mortality rates with thiazide diuretics in treating hypertension
 III. patient's documented allergy to sulfonamide yielding drug–induced Stevens–Johnson syndrome

  A. I only
  B. III only
  C. I and II
  D. II and III
  E. I, II, and III

64. Of the medications that are listed on Mr. Torres' profile, which agent(s) would be (a) concern(s) for causing hyperkalemia?

   I. atenolol
  II. spironolactone
 III. irbesartan

  A. I only
  B. III only
  C. I and II
  D. II and III
  E. I, II, and III

65. As noted on Mr. Torres' profile, he is "status post–acute coronary syndrome." Which of the following represents an example of an acute coronary syndrome?

   I. unstable angina
  II. ST-segment elevated myocardial infarction (STEMI)
 III. non–ST-segment elevated myocardial infarction (NSTEMI)

  A. I only
  B. III only
  C. I and II
  D. II and III
  E. I, II, and III

66. Mr. Torres' profile indicates that he is taking theophylline. Theophylline serum levels are increased by all of the following *except*:

  A. pneumonia.
  B. ciprofloxacin.
  C. heart failure.
  D. smoking.
  E. cor pulmonale.

67. Because Mr. Torres has a secondary diagnosis of asthma, which of the following medications would need to be used cautiously in asthmatic patients?

    I. spironolactone
    II. irbesartan
    III. atenolol

    A. I only
    B. III only
    C. I and II
    D. II and III
    E. I, II, and III

68. Which of the following parameters should be monitored in Mr. Torres based on the fact that he is taking simvastatin?

    A. liver function tests (LFTs)
    B. lipid panel
    C. blood urea nitrogen (BUN)
    D. white blood cell count
    E. both A and B

69. Mr. Torres is taking irbesartan which is a member of which drug class currently available for the treatment of hypertension?

    A. centrally acting α-adrenergic agonist
    B. cardioselective β-adrenergic receptor blocking agent
    C. angiotensin II receptor antagonist
    D. ACE inhibitor
    E. peripheral vasodilator

End of this patient profile; continue with the examination.

70. Which of the following agents slows electrical conduction through the atrioventricular node of the heart and has been used for treating hypertension and tachyarrhythmias as well as angina pectoris?

    A. amlodipine
    B. nifedipine
    C. felodipine
    D. verapamil
    E. isradipine

71. Which of the following represents the medication of choice for the initial therapy of stage I hypertension in an otherwise healthy individual with no compelling indications?

    A. hydrochlorothiazide
    B. spironolactone
    C. doxazosin
    D. hydralazine
    E. clonidine

Use the patient profile below to answer questions 72 to 82.

PATIENT RECORD (INSTITUTION/NURSING HOME)

Patient Name: Eunice Lee
Address: 3549 Lakeside Dr.

Age: 73   Height: 5′2″
Sex: F   Race: White   Weight: 125 lb
Allergies: No known allergies

DIAGNOSIS

Primary	(1)	2-year history of Parkinson disease
Secondary	(1)	Narrow-angle glaucoma
	(2)	30-year history of hypertension
	(3)	GERD

LAB/DIAGNOSTIC TESTS

	Date	Test
(1)	6/20	Na 135 mEq/L; K 3.6 mEq/L; Cl 95 mEq/L; CO_2 24 mEq/L; BUN 18 mg/dL; Cr 1.3 mg/dL
(2)	6/20	Occult blood in stool negative
(3)	6/20	Blood pressure 150/85 mm Hg

MEDICATION ORDERS (Including Parenteral Solutions)

	Date	Drug and Strength	Route	Sig
(1)	6/20	Acetazolamide 250 mg	po	i bid
(2)	6/20	Levodopa/Carbidopa 25/250	po	i tid
(3)	6/20	Pilocarpine 4%	ophthalmic	gtt i ou q6h
(4)	6/20	Reserpine 0.25 mg	po	i qd
(5)	6/20	Diltiazem 30 mg	po	i tid
(6)	6/20	Vitamin B complex w/ vitamin C	po	i qd
(7)	7/20	Entacapone tablets	po	200 mg daily
(8)	12/20	Tolcapone	po	100 mg tid

ADDITIONAL ORDERS

	Date	Comments
(1)	12/20	Baseline LFTs

DIETARY CONSIDERATIONS (Enteral and Parenteral)

	Date	Comments
(1)		None

PHARMACIST NOTES AND OTHER PATIENT INFORMATION

	Date	Comments
(1)	12/20	DC entacapone tablets.

72. Ms. Lee has Parkinson disease, which is a slowly progressive, degenerative, neurologic disease characterized by tremor, rigidity, bradykinesia, and postural instability. Although this disease is primarily idiopathic in origin, secondary parkinsonism may be caused by

    I. dopamine antagonists (e.g., phenothiazines, butyrophenones).
    II. poisoning by chemicals (e.g., carbon monoxide poisoning, manganese, mercury).
    III. infectious diseases (e.g., viral encephalitis, syphilis).

    A. I only
    B. III only
    C. I and II
    D. II and III
    E. I, II, and III

73. Ms. Lee's physician wants to initiate antihistamine therapy to treat the mild tremor that was the initial parkinsonian symptom experienced. Which antihistamines would be suitable?

    I. amantadine
    II. trihexyphenidyl
    III. diphenhydramine

    A. I only
    B. III only
    C. I and II
    D. II and III
    E. I, II, and III

74. The physician selects trihexyphenidyl rather than the antihistamine to treat Ms. Lee's initial symptoms. The usual daily dosage range for trihexyphenidyl is

    A. 1.0 to 6.0 mg.
    B. 1.5 to 4.5 mg.
    C. 6.0 to 10.0 mg.
    D. 300 to 600 mg.
    E. 200 to 1600 mg.

75. Upon the monthly medical record review by the local pharmacist, a notation is made to follow up with the medical staff on the recent order written for entacapone on 7/20. What place does entacapone have in the treatment of Parkinson disease?

    I. Entacapone is indicated as an adjunct to levodopa/carbidopa to treat patients with end-of-dose "wearing-off" symptoms.
    II. Entacapone is an enhancer of the bioavailability of levodopa.
    III. Entacapone is a precursor to dopamine indicated in the treatment of refractory Parkinson disease.

    A. I only
    B. III only
    C. I and II
    D. II and III
    E. I, II, and III

76. The physician has some concerns regarding the use of anticholinergics in Ms. Lee. Of what precautions in their use should the pharmacist inform the physician?

    A. complications of narrow-angle glaucoma
    B. consequences of fluid loss from diarrhea
    C. urinary incontinence
    D. excessive salivation
    E. excessive central nervous system excitation

77. Typical side effects associated with the use of levodopa include

    I. GI effects, such as anorexia, nausea and vomiting, and abdominal distress.
    II. cardiovascular effects, such as postural hypotension and tachycardia.
    III. musculoskeletal effects, such as dystonia or choreiform muscle movements.

    A. I only
    B. III only
    C. I and II
    D. II and III
    E. I, II, and III

78. When using anticholinergic therapy for the treatment of this patient's parkinsonian tremor, which therapeutic considerations are applicable?

  I. Anticholinergic agents are best used in combination to maximize benefits.
 II. Trihexyphenidyl is generally the most effective anticholinergic agent for the treatment of parkinsonian tremor.
III. Changing to another anticholinergic agent may not prove helpful if the therapeutic effect of the first agent is unsatisfactory, but changing to a different drug class may be beneficial.

  A. I only
  B. III only
  C. I and II
  D. II and III
  E. I, II, and III

79. Based on the patient's medical history before admission, the physician concludes that anticholinergic or antihistamine therapy is insufficient. Dopaminergic therapy could be instituted in the form of

  A. chlorpheniramine.
  B. biperiden.
  C. mesoridazine.
  D. amantadine.
  E. perphenazine.

80. Levodopa is metabolized to dopamine by dopa decarboxylase both centrally and peripherally. This metabolism could be a potential complication for this patient because of

  A. concomitant vitamin B complex therapy.
  B. elevated serum creatinine level.
  C. concomitant diltiazem therapy.
  D. concomitant vitamin C therapy.
  E. elevated blood pressure.

81. In choosing dopaminergic therapy for Ms. Lee, the physician considers giving the combination of carbidopa and levodopa therapy. This combination

  I. inhibits peripheral decarboxylation of levodopa to dopamine.
 II. increases the required dose of levodopa by approximately 25%.
III. decreases the amount of levodopa available for transport to the brain.

  A. I only
  B. III only
  C. I and II
  D. II and III
  E. I, II, and III

82. An adjunctive therapeutic regimen for Ms. Lee, relative to her previous "on–off" history, would be

  A. monthly interruption of levodopa therapy (drug holiday) on either an inpatient or an outpatient basis.
  B. addition of bromocriptine in a dosage range of 2.5 to 40.0 mg/day.
  C. addition of amantadine in a dose tailored to the level of renal function.
  D. addition of a monoamine oxidase inhibitor.
  E. addition of haloperidol in a dosage range of 2.5 to 15.0 mg/day.

End of this patient profile; continue with the examination.

83. The effects of food and antacid on the bioavailability of a new antihypertensive agent were studied in 24 men, using a three-way crossover design. The results of this study are summarized in the table below.

Treatment	C_{max} (μg/mL)[a]	AUC (0–24 hr; μg × hr/mL)[a]	T_{max} (hr)[a]
Fasting	95 ± 10	450 ± 115	1.5 ± 1.1
With antacid	106 ± 18	498 ± 123	1.0 ± 1.2
With high-fat breakfast	75 ± 11[b]	423 ± 110	2.4 ± 1.3

[a]Results are expressed as the mean ± SD.
[b]Compared with fasting, $P \leq .05$.

Compared with fasting, what results did the study show?

   I. The high-fat breakfast had no significant effect on the bioavailability of the drug.
   II. The antacid significantly increased the extent of systemic drug absorption.
   III. The high-fat breakfast treatment decreased the rate of systemic drug absorption.

   A. I only
   B. III only
   C. I and II
   D. II and III
   E. I, II, and III

84. An example of a nitrogen mustard is

   A. chlorambucil.
   B. busulfan.
   C. melphalan.
   D. mechlorethamine.
   E. doxorubicin.

85. A controlled-release dosage form by which the mechanism for drug release is the result of an osmotically active drug core is known as

   A. Dospan.
   B. OROS.
   C. TDDS.
   D. Pennkinetic.
   E. HBS.

86. All of the following are quinolone antimicrobials *except*

   A. moxifloxacin.
   B. levofloxacin.
   C. clarithromycin.
   D. ciprofloxacin.
   E. gemifloxacin.

87. Which immunosuppressive agents are used after kidney transplantation?

   I. azathioprine
   II. basiliximab
   III. cyclosporine

   A. I only
   B. III only
   C. I and II
   D. II and III
   E. I, II, and III

Use the patient profile below to answer questions 88 to 93.

PATIENT RECORD (INSTITUTION/NURSING HOME)

Patient Name: Joel Melvin
Address: 345 Bimini Ct.
Age: 54   Height: 5′8″
Sex: M   Race: Caucasian   Weight: 190 lb
Allergies: Penicillin: rash

DIAGNOSIS

Primary   (1)   Acute myocardial infarction
Secondary   (1)   Hypertension
             (2)   Chronic kidney disease

LAB/DIAGNOSTIC TESTS

	Date	Test
(1)	3/20	EKG stat and then at completion of TNKase therapy; baseline ST segment increase in II, III, and aVF
(2)	3/20	CBC: WBC count 12,000/mm^3
(3)	3/20	Platelet count 240,000 µL
(4)	3/20	Chem 20
(5)	3/20	Cardiac enzymes stat and q 8 h × 3; results: CK 320 IU/L, CK MB% 18; CK MB 57 IU/L. Troponin 6ng/ml
(6)	3/20	INR, aPTT stat, and then at 6 and 12 hours after completion of TNKase; aPTT at baseline 30 sec, 6 hour > 120 sec; INR at baseline is 1
(7)	3/20	Urinalysis stat and then at 6 hours; baseline within normal limits
(8)	3/23	+ S$_3$, short of breath, bradycardia (55), fatigued

MEDICATION ORDERS (Including Parenteral Solutions)

	Date	Drug and Strength	Route	Sig
(1)	3/20	Chewable ASA 81 mg		Chew 4 tablets and swallow ASAP
(2)	3/20	Heparin 5000 U	IV	as one-time only bolus
(3)	3/20	Heparin 1000 U	IV	continuous infusion
(4)	3/20	TNKase 50 mg	IVP	over 5 sec
(5)	3/20	Metoprolol 5 mg	IV	every 2 min for 3 doses
(6)	3/20	Metoprolol 50 mg	po	15 min after last IV dose and q6h for 48 hours
(7)	3/20	Lisinopril 5 mg	po	i qd
(8)	3/20	Docusate 100 mg capsules	po	ii hs
(9)	3/20	Reduce heparin infusion to 800 U	IV	continuous infusion
(10)	3/23	Discontinue lisinopril 5 mg; start lisinopril 10 mg	po	i qd
(11)	3/23	Metoprolol 25 mg	po	i bid

DIETARY CONSIDERATIONS (Enteral and Parenteral)

	Date	Comments
(1)	3/20	Low-salt, low-fat diet
(2)	3/22	Extra fiber

PHARMACIST NOTES AND OTHER PATIENT INFORMATION

	Date	Comments
(1)	3/20	BP 150/100, pulse 120, respirations 20/min.
(2)	3/20	ST-segment elevation in II, III, and aVF.
(3)	3/20	aPTT at 6 hours > 120 sec.
(4)	3/20	aPTT at 12 hours 65 sec.
(5)	3/21	Urine output OK.
(6)	3/22	Pulmonary rales, S_3.
(7)	3/23	BP 140/90, P 55.
(8)	3/24	Appears well, good color, no chest pain, shortness of breath.

88. From the medication orders written for Mr. Melvin, it appears that lisinopril was prescribed shortly after the acute period of the heart attack. Based on the patient's profile, what is the primary reason for including lisinopril in this setting?

    I. adjunctive therapy to prevent left ventricular dysfunction after acute MI
    II. additive therapy to help bring the patient's blood pressure down
    III. treatment of suspected renal dysfunction

    A. I only
    B. III only
    C. I and II
    D. II and III
    E. I, II, and III

89. Mr. Melvin's estimated creatinine clearance may be calculated from serum creatinine by using

    A. Cockcroft and Gault equation.
    B. Fick's law.
    C. law of mass action.
    D. Henderson–Hasselbalch equation.
    E. Noyes–Whitney equation.

90. On 3/23, Mr. Melvin appears to be demonstrating signs and symptoms consistent with cardiac decompensation. On examination, his heart rate is found to be 55, he is short of breath, and fatigued. Which of the following might be contributing to these symptoms?

    I. metoprolol
    II. heart failure post-MI
    III. lisinopril

    A. I only
    B. III only
    C. I and II
    D. II and III
    E. I, II, and III

91. Mr. Melvin received TNKase. Which of the following is/are true regarding the use of this agent?

    I. It is a thrombolytic used to dissolve a clot when given within 12 hours of symptom onset.
    II. It is contraindicated if the patient is at risk of an intracranial hemorrhage.
    III. It should be administered within a 30 minute window after arrival to hospital for NSTEMI or STEMI.

    A. I only
    B. II only
    C. I and II
    D. I and III
    E. I, II, and III

92. Metoprolol is prescribed for the acute management of Mr. Melvin's MI for which of the following reasons?

    I.   It is used as an adjunctive treatment that prevents angina pectoris and potentially significant atrial tachyarrhythmias.

   II.   It is used in this patient to decrease the patient's blood pressure.

  III.   β-Adrenergic blockers have been shown to be effective in post-MI patients in the prevention of mortality owing to sudden cardiac death.

    A. I only
    B. III only
    C. I and II
    D. II and III
    E. I, II, and III

93. All of the following laboratory tests should be monitored in Mr. Melvin while he is on heparin *except*:

    A. aPTT.
    B. hemoglobin and hematocrit.
    C. serum potassium.
    D. neutrophils.
    E. platelets.

End of this patient profile; continue with the examination.

94. The half-life of amiodarone is

    A. 1 hour.
    B. 6 hours.
    C. 24 hours.
    D. 50 hours.
    E. up to 50 days.

95. Propranolol is administered to patients with hyperthyroidism because it

    I.   helps reduce tachycardia, sweating, and tremor associated with the condition.

   II.   inhibits the conversion of thyroxine (T_4) to triiodothyronine (T_3) in high doses.

  III.   suppresses the production of T_4.

    A. I only
    B. III only
    C. I and II
    D. II and III
    E. I, II, and III

Use the patient profile below to answer questions 96 to 108.

MEDICATION PROFILE (COMMUNITY)

Patient Name: Jon Rones
Address: 11 Cherry Ln.
Age: 65   Height: 5'10"
Sex: M   Race: White   Weight: 230 lb
Allergies: Sulfonamides, penicillin: both cause rash

DIAGNOSIS

Primary	(1)	Acute renal failure
	(2)	Hyperkalemia
Secondary	(1)	Hypertension
	(2)	Heart failure
	(3)	Sinus congestion

MEDICATION RECORD (Prescription and OTC)

	Date	Rx No.	Physician	Drug and Strength	Quan	Sig	Refills
(1)	6/8	245320	Sadler	Hydrochlorothiazide 50 mg	30	i qd	6
(2)	6/8	245321	Sadler	Moexipril 7.5 mg	30	i qd	6
(3)	6/8	245322	Sadler	Slow-K 8 mEq	100	i tid	6
(4)	6/15	246100	Frisch	Sudafed 60 mg	100	i q6h	12
(5)	11/7	278900	Sadler	Isoptin SR 120 mg	60	i bid	0
(6)	11/7	278901	Sadler	Tenormin 50 mg	60	i bid	0
(7)	11/7	278902	Sadler	Isordil Titradose 40 mg	120	i qid	5
(8)	11/7	278903	Sadler	Lanoxin 0.25 mg	30	i qd	0
(9)	2/5	280001	Sadler	Capoten 25 mg	100	i tid	1
(10)	2/5	280002	Sadler	Aldactone 25 mg	100	i tid	1
(11)	3/15	290016	Sadler	Vasotec 5 mg	60	i bid	6
(12)	3/15	290017	Sadler	Lanoxin 0.125 mg	30	i qd	6

PHARMACIST NOTES AND OTHER PATIENT INFORMATION

	Date	Comments
(1)	11/7	DC HydroDIURIL 50 mg.
(2)	11/7	DC Moexipril 7.5 mg.
(3)	11/7	DC Slow-K 8 mEq.
(4)	2/5	DC Lanoxin 0.25 mg.
(5)	2/5	DC Isoptin SR 120 mg.
(6)	2/5	DC Tenormin 50 mg.
(7)	3/5	DC Capoten 25 mg.
(8)	3/5	DC Aldactone 25 mg.
(9)	3/5	DC Sudafed.

96. Based on the patient's medication profile, which condition(s) are potential underlying causes of the acute renal failure (ARF) in Mr. Rones?

    I. heart failure
   II. hypertension
 III. hyperkalemia

  A. I only
  B. III only
  C. I and II
  D. II and III
  E. I, II, and III

97. Based on Mr. Rones' allergies, which medication can he receive safely?

  A. hydrochlorothiazide
  B. V-Cillin-K
  C. Bactrim
  D. Septra
  E. None of the above

98. Based on the patient information, which medications would warrant a call to the physician before the pharmacist dispensed them to Mr. Rones?

    I. Slow-K
   II. Sudafed
 III. moexipril

  A. I only
  B. III only
  C. I and II
  D. II and III
  E. I, II, and III

99. According to the guidelines from JNC-7, which agents are suitable alternatives to a thiazide diuretic for the initial treatment of stage I hypertension in this patient?

    I. atenolol
   II. ramipril
 III. candesartan

  A. I only
  B. III only
  C. I and II
  D. II and III
  E. I, II, and III

100. All of the following measures can be used in the prevention and treatment of digoxin-induced toxicity *except*

  A. maintaining normal concentrations of potassium in the serum.
  B. routinely monitoring renal function to determine digoxin elimination.
  C. administering Kayexalate solutions.
  D. administering lidocaine.
  E. none of the above.

101. Which of the following accurately describes the agents listed and the drug class they belong to?

    I. felodipine: β-adrenergic receptor blocker; ramipril: ACE inhibitor; losartan: calcium-channel blocker; propranolol: β-adrenergic receptor blocker
   II. felodipine: calcium-channel blocker; losartan: angiotensin II receptor antagonist; ramipril: ACE inhibitor; enalapril: ACE inhibitor
 III. atenolol: β-adrenergic receptor blocker; carvedilol: β-adrenergic receptor blocker; isradipine: calcium-channel blocker; enalapril: ACE inhibitor

  A. I only
  B. III only
  C. I and II
  D. II and III
  E. I, II, and III

102. Which of the following would not be considered appropriate treatment for this patient's hyperkalemia?

  A. dialysis
  B. calcium chloride or calcium gluconate
  C. regular insulin with dextrose
  D. sodium polystyrene sulfonate
  E. spironolactone

103. When dispensing the prescription for Isoptin and Tenormin, the pharmacist should advise Mr. Rones to

    I. check his heart rate regularly for bradycardia.
   II. report swelling, shortness of breath, and fatigue.
 III. report orthopnea, dyspnea on exertion, and paroxysmal nocturnal dyspnea.

  A. I only
  B. III only
  C. I and II
  D. II and III
  E. I, II, and III

104. Which reference text could a pharmacist use to determine the indications and dosage for a relatively newly released medication for the treatment of hypertension?

    A. *Merck Index*
    B. Facts and Comparisons eAnswers
    C. *Trissel's*
    D. *Hansten's*
    E. *AHFS*

105. The use of Lanoxin 0.125 mg for Mr. Rones centers around its ability to

    A. decrease the chronotropic actions of the heart, thereby reducing blood pressure.
    B. increase the chronotropic actions of the heart, thereby reducing blood pressure.
    C. increase renal blood flow, thereby improving urinary output.
    D. increase the inotropic actions of the heart, thereby increasing cardiac output.
    E. decrease the inotropic actions of the heart, thereby decreasing cardiac output.

106. Digoxin has an elimination half-life of 36 hours and 4.5 days in patients who have normal renal function and in those who are anephric, respectively. If no loading doses were used in Mr. Rones and he is anephric, the time to reach steady-state serum digoxin (Lanoxin) concentrations would be

    A. 2 to 3 days.
    B. 3 to 5 days.
    C. 6 to 8 days.
    D. 10 to 15 days.
    E. 15 to 20 days.

107. Which medication might provide benefit as an alternative to Inderal in a hypertensive patient who also suffers from bronchospastic lung disease and noncompliance?

    A. Inderal LA
    B. Coreg
    C. Brevibloc
    D. Corgard
    E. Sectral

108. Which statements about the treatment of heart failure in Mr. Rones are correct?

    I. Isordil is probably being used as a preload reducing agent.
    II. Dopamine would be an appropriate alternative to Lanoxin in this patient.
    III. Dobutamine would be an appropriate alternative to Lanoxin in this patient.

    A. I only
    B. III only
    C. I and II
    D. II and III
    E. I, II, and III

End of this patient profile; continue with the examination.

109. A patient has just returned from England, where she received a drug to treat her asthma. She asks for the U.S. equivalent for this drug. What is the best resource for identifying this drug?

    A. *Facts and Comparisons*
    B. *Martindale: The Complete Drug Reference*
    C. *Trissel's Stability of Compounded Formulations*
    D. *Physicians' Desk Reference* (PDR)
    E. *AHFS*

110. Peritoneal dialysis is useful for removing drugs from an intoxicated person if the drug

    A. is polar.
    B. is lipid soluble.
    C. is highly bound to plasma proteins.
    D. is nonpolar.
    E. has a large apparent volume of distribution.

111. Which of the following groups of herbal medicines are considered unsafe by the U.S. Food and Drug Administration (FDA) because of their ability to cause damage to various organ systems?

    I. tonka bean, heliotrope, and periwinkle, causing hepatotoxicity
    II. mistletoe, spindle tree, and wahoo, causing seizures
    III. jimson weed and sweet flag, causing hallucinations

    A. I only
    B. III only
    C. I and II
    D. II and III
    E. I, II, and III

112. The percentage of elemental iron in ferrous gluconate is

    A. 10%.
    B. 12%.
    C. 20%.
    D. 30%.
    E. 33%.

113. In the extemporaneous compounding of an ointment, the process of using a suitable nonsolvent to reduce the particle size of a drug before its incorporation into the ointment is known as

    A. geometric dilution.
    B. levigation.
    C. pulverization by intervention.
    D. spatulation.
    E. trituration.

114. An antibiotic for IV infusion is supplied in 50-mL vials at a concentration of 5 mg/mL. How many vials are required for an 80-kg patient who needs an adult dose at a suggested infusion rate of 2.5 mg/kg/hr for 6 hours?

    A. 1
    B. 2
    C. 3
    D. 4
    E. 5

115. The bioavailability of a drug from an immediate-release tablet dosage form is most often related to the

    A. disintegration of the tablet.
    B. dissolution of the drug.
    C. elimination half-life of the drug.
    D. plasma protein binding of the drug.
    E. size of the tablet.

116. Which of the following is a list of protease inhibitors used in the treatment of HIV?

    I. atazanavir, indinavir, nelfinavir
    II. abacavir, stavudine, lamivudine
    III. delavirdine, efavirenz, nevirapine

    A. I only
    B. III only
    C. I and II
    D. II and III
    E. I, II, and III

117. The rate of dissolution of a weak acid drug may be increased by

    I. increasing the pH of the medium.
    II. increasing the particle size of the solid drug.
    III. increasing the viscosity of the medium.

    A. I only
    B. III only
    C. I and II
    D. II and III
    E. I, II, and III

Use the patient profile below to answer questions 118 to 128.

PATIENT RECORD (INSTITUTION/NURSING HOME)

Patient Name: Calvin Jorgenson
Address: 19822 Weyher St.
Age: 35   Height: 6′1″
Sex: M   Race: African American   Weight: 210 lb
Allergies: Reaction to contrast media, shellfish: local hives

DIAGNOSIS

Primary   (1)   Bipolar disorder
Secondary   (1)   Prehypertension
               (2)   History of epilepsy

LAB/DIAGNOSTIC TESTS

	Date	Test
(1)	8/10	Lithium 0.9 mEq/L
(2)	8/10	WBC 14,000/mm
(3)	8/11	Basic metabolic panel
(4)	8/11	Lipid panel to include total cholesterol, LDL, HDL
(5)	8/11	12-lead standard EKG

MEDICATION ORDERS (Including Parenteral Solutions)

	Date	Drug and Strength	Route	Sig
(1)	8/10	Lithium carbonate 300 mg	po	i q12h
(2)	8/10	Hydrochlorothiazide 25 mg	po	i q A.M.
(3)	8/10	Zolpidem 10 mg	po	i q hs prn
(4)	8/10	Acetaminophen 500 mg	po	i–ii q4h prn
(5)	8/10	Multivitamin	po	i q d
(6)	8/11	Olanzapine 10 mg	po	i q d

ADDITIONAL ORDERS

	Date	Comments
(1)	8/11	Accurate height and weight

DIETARY CONSIDERATIONS (Enteral and Parenteral)

	Date	Comments
(1)	8/10	Salt-restricted diet

PHARMACIST NOTES AND OTHER PATIENT INFORMATION

	Date	Comments
(1)		None

118. Which of the following statements is/are correct concerning Mr. Jorgenson's primary diagnosis?

  I. This condition is also known as manic depression.
  II. Bipolar disorder may be classified as bipolar I disorder, bipolar II disorder, cyclothymia, and rapid cycling.
  III. Mood stabilizers have historically been the mainstays of therapy for this condition.

  A. I only
  B. III only
  C. I and II
  D. II and III
  E. I, II, and III

119. Which statement concerning lithium is true?

  A. It is the drug of choice for the acute and maintenance treatment of mania and hypomania.
  B. It is classified as an anxiolytic.
  C. It is a serum electrolyte similar to sodium and is relatively free of serious adverse effects and drug interactions.
  D. It is commonly used as an antidepressant.
  E. It is similar to haloperidol in neuroleptic activity.

120. The molecular weight of lithium carbonate, Li_2CO_3, is 73.89. How many milliequivalents of lithium are there in a 300-mg tablet of lithium carbonate?

  A. 1.24
  B. 2.46
  C. 4.06
  D. 8.12
  E. 12.18

121. The admitting physician had suspected that the patient was noncompliant with lithium therapy before admission. When interpreting the admission lithium level, the physician should consider

  I. the sample draw time with respect to the time of the last scheduled lithium dose.
  II. concomitant drug therapy.
  III. the acute manic condition of the patient.

  A. I only
  B. III only
  C. I and II
  D. II and III
  E. I, II, and III

122. For monitoring this patient's serum lithium concentrations, the most appropriate serum drug concentration that can be conveniently sampled is the

  I. minimum (trough) serum drug concentration.
  II. average serum drug concentration.
  III. peak serum drug concentration.

  A. I only
  B. III only
  C. I and II
  D. II and III
  E. I, II, and III

123. On the second day of admission (8/11), laboratory tests for lipids, basic metabolic panel, and EKG were ordered along with accurate height and weight. Which of the following best represents the orders documented during the second day of admission?

  I. The laboratory tests ordered are paramount to patients receiving lithium.
  II. Olanzapine, as a nontraditional antipsychotic, is indicated as combination therapy to lithium patients who have not obtained a desired therapeutic response.
  III. Baseline blood glucose, lipid profile, EKG for those with cardiovascular risk factors, and weight and height at the start of antipsychotic.

  A. I only
  B. III only
  C. I and II
  D. II and III
  E. I, II, and III

124. The hydrochlorothiazide order for Mr. Jorgenson might affect his serum lithium concentration by

  A. altering the glomerular filtration of lithium.
  B. increasing the absorption of lithium in the loop of Henle.
  C. increasing the absorption of lithium and sodium in the GI tract.
  D. interfering with sodium reabsorption in the kidney.
  E. decreasing lithium reabsorption in the distal tubule.

125. Assuming Mr. Jorgenson was already taking each of the agents noted on his profile at admission, what drug would likely explain the white blood cell (WBC) count reported on admission?

  A. acetaminophen
  B. hydrochlorothiazide
  C. zolpidem
  D. lithium
  E. multiple vitamins

126. Which of the following groups of agents have been shown to be effective in addition to the current agents being used in Mr. Jorgenson for bipolar disorders?

    I. valproate, carbamazepine, lamotrigine
    II. aripiprazole, quetiapine, ziprasidone
    III. amitriptyline, nortriptyline, protriptyline

    A. I only
    B. III only
    C. I and II
    D. II and III
    E. I, II, and III

127. Recent literature has supported the use of atypical antipsychotics as monotherapy or adjunctive treatment in bipolar mania. Which of the following is *not* an atypical antipsychotic?

    A. olanzapine (Zyprexa)
    B. quetiapine (Seroquel)
    C. aripiprazole (Abilify)
    D. chlorpromazine
    E. risperidone (Risperdal)

128. Symbyax is the trade name of a combination product of an atypical antipsychotic with an SSRI and is approved for depressive episodes in bipolar disorder. What are the two agents that make up this product?

    A. olanzapine/fluoxetine
    B. aripiprazole/amitriptyline
    C. chlorpromazine/fluoxetine
    D. quetiapine/paroxetine
    E. perphenazine/amitriptyline

End of this patient profile; continue with the examination.

129. Methotrexate is used alone or in combination for the treatment of various neoplastic diseases. A recommended IV loading dose of methotrexate for the treatment of acute lymphoblastic leukemia is 200 mg/m^2 for the pediatric patient. What would be the loading dose for an 8-year-old patient whose body surface area is 0.89 m^2?

    A. 224 mg
    B. 150 mg
    C. 178 mg
    D. 200 mg
    E. 295 mg

130. The diuretic action of furosemide is the result of

    A. osmotic activity within the renal tubules.
    B. inhibition of sodium and chloride reabsorption at the distal segment of the nephron.
    C. inhibition of carbonic anhydrase at the nephron.
    D. inhibition of sodium reabsorption at the ascending limb of the loop of Henle.
    E. inhibition of aldosterone at the distal segment of the nephron.

131. Nonprescription decongestants used for topical application to the nasal passages include

    I. phenylephrine.
    II. oxymetazoline.
    III. pseudoephedrine.

    A. I only
    B. III only
    C. I and II
    D. II and III
    E. I, II, and III

132. According to JNC-7, first-line drugs in the treatment of stage I hypertension, in the absence of other disease states, include

    I. hydrochlorothiazide.
    II. atenolol.
    III. clonidine.

    A. I only
    B. III only
    C. I and II
    D. II and III
    E. I, II, and III

133. To minimize the risk of tardive dyskinesia in a patient receiving antipsychotic drug therapy, a patient should be

   I. given the lowest possible dose of antipsychotic agent for the shortest duration possible.
   II. monitored closely for signs or symptoms of tardive dyskinesia.
   III. given second-generation agents (atypical antipsychotics) as first-line therapy.

   A. I only
   B. III only
   C. I and II
   D. II and III
   E. I, II, and III

134. Which of these agents would produce a significant drug–drug interaction in a patient who is taking Parnate?

   I. meperidine
   II. morphine
   III. ketorolac

   A. I only
   B. III only
   C. I and II
   D. II and III
   E. I, II, and III

135. Which agent is a selective antagonist of serotonin and has been shown to prevent the nausea and vomiting caused by highly emetogenic cancer chemotherapy?

   A. bupropion (Zyban)
   B. sertraline (Zoloft)
   C. linezolid (Zyvox)
   D. ondansetron (Zofran)
   E. simvastatin (Zocor)

136. Which of the following drugs is an antipsychotic agent?

   A. aripiprazole (Abilify)
   B. rabeprazole (Aciphex)
   C. butoconazole (Gynazole-1)
   D. clotrimazole
   E. carbamazepine (Tegretol)

137. Which vitamin or other agent is often given along with a calcium supplement to aid in its absorption?

   A. thiamine
   B. vitamin D
   C. ascorbic acid
   D. vitamin E
   E. pantothenic acid

Use the patient profile below to answer questions 138 to 148.

MEDICATION PROFILE (COMMUNITY)

Patient Name: Kelley Trombley
Address: 615 Elsinore Ct.
Age: 40   Height: 5'7"
Sex: F   Race: White   Weight: 145 lb
Allergies: Penicillin: anaphylaxis; codeine: local hives

DIAGNOSIS

Primary	(1)	Rheumatoid arthritis (RA), diagnosed 1/5
Secondary	(1)	Community-acquired pneumonia, 1/15
	(2)	Urinary tract infection, 6/5

MEDICATION RECORD (Prescription and OTC)

	Date	Rx No.	Physician	Drug and Strength	Quan	Sig	Refills
(1)	1/5	209356	Cook	Ibuprofen 800 mg	90	i tid	2
(2)	1/15	209357	Cook	Moxifloxacin 400 mg	14	i po qd	0
(3)	2/1	211323	Cook	Hydroxychloroquine 200 mg	60	ii qd	3
(4)	2/1	211324	Cook	Prednisone 5 mg	30	i qd	3
(5)	2/1	211324	Cook	Doxycycline 100 mg	7	i qd	0
(6)	5/1	280333	Cook	Hydroxychloroquine 200 mg	90	iii qd	0
(7)	5/1	280334	Cook	Vitamin B$_{12}$ 250 μg	30	i q A.M.	0
(8)	5/1	280335	Cook	Folic acid 1 mg	30	i q A.M.	0
(9)	5/1	280336	Cook	Ferrous sulfate 325 mg	90	i q tid	0
(10)	5/1	280337	Cook	Arthrotec 75/0.2 mg	90	i tid	0
(11)	6/5	310444	Cook	Ciprofloxacin 250 mg	6	i bid	0
(12)	7/5	325001	Cook	Etanercept 50 mg	Office SQ injection		4
(13)	7/5	325002	Cook	Methotrexate 2.5 mg	12	iii po q wk	4

PHARMACIST NOTES AND OTHER PATIENT INFORMATION

	Date	Comments
(1)	1/15	Pneumonia.
(2)	2/1	Spoke to patient about the need for routine tests to monitor disease modifying drug added for treatment of rheumatoid arthritis.
(3)	5/1	Called MD to discuss rationale for anemia medications; he agreed that these should not be filled at this time and instead would initiate Arthrotec therapy and DC Motrin.
(4)	6/5	UTI; contacted Dr. Cook for instructions for the hydroxychloroquine prescription; patient to start Enbrel next month after a final month of hydroxychloroquine.
(5)	7/5	Prescription for hydroxychloroquine no longer active; with initiation of etanercept and methotrexate prescriptions.

138. Which of the agents listed in the patient profile is considered a respiratory quinolone antibiotic?

    I. moxifloxacin (Avelox)
    II. ciprofloxacin (Cipro)
    III. doxycycline (Vibramycin)

    A. I only
    B. III only
    C. I and II
    D. II and III
    E. I, II, and III

139. Pharmacists will encounter patients with various types of arthritis. The American College of Rheumatology identified the need for at least four of seven criteria they had identified, in order to make the diagnosis. Which of the following would Ms. Trombley have likely experienced?

    I. morning stiffness in and around the joint lasting at least 1 hour before improvement
    II. arthritis of at least one joint in the wrist, hands, or fingers
    III. asymmetric involvement of the body joints

    A. I only
    B. III only
    C. I and II
    D. II and III
    E. I, II, and III

140. Which of the following arthritis medications in Ms. Trombley's profile require(s) close monitoring by an ophthalmologist to prevent adverse effects on the eyes?

    I. ibuprofen (Motrin)
    II. diclofenac/misoprostol (Arthrotec)
    III. hydroxychloroquine (Plaquenil)

    A. I only
    B. III only
    C. I and II
    D. II and III
    E. I, II, and III

141. All of the following agents could be used to replace hydroxychloroquine *except*

    A. clopidogrel (Plavix).
    B. sulfasalazine (Azulfidine).
    C. methotrexate (Rheumatrex).
    D. penicillamine (Cuprimine).
    E. gold sodium thiomalate (Myochrysine).

142. Which agent(s) would be (an) appropriate alternative(s) for ibuprofen (Motrin) when it was originally prescribed (1/5) for Ms. Trombley?

    I. celecoxib (Celebrex)
    II. naproxen (Naprosyn)
    III. nabumetone

    A. I only
    B. III only
    C. I and II
    D. II and III
    E. I, II, and III

143. Which of the following NSAIDs are correctly matched by brand and generic names?

    I. Clinoril/sulindac
    II. Voltaren-XR/diclofenac
    III. Ansaid/flurbiprofen

    A. I only
    B. III only
    C. I and II
    D. II and III
    E. I, II, and III

144. Which of the following apply to Ms. Trombley's prescriptions written on 2/1?

    I. The prednisone is likely used as a bridge therapy as Ms. Trombley is begun on a disease-modifying antirheumatic drug (DMARD).
    II. The prednisone appears to be dosed appropriately (lowest effective dose to minimize adverse effects).
    III. Hydroxychloroquine (Plaquenil) was begun within the recommended time frame after diagnosis of rheumatoid arthritis (RA).

    A. I only
    B. III only
    C. I and II
    D. II and III
    E. I, II, and III

145. On 5/1, Ms. Trombley was given prescriptions for three medications used to treat anemia. Patients with rheumatoid arthritis may have an anemia associated with their disease, which is unrelated to drug therapy. Would any of these medications be appropriate for this anemia?

    A. Yes
    B. No

146. The non-anemia prescription that Dr. Cook wrote for Ms. Trombley on 5/1 was most likely given

    I. for treatment of her constipation.
    II. as an additional DMARD.
    III. because of concern about potential GI damage caused by Motrin.

    A. I only
    B. III only
    C. I and II
    D. II and III
    E. I, II, and III

147. On 6/5, Ms. Trombley was placed on ciprofloxacin for a documented urinary tract infection (UTI). However, after contacting Dr. Cook, the decision was made for one final month of hydroxychloroquine. Which of the following responses accurately reflects the final treatments for Ms. Trombleys' rheumatoid arthritis?

    I. Ms. Trombley was not responding to the hydroxychloroquine, which prompted a change in therapy to etanercept.
    II. Etanercept is a tumor necrosis factor (TNF) inhibitor which can increase the risk of infections and should not be used in patients with active infections.
    III. TNF-inhibitors have been shown to be more effective when combined with methotrexate.

    A. I only
    B. III only
    C. I and II
    D. II and III
    E. I, II, and III

148. Finally, Ms. Trombley was placed on etanercept (Enbrel). All of the following are correct statements concerning the use of this agent *except* which one?

    A. It is a biological response modifier for slowing the progression of rheumatoid arthritis.
    B. It is an agent that inhibits only the cyclooxygenase 2 receptor.
    C. The agent is given by subcutaneous injection.
    D. Agents such as this can be used when other traditional DMARDs fail.
    E. Baseline laboratory tests should include HBsAg, PPD, and signs and symptoms of HBV.

End of this patient profile; continue with the examination.

---

149. Pyrantel pamoate is indicated for the treatment of pinworms. Besides treatment with this agent, other precautions must be used when a child has pinworms. Related to the treatment of this condition, all of the following are correct *except* which one?

    A. Pyrantel pamoate paralyzes the worms through depolarization of muscle.
    B. All household members should be treated.
    C. All bedrooms should be thoroughly swept with a broom.
    D. Clothes and linens should be washed in hot water.
    E. Children should take showers rather than baths.

150. Sally, a regular customer in your pharmacy, wants some advice on an OTC treatment for itchy, odorous feet. Upon questioning, you discover that in between her toes, the skin is whiter than usual, thick, and scaly. She tells you that she swims competitively and often uses public showers at the pool. What condition is Sally most likely suffering from?

    A. tinea cruris
    B. tinea capitis
    C. tinea pedis
    D. tinea corporis
    E. tinea unguium

151. All of the following OTC agents are considered safe and effective for treating Sally's condition (see question 150) *except*

    A. terbinafine.
    B. clotrimazole.
    C. tolnaftate.
    D. hexylresorcinol.
    E. miconazole.

152. What are the two OTC antihistamines approved by the FDA for insomnia?

    A. diphenhydramine and doxylamine
    B. chlorpheniramine and loratadine
    C. doxylamine and brompheniramine
    D. thonzylamine and pheniramine
    E. dexbrompheniramine and chlorpheniramine

153. Mr. Conway, a 45-year-old who drives cross-country for a trucking company, complains of a runny nose, sneezing, and watery eyes that typically occur about this time of year. He knows it is allergies but cannot remember what medication he took for his allergies last year. Which of the following would be the best initial OTC recommendation for Mr. Conway to take for this condition this year?

    A. pseudoephedrine 60 mg twice a day
    B. loratadine 10 mg every day
    C. diphenhydramine 25 mg every 6 hours
    D. doxylamine 25 mg three times daily
    E. no OTC recommendation; refer the patient to a physician for a prescription for a nonsedating antihistamine

154. On a slow Sunday afternoon, you spot a teenager in the analgesic aisle and ask if there's anything you can help her find. She blushes a bit and blurts, "I just started my period and I think I'm going to die if I don't take something pretty quick here!" You hide your surprise (after all, this is the 12-year-old daughter of one of your friends at church) and offer to help. Which of the following medications is *not* an option for this girl?

    A. ketoprofen
    B. acetaminophen
    C. ibuprofen
    D. naproxen
    E. aspirin

155. Your pharmacy student pulls you aside and says, "I'm trying to counsel Mrs. Pound on the nonprescription medication treatment options to take care of her daughter's head lice." Which of the following products could be recommended OTC?

    I. a synergized pyrethrins product
    II. a product containing permethrin
    III. a product containing lindane

    A. I only
    B. III only
    C. I and II
    D. II and III
    E. I, II, and III

156. There are a large number of insulin products. What is the composition of Novolin 70/30?

    A. 70% regular insulin, 30% NPH insulin
    B. 70% Humalog insulin, 30% NPH insulin
    C. 70% NPH insulin, 30% regular insulin
    D. 70% NPH insulin, 30% Humalog insulin
    E. 70% regular insulin, 30% Humalog insulin

Use the patient profile below to answer questions 157 to 162.

MEDICATION PROFILE (SKILLED NURSING FACILITY)

Patient Name: Fanny Urmeister
Address: 24555 Colonial Estates
Age: 79   Height: 5′2″
Sex: F   Race: African American   Weight: 178 lb
Allergies: Aspirin, ciprofloxacin

DIAGNOSIS

Primary	(1)	UTI
Secondary	(1)	Atrial fibrillation
	(2)	History of smoking
	(3)	Obesity
	(4)	Hyperlipidemia

MEDICATION RECORD (Prescription and OTC)

	Date	Physician	Drug and Strength	Quan	Sig	Refills
(1)	10/5	Lamb	Zocor 40 mg	60	i qhs	6
(2)	10/5	Lamb	Docusate 100 mg	60	ii hs	6
(3)	10/5	Lamb	Coumadin 2.5 mg	30	i daily	6
(4)	10/5	Lamb	Metoprolol 25 mg	60	i bid	6
(5)	10/5	Lamb	Omeprazole 20 mg	30	i daily	6

LABS

10/5	WBC	17.2 K/μL
10/5	Urinalysis	Bacteria present, nitrite negative, 2+ leukocytes, negative for ketones, specific gravity 1.003, negative glucose, 0 red blood cells present, few epithelial cells, leukocyte esterase positive
10/5		Chem 7 performed; BUN 27, SCr 1.5
10/5		BP 136/74, HR 72

PHARMACIST NOTES AND OTHER PATIENT INFORMATION

	Date	Comments
(1)	10/5	Patient complained to nurse of burning upon urination and hard stools.
(2)	10/5	Urinalysis, Chem 7 ordered.
(3)	10/5	Results of U/A reviewed.

157. Based on Ms. Urmeister's laboratory and urinalysis results, which of the following statements is/are true?

    I. Her Chem 7 results indicate that she likely has some renal impairment.
    II. Her WBC count is an indicator that she may have an infection.
    III. The urinalysis was nitrite negative, therefore, the bacteria causing the UTI is likely gram-positive.

    A. I only
    B. III only
    C. I and II
    D. II and III
    E. I, II, and III

158. What medication would be the most appropriate option to treat Ms. Urmeister's UTI based on the patient's profile?

    A. sulfamethoxazole/trimethoprim
    B. nitrofurantoin
    C. amoxicillin
    D. ciprofloxacin
    E. metronidazole

159. Ms. Urmeister is currently taking warfarin related to her atrial fibrillation. Warfarin works as an anticoagulant in the following way(s):

    A. It inhibits the production of the vitamin K–dependent clotting factors II, VII, IX, and X.
    B. It inhibits the production of proteins C and S.
    C. It inhibits the activity of antithrombin III.
    D. It directly inhibits thrombin.
    E. Both A and B.

160. Based on the fact that Ms. Urmeister is on warfarin therapy, all of the following parameters would be appropriate to monitor *except*:

    A. serum ketones.
    B. prothrombin time.
    C. INR.
    D. stool guaiac.
    E. hematocrit.

161. Which of the following medications in Ms. Urmeister's current profile does not have an indication noted?

    A. warfarin
    B. omeprazole
    C. simvastatin
    D. metoprolol
    E. docusate

162. All of the following are components of the CHADS(2) score that could be used to calculate Ms. Urmeister's risk for having a stroke *except*:

    A. congestive heart failure.
    B. age.
    C. diabetes mellitus.
    D. renal function.
    E. hypertension.

End of this patient profile; continue with the examination.

163. Which of the following medications does not match with its corresponding major mechanism of action as an antiarrhythmic?

    A. dofetilide – sodium channel blocker
    B. amiodarone – potassium channel blocker
    C. atenolol – β blocker
    D. procainamide – sodium channel blocker
    E. diltiazem – calcium-channel blocker

164. All of the following are major adverse effects associated with the drug amiodarone *except*

    A. pulmonary fibrosis.
    B. hypertension.
    C. hypothyroidism.
    D. corneal microdeposits.
    E. hepatotoxicity.

165. Which agent is effective in reducing pain, anxiety, and cardiac workload in the myocardial infarction patient?

    A. aspirin
    B. morphine
    C. furosemide
    D. digoxin
    E. lidocaine

166. All of the following are correctly matched by brand and generic names *except* which one?

    A. cholestyramine/Questran
    B. warfarin/Coumadin
    C. nitroglycerin patches/NicoDerm CQ
    D. disopyramide/Norpace
    E. diltiazem/Cardizem

167. Isosorbide dinitrate can be used to treat

    I. heart failure.

    II. angina pectoris.

    III. acute treatment of hypertension.

    A. I only

    B. III only

    C. I and II

    D. II and III

    E. I, II, and III

168. All of the following medications would be appropriate during the first several hours after a NSTEMI *except*

    A. reteplase.

    B. metoprolol.

    C. aspirin.

    D. morphine.

    E. nitroglycerin.

169. A 30-year-old man comes into your pharmacy complaining of difficulty falling asleep at night. He hands you a list of all the drugs he is currently taking. Which one of these medications is the *most likely* culprit responsible for this sleep problem?

    A. Metamucil

    B. Sudafed

    C. Flonase

    D. Benadryl

    E. aspirin

170. Which of the following conditions can be treated with nonprescription products?

    A. water-clogged ears

    B. otitis media

    C. swimmer's ear

    D. impacted cerumen

    E. both A and D

171. Which of the following topical nasal decongestant agents has a 12-hour duration of action and, therefore, is administered twice daily for adult patients?

    A. oxymetazoline

    B. naphazoline

    C. phenylephrine

    D. ephedrine

    E. xylometazoline

172. Jim, a technician working in your pharmacy, asks you to recommend a sunscreen for him to take to the beach for spring break. He has fair skin and states that he usually gets some minimal redness on his skin after only 10 minutes in the sun. If you recommend a sun protection factor (SPF) product of 15 and assume Jim applies this product correctly, for how long will Jim be able to stay in the sun before he gets the same minimal degree of redness on his skin as noted above?

    A. 30 minutes

    B. 2.5 hours

    C. 6 hours

    D. 45 minutes

    E. 1.5 hours

173. A 21-year-old man walks up to you at the counter with a bottle of 5% minoxidil topical solution in hand. He proceeds to ask you about how to effectively apply this product. All of the following are appropriate points to cover in counseling this patient *except* which one?

    A. Double the dose if you miss an application.

    B. Rub about 1 mL of the product onto the affected area of the scalp twice daily.

    C. This strength is indicated for men only, not women.

    D. This product must be used continuously to maintain any hair regrowth.

    E. Allow 2 to 4 hours for the drug to penetrate the scalp before showering or going swimming.

174. Which of the following nonprescription ingredients does *not* have proven safety/efficacy for the treatment of acne?

    A. benzoyl peroxide

    B. sulfur

    C. triclosan

    D. salicylic acid

    E. sulfur and resorcinol

175. A teenage girl and her mother are at your counseling window in the pharmacy. The mother explains that her daughter has had acne for a few months now and has used a couple of OTC agents (benzoyl peroxide cream and face wash) and asks you to recommend a product to help treat the acne. You examine the girl's face and count over a dozen papules and pustules along with some mild scarring. The girl says she has a few more on her trunk. What do you recommend for this patient?

A. Use Oxy Daily Wash Acne Treatment (benzoyl peroxide 10%) each evening.
B. Use Clearasil Stayclear adult acne treatment cream (resorcinol 2%; sulfur 8%) each morning.
C. Wash face at least four to five times daily with a soap containing salicylic acid.
D. No further OTC product recommendations can be made at this time; advise the girl to see a physician or dermatologist.
E. Use Gly Derm (glycolic acid) twice daily.

176. Which one of the following best describes the mechanism of action of benzoyl peroxide for acne?

A. pyrolytic—allows the pores to "open up"
B. keratolytic only
C. antibacterial only
D. generates free radicals that oxidize protein in the cell membranes plus a keratolytic action
E. dries out lesions by decreasing sebum production by sebaceous glands

177. Rhinitis medicamentosa is an adverse effect associated with overuse of which agents?

A. oral decongestants
B. antihistamines
C. topical decongestants
D. expectorants
E. cough suppressants

178. The pharmacist should advise a patient not to crush Coreg CR because crushing this tablet:

   I. destroys the active drug in this dosage form.
  II. allows immediate absorption of the active drug.
 III. destroys the integrity of the delivery system.

A. I only
B. III only
C. I and II
D. II and III
E. I, II, and III

179. A first-order reaction is characterized by:

   I. $da/dt = -k$.
  II. $A = A_0 e^{-kt}$.
 III. $t_{1/2} = 0.693/k$.

A. I only
B. III only
C. I and II
D. II and III
E. I, II, and III

180. FluMist is approved for use in:

   I. children < 2 years of age.
  II. children aged 2 to 17.
 III. adults aged 18 to 49.

A. I only
B. III only
C. I and II
D. II and III
E. I, II, and III

181. Calcium is available for oral administration in all of the following salt forms *except*:

A. chloride.
B. lactate.
C. gluconate.
D. phosphate.
E. carbonate.

182. All of the following are side effects of prednisone *except*:

A. osteoporosis.
B. hyperglycemia.
C. leukopenia.
D. fluid retention.
E. cataracts.

183. Which of the following is *not* a protease inhibitor for treatment of HIV infection?

A. saquinavir
B. ritonavir
C. cidofovir
D. indinavir
E. atazanavir

184. Pyrogen testing of parenteral solutions is a quality control procedure used to check that the product

    I. does not contain fever-producing substances.
    II. is sterile.
    III. does not contain particulate matter.

    A. I only
    B. III only
    C. I and II
    D. II and III
    E. I, II, and III

185. Common laboratory tests to assess kidney disease include

    I. BUN and serum creatinine.
    II. lactic dehydrogenase (LDH), aspartate aminotransferase (AST; formerly SGOT), and alanine aminotransferase (ALT; formerly SGPT).
    III. red blood count (RBC) and white blood count (WBC).

    A. I only
    B. III only
    C. I and II
    D. II and III
    E. I, II, and III

186. Treatment of chemotherapy-induced nausea and vomiting includes all of the following drugs *except*:

    A. ondansetron.
    B. metoclopramide.
    C. aprepitant.
    D. cimetidine.
    E. dronabinol.

187. Laboratory findings in acute renal failure (ARF) may include all of the following conditions *except*

    A. hypophosphatemia.
    B. hyperuricemia.
    C. hyperkalemia.
    D. metabolic acidosis.
    E. hypocalcemia.

188. Which trace element, if deficient, is responsible for cretinism in children?

    A. zinc
    B. copper
    C. chromium
    D. selenium
    E. iodine

189. Which vitamin below must be given in sufficient quantities during pregnancy to prevent neural tube defects in the baby?

    A. vitamin B_{12}
    B. niacin
    C. thiamine
    D. folic acid
    E. vitamin C

190. All of the following would be good recommendations to prevent poison ivy contact dermatitis *except* which one?

    A. Wash hands with soap and water within 10 minutes of exposure to poison ivy.
    B. Apply bentoquatam 5% solution at least 15 minutes before possible plant contact.
    C. Apply bentoquatam 5% solution immediately after contact with the poison ivy plant to exposed area of skin.
    D. Wear protective clothing to cover exposed areas.
    E. Identify the poison ivy plant in books, via internet sites, etc. so the patient will know what it looks like and how to avoid it.

Test 1 Answers and Explanations

1. The answer is C (I and II). The potential problem is the drug interaction between gemfibrozil and simvastatin. The combination of gemfibrozil and simvastatin has been associated with an increased risk of myopathy and rhabdomyolysis. One would need to know the lipid panel results to determine the necessity of both agents being used together due to the marked severity of this interaction.

2. The answer is A (I only). Doxazosin in doses of 2 to 8 mg/day was one of the treatment arms in ALLHAT, and the treatment was discontinued prematurely owing to an apparent 25% increase in the incidence of combined cardiovascular disease outcomes compared to patients in the control group receiving the diuretic chlorthalidone. The added risks for heart failure, stroke, and coronary heart disease were the major outcomes of the doxazosin arm.

3. The answer is E (I, II, and III). The JNC-7 provided a table of compelling indications that suggested specific drug therapy in select patients rather than the use of standard suggested guidelines. Included as compelling indications, and their respective therapy, are heart failure (diuretics, β-blockers, ACE inhibitors, ARBs, aldosterone antagonists), post-MI (β-blockers, ACE inhibitors, aldosterone antagonists), high coronary disease risk (diuretics, β-blockers, ACE inhibitors, calcium-channel blockers), diabetes (diuretics, β-blockers, ACE inhibitors, ARBs, calcium-channel blockers), chronic kidney disease (ACE inhibitors, ARBs), and recurrent stroke prevention (diuretics, ACE inhibitors).

4. The answer is C (I and II). β-Adrenergic blockers such as metoprolol are indicated in post-MI patients, where they have been shown to significantly reduce sudden death and overall mortality. In addition, they have been suggested by the JNC-7 guidelines as therapeutic options in hypertensive patients with the following compelling indications for their use instead of standard suggested therapy: heart failure, post-MI, high-risk coronary disease patients, and diabetes. Ms. Honors, as a post-MI patient with hypertension, would be a candidate for metoprolol.

5. The answer is E (I, II, and III). Thrombolytic agents (rt-PA, r-PA, TNKase) have been used in patients with STEMI who have had chest pain for < 6 to 12 hours. Successful early reperfusion has been shown to reduce infarct size, improve ventricular function, and improve mortality. Benefits may be seen in patients using thrombolytic therapy as late as 12 hours after pain starts. The use of thrombolytics may restore blood flow in an occluded artery if administered within 12 hours of an acute MI, although < 6 hours is optimal. The goal of treatment of STEMI patients is to initiate thrombolytic therapy within 30 to 60 minutes of arrival in an emergency room. Most studies have shown that each agent, when used early, can reopen (reperfuse) occluded coronary arteries and reduce mortality from STEMI. However, considerations such as ease of use, onset of action, incidence of bleed, and cost are important in determining which agent is used in a given hospital and given patient.

6. The answer is B (III only). Clopidogrel possesses antithrombotic effects and is recommended to prevent the development of acute coronary syndromes. I and II are incorrect.

7. The answer is B. Rabeprazole (Aciphex) is a proton pump inhibitor (PPI), which among other indications (duodenal ulcer, erosive gastritis, hypersecretory conditions, and treatment of *Helicobacter pylori* infections) is primarily indicated for the treatment of GERD. Current recommendations suggest a dosage of 20 mg by mouth daily.

8. The answer is B (III only). Sublingual nitroglycerin is indicated for the acute treatment of angina pectoris as well as for the prophylaxis of angina pectoris. The tablets are to be placed under the tongue, where they dissolve and demonstrate a quick onset of action of 2 to 5 minutes. Sublingual nitroglycerin tablets are not to be swallowed or placed in easy-to-open plastic containers and should remain in the manufacturer's bottle to reduce loss of potency. Patients should also be warned that they may become light-headed or dizzy after taking a tablet and should either sit down or support themselves against a solid object to prevent falls. Patients should also be informed that nitroglycerin tablets can cause a headache and routinely cause a slight burning sensation when placed under the tongue.

9. The answer is C. She has stage II hypertension. JNC-7 guidelines include four blood pressure classes (normal, prehypertension, stage I hypertension, and stage II hypertension); the classes are based on patient's blood pressure readings and are linked to current treatment recommendations. Normal (systolic < 120 and diastolic < 80 mm Hg) requires no treatment. Prehypertension (systolic 120 to 139 or diastolic of 80 to 89 mm Hg) again requires no antihypertensive treatment unless the patient has a compelling indication. In stage I hypertension (systolic 140 to 159 or diastolic 90 to 99 mm Hg), thiazide-type diuretics are indicated for most patients, although patients with compelling indications would be candidates for other agents. In stage II hypertension (systolic ≥ 160 or diastolic ≥ 100 mm Hg), two-drug combinations are indicated for most patients (thiazide-type diuretic and ACE inhibitor, ARB, β-blocker, or calcium-channel blocker). Ms. Honors' BP (162/104) indicates that she has stage II hypertension and she is receiving a diuretic, a β-blocker, and an ACE inhibitor.

10. The answer is D (II & III). There is not any information in the profile that would prevent the use of acetaminophen. NSAIDs (ibuprofen and celecoxib) may decrease the effectiveness of her antihypertensive therapy and may cause an increased risk of myocardial infarction in this patient.

11. The answer is E (I, II, and III). Untreated hypertension has been shown to cause target organ damage to four major organ systems. *Cardiac effects:* left ventricular hypertrophy compensates for the increased cardiac workload, resulting in signs and symptoms of heart failure, and increased oxygen requirements of the enlarged heart may produce angina pectoris. Hypertension can be caused by accelerated atherosclerosis. Atheromatous lesions in the coronary arteries lead to decreased blood flow, resulting in angina pectoris and MI; sudden death may ensue. *Renal effects:* decreased blood flow leads to an increase in renin-aldosterone secretion, which heightens the reabsorption of sodium and water and increases blood volume. Accelerated atherosclerosis decreases the oxygen supply, leading to renal parenchymal damage, with decreased filtration capability and azotemia. The atherosclerosis also decreases blood flow to the renal arterioles, leading to nephrosclerosis and, ultimately, renal failure (acute as well as chronic). *Cerebral effects:* decreased blood flow, decreased oxygen supply, and weakened blood vessel walls lead to transient ischemic attacks, cerebral thromboses, and the development of aneurysms with hemorrhage. There are alterations in mobility along with weakness, paralysis, and memory deficits. *Retinal effects:* decreased blood flow with retinal vascular sclerosis and increased arteriolar pressure with the appearance of exudates and hemorrhage result in visual defects (e.g., blurred vision, spots, blindness).

12. The answer is A. Amiloride. In an otherwise healthy patient with stage I hypertension, thiazide diuretics are considered the first-line treatment of choice for most patients. In patients who might have a compelling indication, such as renal disease, stroke, high-risk cardiovascular disease, or diabetes mellitus, other agents have been recommended. Amiloride is a potassium-sparing diuretic and is not indicated over thiazide diuretics as first-line therapy. Chlorthalidone, chlorothiazide, indapamide, and hydroclothiazide are all thiazide diuretics; and although they may have different pharmacokinetic profiles and different costs, they should all be considered first-line antihypertensives.

13. The answer is B. Isotonic and isoosmotic solutions have osmotic pressures that are equal to blood. Normal saline solution, 0.9% sodium chloride, usually is given as an example of an isotonic solution. Hypertonic solutions have osmotic pressures greater than blood (e.g., high concentrations of dextrose used in total parenteral therapy). Half-normal saline solution (0.45% sodium chloride) has an osmotic pressure less than that of blood and is referred to as a hypotonic solution.

14. The answer is B. Anemia is a common complication of chronic kidney disease caused by a decrease in erythropoietin, an endocrine product produced in the kidney. Erythropoietin, stimulates red blood cell production in the bone marrow. This is reflected by an increase in hematocrit and hemoglobin and a decrease in the need for blood transfusions.

15. The answer is D (II and III). Insulin resistance can occur in both type 1 and type 2 diabetes patients so statement I is incorrect. The other two statements about insulin resistance are correct.

16. The answer is C (I and II). Lanolin is the waxy substance that is secreted by the sebaceous glands of sheep and deposited onto the sheep wool fibers. It is found in many OTC moisturizing products and serves as an emollient occlusive film that can prevent water loss from the skin through evaporation.

17. The answer is A. Both bismuth subsalicylate and loperamide are considered safe and effective. Adsorbents (pectin and attapulgite) that have been used in OTC antidiarrheal products in the past have not been shown to be effective. Kaolin, another adsorbent, has been shown to be safe and effective by itself, but there are no OTC products on the market that contain only kaolin.

18. The answer is E (I, II, and III). Levodopa crosses the blood–brain barrier. It is converted to dopamine where it exerts its effects in Parkinson disease. Levodopa is metabolized centrally and peripherally to dopamine by dopa decarboxylase. Carbidopa does not cross the blood–brain barrier and inhibits peripheral decarboxylation of levodopa. Therefore, more levodopa is available for transport to the brain, and the peripheral side effects are reduced. Sinemet combines the antiparkinsonian effects of levodopa with the dopamine metabolism-inhibiting effects of carbidopa.

19. The answer is E (I, II, and III). Drugs that are highly bound to albumin will have higher concentrations of free drug circulating in the blood if albumin levels are reduced. Hypoalbuminemia, liver (hepatic) disease, malnutrition, and cancer are several of the more common conditions that result in decreased albumin levels, which necessitate alterations in dosage in highly albumin-bound drugs.

20. The answer is A. The action of salmeterol is that of a sympathomimetic agonist with high β_2 selectivity. The lung contains β_2-receptors, which are responsible for the relaxation of tracheal and bronchial muscles. In contrast, β_1-receptors are in the heart and are responsible for chronotropic (rate) and inotropic (contraction force) effects. Salmeterol gives the asthmatic patient maximal bronchodilation with minimal stimulation of cardiac receptors.

21. The answer is A (I). Different age groups have common underlying causes for the development of heart failure. The patient in this case is 54 years of age and has no history of MI as a possible cause, which is a leading cause of heart failure in people aged 40 to 50 years. Drugs such as corticosteroids have been implicated as causative agents in the development of heart failure owing to their ability to cause sodium and water retention. In both of these cases, metabolic demands placed on the heart normally do not increase; however, the heart is still unable to meet them (low output). Mr. Mutrick has a secondary diagnosis of anemia (possibly caused by steroid use), which increases the metabolic demands placed on a heart that is already unable to meet such demands (high output).

22. The answer is D (II and III). On receiving the prescriptions on 8/10, the pharmacist should have called the physician's office for assurance that the potassium supplement was truly warranted owing to the documentation of chronic kidney disease. Potassium elimination depends on the kidney, and declining function means the ability to excrete potassium is reduced. In addition, based on updated treatment guidelines, the pharmacist would be justified in discussing the potential role for a β-adrenergic blocker in this type of patient. Its merits may very well extend beyond those appreciated in heart failure, including hypertension as compelling condition.

23. The answer is D (II and III). Carvedilol (Coreg) is a β-adrenergic receptor blocker that is indicated in the treatment of hypertension and heart failure. When used in the treatment of heart failure, as in Mr. Mutrick, doses must be slowly and closely titrated up to the maximal dosage every 2 weeks as tolerated. The pharmacist was able to identify that there were no prescriptions on file for Mr. Mutrick for Coreg and there were no refills provided with the initial prescription of Coreg 3.125 mg. This has the potential for leaving the patient without his medication at the end of the 2-week period. Cardiac patients receiving β-adrenergic receptor blockers should not have their β-blocker discontinued abruptly, as this may induce an acute coronary event caused by the lack of β-blockade.

24. The answer is A. A patient with left-sided heart failure presents with symptoms and signs of fluid backing up behind a failed left ventricle. Mr. Mutrick would initially present with complaints involving the pulmonary system (e.g., rales, shortness of breath, paroxysmal nocturnal dyspnea). Peripheral signs and symptoms (e.g., jugular venous distention, hepatojugular reflux, pedal edema, abdominal distention, and hepatomegaly) are more the consequence of the backup of fluid behind the failing right ventricle, characteristically seen in right-sided heart failure. It is important to recognize that, because the circulatory system is closed, patients rarely present with strictly left-sided signs or right-sided signs; rather, they present with a combination of signs and symptoms that reflect global circulatory problems.

25. The answer is E (I, II, and III). Ramipril (Altace) is an ACE inhibitor. Recent clinical guidelines recommend the use of ACE inhibitors in all patients with heart failure owing to left ventricular systolic dysfunction, unless they have a contraindication to their use or have demonstrated intolerance to their use. Currently, these drugs are considered the first-line agents in the treatment of heart failure and have been shown to have a beneficial effect on cardiac remodeling. The Heart Outcomes Prevention Evaluation (HOPE) trial demonstrated that the ACE inhibitor ramipril (10 mg/day) reduced cardiovascular death, MI, and stroke in patients > 55 years of age who were at high risk for or had vascular disease in the absence of heart failure. ACE inhibitors have also been shown to be beneficial in patients who have chronic kidney disease, in whom they can reduce the onset of deteriorating renal function. Each of the three conditions—hypertension, heart failure, and chronic kidney disease—have now been shown to benefit from the use of ACE inhibitors such as ramipril. However, caution is still required; patients should be monitored for elevations in potassium levels and a potential reduction in renal function indicators (serum creatinine).

26. The answer is B. Ferrous sulfate is available in the hydrous form as a 325-mg tablet. The preparation contains 20% elemental iron. Consequently, 325 mg given three times a day would equal $0.20 \times 3 \times 325$ mg, or 195 mg per day. Other available salts that contain varying degrees of elemental iron are ferrous gluconate, 12%; ferrous fumarate, 33%; and ferrous sulfate (desiccated), 30%.

27. The answer is C (I and II). Clopidogrel is a thienopyridine derivative related to ticlopidine, but it possesses antithrombotic effects greater than those of ticlopidine. The most recent national guidelines for ST-segment elevated myocardial infarction (STEMI) state that clopidogrel should be added to aspirin in STEMI patients regardless of whether they undergo reperfusion with fibrinolytics or do not receive reperfusion. Doses of 75 mg by mouth daily should be administered and treatment should continue for at least 14 days. However, long-term maintenance therapy for up to 1 year can be used as well.

28. The answer is C (I and II). Enalapril (Vasotec), captopril (Capoten), lisinopril (Zestril and Prinivil), benazepril (Lotensin), fosinopril (Monopril), quinapril (Accupril), ramipril (Altace), moexipril (Univasc), and trandolapril (Mavik) are the ACE inhibitors currently on the market.

The agents as a group have the same general pharmacologic effects by blocking the actions of the converting enzyme, which converts angiotensin I to angiotensin II (a potent vasoconstrictor), thereby reducing afterload and inhibiting aldosterone release from the adrenal gland. Currently, ACE inhibitors are considered the first-line agents in the treatment of heart failure and have been shown to have a beneficial effect on cardiac remodeling.

29. The answer is E (I, II, and III). Digoxin is excreted by the renal route, with 60% to 80% of bioavailable digoxin excreted unchanged by glomerular filtration and active tubular secretion. The half-life for digoxin in patients with normal renal function is approximately 1.6 days, whereas renal function may significantly increase the elimination half-life. In congestive heart failure patients, renal clearance of digoxin may be reduced enough to allow for significant accumulation of drug if dose is not altered. Potassium-losing diuretics such as furosemide (Lasix) may increase binding of digoxin to target organ myocardial tissues, which may help explain why reduced potassium levels potentiate digoxin toxicity. Potassium levels need to be evaluated prior to initiating therapy.

30. The answer is A. Hydralazine (Apresoline) is an arteriole dilator that has been used in hypertension. However, by decreasing peripheral vascular resistance, it also has been shown to reduce afterload in patients with heart failure. A Veterans Administration study has shown that the combination of hydralazine and isosorbide dinitrate significantly reduced mortality in heart failure patients unresponsive to digitalis and diuretics. Long-term therapy with hydralazine has been associated with the development of systemic lupus erythematosus, which presents as fatigue, malaise, low-grade fever, and joint aches and pains. Baseline and serial blood counts for antinuclear antibody titers should be performed; if systemic lupus erythematosus develops, discontinuation of the drug results in reversal of the symptoms over time.

31. The answer is E (I, II, and III). Inamrinone, dobutamine, and dopamine are inotropic agents. Inotropic agents have been used in the emergency treatment of patients with heart failure and in patients refractory to, or unable to take, digitalis. However, current guidelines provide a Class III recommendation for these drugs. In addition, current guidelines provide a Class IIb recommendation—"conditions for which there is conflicting evidence and/or a divergence of opinion about the usefulness/efficacy of performing the procedure/therapy and that the usefulness/efficacy is less well established by evidence/opinion"—for the use of continuous intravenous infusion of a positive inotropic agent for palliation of heart failure symptoms.

32. The answer is A (I). NSAIDs have been reported to cause GI erosions and ulcers. This patient could have a major problem because of a report of anemia. In addition, the

physician should be given an update from the pharmacist regarding the current disease conditions to reinforce caution for such agents owing to the patient's history of hypertension and chronic kidney disease.

33. The answer is E. Similar to ACE inhibitors, β-adrenergic blockers work through actions of the endogenous neurohormonal system. Unlike ACE inhibitors, which work strictly by blocking the effects of the renin–angiotensin system, β-adrenergic blockers work by interfering with the sympathetic nervous system. This has prompted the use of three different types of β-adrenergic blockers: those that are relatively selective toward β_1-receptors (e.g., metoprolol); those that are selective to both β_1- and β_2-receptors (e.g., propranolol and bucindolol); and those that are selective to β_1-, β_2-, and α_1-receptors (e.g., carvedilol). β-Adrenergic blockers, similar to ACE inhibitors, have been shown to decrease the risk of death and hospitalization as well as improve the clinical status of heart failure patients. Current guidelines recommend the use of a β-adrenergic blocker in all patients with stable heart failure owing to left ventricular dysfunction, unless they have a contraindication to their use or are unable to tolerate their effects because of hypotension, bradycardia, bronchospasm, and the like.

34. The answer is C. Atropine in therapeutic doses inhibits cholinergic impulses and increases the heart rate. When treatment is initiated in a patient with sinus bradycardia, initial small doses may actually stimulate cholinergic receptors and therefore increase the degree of bradycardia. Constipation, dry mouth, decreased secretions, and pupillary dilation are all side effects associated with anticholinergic drugs. Rarely do single doses of atropine cause constipation.

35. The answer is E (I, II, and III). Although the branded version of Quinaglute is no longer available, currently there are several extended-release generic quinidine gluconate products on the market to fill this gap. Quinidine is a class I_A antiarrhythmic agent, with GI intolerance as one of its more troubling side effects. The extended-release quinidine gluconate products have been marketed as a way to reduce the GI effects while providing a more sustained, consistent quinidine level with less fluctuations and lower peak effects. Carvedilol (Coreg) is a β-adrenergic blocker and is indicated in the treatment of heart failure and is currently available as a rapid-release product (Coreg) and an extended-release product (Coreg CR). Felodipine (Plendil) is considered an extended-release product and is used in the treatment of hypertension. It is one of the second-generation calcium-channel blocking agents and is not indicated as an antiarrhythmic agent.

36. The answer is D. Inamrinone is a bipyridine agent that has both positive inotropic effects and vasodilating effects. It does offer an alternative to dopamine and dobutamine and is given as an IV infusion of 5 to 10 μg/kg/min. Timolol and atenolol are β-adrenergic blockers, verapamil is a calcium-channel blocker, and disopyramide is a class I_A antiarrhythmic agent—all have negative inotropic activities. Their use could create a problem in a patient who requires inotropic support. β-Adrenergic blockers are currently recommended as first-line agents in patients with stable heart failure, unless they have a contraindication to their use or cannot tolerate their effects because of hypotension, bradycardia, bronchospasm, and the like.

37. The answer is D. Lansoprazole (Prevacid) is a PPI used for the short-term treatment of refractory duodenal ulcer, severe erosive esophagitis, and poorly responsive gastroesophageal reflux disease. Cimetidine (Tagamet) and famotidine (Pepcid) are H_2-receptor antagonists that work by inhibiting the actions of histamine at the parietal cell receptor sites. Sucralfate (Carafate) is a nonabsorbable mucosal protectant that adheres to the base of ulcer craters. Octreotide (Sandostatin) is a long-acting synthetic octapeptide that works like somatostatin by inhibiting serotonin, gastrin, vasoactive intestinal polypeptide, insulin, glucagon, growth hormone, and other agents.

38. The answer is A. Creatinine is formed during muscle metabolism, and creatinine clearance is the most common method for the measurement of GFR. When only the serum creatinine level and the patient's age, weight, and gender are known, creatinine clearance may be determined by the Cockcroft and Gault equation.

39. The answer is E (I, II, and III). Low doses of aspirin and other salicylates inhibit the tubular secretion of uric acid, which may result in uric acid accumulation and gout. Nicotinic acid competes with uric acid for excretion in the kidney tubule, resulting in greater retention of uric acid and the possibility of a gout attack. Cytotoxic drugs, by nature of their ability to increase nucleic acid turnover (uric acid is a by product of nucleic acid), cause an increase in uric acid and the potential for a gout attack.

40. The answer is C (I and II). Oxymetazoline is a sympathomimetic vasoconstrictor; its effect lasts up to 12 hours. This agent is administered twice daily for up to 3 days.

41. The answer is E. For any first-order process, 50% of the initial amount of drug is eliminated at the end of the first half-life, and 50% of the remaining amount of drug (i.e., 75% of the original amount) is eliminated at the end of the second half-life. Because the half-life of the drug is 2 hours, in 2 hours 50.0% is eliminated, at 4 hours (an additional half-life) 75.0%, and at 6 hours (a third half-life) 87.5% of the drug is eliminated.

42. The answer is C. The MIC for an antimicrobial indicates the lowest concentration of antibiotic that prevents microbial growth after 18 to 24 hours of incubation. The report states that the antimicrobial agent cefepime, at a concentration of 1 μg/mL is able to prevent such growth. This is in contrast to ciprofloxacin, which requires a concentration of 32 μg/mL, ceftazidime (8 μg/mL), gentamicin (4 μg/mL), and meropenem (2 μg/mL). Typically, for antimicrobials that demonstrate concentration-dependent antimicrobial activity, the peak antibiotic concentration at the site of infection must be four to five times the MIC to be considered therapeutic and effective.

43. The answer is C. Four clinical classes have been described for diabetes mellitus and include type 1, type 2, gestational diabetes mellitus, and secondary diabetes. However, the three major classes include type 1, type 2, and gestational. Hyperglycemia is elevated blood sugar but is not identified as a clinical class of diabetes mellitus. Hyperosmolar hyperglycemic state (HHS) can occur in type 2 diabetes, when blood glucose levels increase but without the breakdown of fats because some insulin is present. Diabetic ketoacidosis may occur in patients with type 1 diabetes. This results in hyperglycemia and the breakdown of fats because of insulin insufficiency. Ketonemia (accumulation of ketone bodies in the blood) results from the breakdown of adipose tissue when there is insulin deficiency in type 1 diabetes. Thiazide diuretics and Cushing syndrome may result in hyperglycemia (secondary diabetes). There is no such thing as type 3 diabetes.

44. The answer is C (I and II). Choices I and II describe the diagnostic criteria for nonpregnant adults. As documented by the pharmacist in the notes section, the patient had a hemoglobin $A_{1C} \geq 6.5\%$ at 7.3%, and a random blood glucose level ≥ 126 mg/dL at 140 mg/dL. Additional diagnostic criteria would include a plasma glucose level 2 hours after a glucose load (postprandial) ≥ 200 mg/dL. Mr. Farmer's postprandial glucose level was 175 mg/dL.

45. The answer is E (I, II, and III). Hemoglobin A_{1C} is a useful long-term monitoring tool to measure glycemic control. It is usually tested at least once or twice per year in patients under good control and at least quarterly for therapy changes and for those who are in poor control. The value of < 7% (based on 6.5% as the upper limit of normal) is a desired therapeutic endpoint per the American Diabetes Association standards of medical care.

46. The answer is E (I, II, and III). Glyburide is chemically classified as a sulfonylurea. These agents stimulate the pancreatic secretion of insulin (insulin secretagogue) and, therefore, result in lowered blood glucose (hypoglycemic agent) levels.

47. The answer is B (III). Celecoxib is classified as an NSAID, which was added by Dr. Wilson to help Mr. Farmer with his osteoarthritis. However, the patient has a history of peptic ulcer disease, and the use of an NSAID in this patient population should be avoided. Ramipril is an ACE inhibitor, which would be a rational initial choice in the treatment of the patient's hypertension with diabetes as a comorbidity. Metformin is considered within several national guidelines as the initial therapy. Key benefits include consistent lowering of blood glucose levels, lack of substantial weight gain associated with its use, low cost, and a high level of patient acceptance.

48. The answer is E (I, II, and III). Currently, there are several combination products available on the market which combine metformin along with other hypoglycemic classes (sulfonylureas, thiazolidinediones, and gliptins): glipizide/metformin (Metaglip), glyburide/metformin (Glucovance), pioglitazone/metformin (ACTOplus met), saxagliptin/metformin (Kombiglyze XR), repaglinide/metformin (Prandimet) etc. The combinations have been used successfully to treat type 2 diabetes. Metformin has several mechanisms of action, but it is generally recognized as an insulin sensitizer. Situations such as renal dysfunction and chronic or binge alcohol ingestion can increase the risk for developing lactic acidosis and need to be avoided.

49. The answer is A (I). Acarbose is an α-glucosidase inhibitor in the intestine and acts by reducing the absorption of carbohydrates (complex carbohydrate absorption requires the action of α-glucosidase). Postprandial blood glucose levels are, therefore, lower. This agent has little effect on preprandial or fasting blood glucose levels, and it has an entirely different mechanism of action from metformin.

50. The answer is D (II and III). Alternative test sites such as the forearm, upper arm, thigh, calf, and other areas of the hand should not be used when a patient feels an episode of hypoglycemia coming on or immediately after a meal. Such alternative sites are approved for glucose testing in the fasting state, 2 hours after a meal, or 2 hours after exercise. Blood flow to the fingers is three to five times faster than any other site, and consequently the alternate sites are unable to detect rapid changes in blood glucose.

51. The answer is C (I and II). Osteoarthritis, formerly known as degenerative joint disease, is the most common form of arthritis. There is little, if any, inflammation in the osteoarthritic joint.

52. The answer is C (I and II). The product contains the antihistamine diphenhydramine. Diphenhydramine and doxylamine are the two FDA-approved OTC agents indicated for insomnia. Doxylamine may produce adverse central anticholinergic effects in the elderly, including confusion, disorientation, impaired short-term memory, and sometimes visual and tactile hallucinations. Because of its anticholinergic properties, doxylamine may cause restriction

in the urinary outflow in a male patient with an enlarged prostate and should be avoided in this situation. It would not cause polyuria.

53. The answer is A (I). Sulfonylureas are not associated with weight loss, but instead have shown to cause weight gain, which is one of the most undesirable side effects associated with sulfonylureas. Hypoglycemia is probably the most troublesome of side effects and can represent a medical emergency. Sulfonylureas were the first orally available agents introduced in the late 1950s for the treatment of type 2 diabetes and an alternative to the routine use of injectable insulin.

54. The answer is B. In late 2010, the FDA arrived at the conclusion that rosiglitazone had demonstrated an increased risk of MI in diabetic patients taking the drug. This resulted in a decision during late 2010 to restrict the availability of rosiglitazone to patients who are already taking the drug after being advised of the increased risk, or those who are unable to take alternative drugs in the treatment of type 2 diabetes mellitus. Celecoxib has been given a Black Box Warning as well for an increased risk of serious cardiovascular events, MI, and stroke, but has not yet been restricted, as rosiglitazone.

55. The answer is E (I, II, and III). Exenatide (Byetta) activates glucagon-like peptide-1 (GLP-1) receptor, resulting in the increase in insulin secretion, while decreasing glucagon secretion and delaying gastric emptying. Exenatide is a synthetic version of the hormone substance, exendin-4, which is found in the saliva of the Gila monster. Studies have shown that exenatide causes a rapid increase in insulin release after subcutaneous administration within 10 minutes, but the effect quickly declines over the next 1 to 2 hours. Doses administered after meals have a smaller effect on sugar levels as compared to doses given within 60 minutes of meals.

56. The answer is E (I, II, and III). Dr. Drake identified the need to add a second agent to the previous metformin regimen for Mr. Farmer and added pioglitazone for an additive effect. After 3 months of the combination treatment, Dr. Drake opted to introduce the combination product by titrating the dose of pioglitazone/metformin in order to simplify the regimen.

57. The answer is E (I, II, and III). Alka-Seltzer Plus Day Cold Liquid-Gel Capsules contains acetaminophen, phenylephrine, and dextromethorphan. Before recommending an OTC product for the treatment of the common cold, it is important to know what symptoms the patient is experiencing and then target the therapy to those symptoms—most likely with a single-ingredient product. Phenylephrine administration may result in increasing Mr. Farmer's blood sugar, so this agent should be used cautiously (if at all) in patients with diabetes. Additionally, the product does contain 325 mg acetaminophen, which may push Mr. Farmer over the 4 g maximum daily allotment of acetaminophen.

58. The answer is A. Glyburide (DiaBeta) represents the sulfonylurea hypoglycemic class of drugs, which have been described as having both primary and secondary failure rates, which are not consistent with long-term use in type 2 diabetes. It has been estimated that 10% to 20% of patients started on a sulfonylurea agent will not obtain a therapeutic benefit upon maximizing initial therapy (primary failure), and as many as 5% to 10% of those initially responding subsequently failing each year (secondary failure).

59. The answer is D. Massaging with oil and shampooing treat this form of seborrhea of the scalp in the newborn. This procedure will gently remove the accumulated scaly skin.

60. The answer is C. It is generally believed that the absorptive characteristics of the skin in children < 6 months of age are different from those of adults. The metabolic and excretory systems of these young children may not be able to handle the sunscreen agent that does get absorbed.

61. The answer is B. Salicylic acid is a keratolytic agent and is considered safe and effective for the treatment of warts by the FDA. It is also used for the treatment of corns and calluses.

62. The answer is E. Human papillomavirus is the cause of common warts. Herpes simplex virus 1 (HSV-1) is responsible for cold sores; HSV-2, for genital herpes. The Epstein-Barr virus is the usual cause of infectious mononucleosis. Coronavirus is one of the viruses responsible for the common cold. HIV is the human immunodeficiency virus.

63. The answer is B (III). The individual reviewing the orders identified that HCTZ is a sulfonamide derivative and, because of the nature of the previously documented allergy—specifically Stevens–Johnson syndrome (a type of erythema multiforme reaction)—was able to inform the prescriber, so that spironolactone, which is not a sulfonamide derivative (although it is considerably less potent than HCTZ for hypertension), was prescribed. Previous studies have demonstrated the benefit of thiazide diuretics on mortality rates in hypertensive patients. However, additional considerations in the current patient should include the potential use of ACE inhibitors, ARBs, β-adrenergic receptor blockers, and/or calcium-channel blockers because this patient cannot take a thiazide diuretic.

64. The answer is D (II and III). Irbesartan is an ARB and spironolactone is a potassium-sparing diuretic. If used together, these agents could lead to significant increases in serum potassium. Mr. Torres' serum potassium should,

therefore, be monitored. Atenolol generally does not increase the serum potassium to any extent.

65. The answer is E (I, II, and III). Acute ischemic (coronary) syndromes is a term that has evolved as a way to describe a group of clinical symptoms representing acute myocardial ischemia. The clinical symptoms include acute MI, which might be STEMI or NSTEMI, and unstable angina. Current terminology has not included angina pectoris as one of the acute coronary syndromes.

66. The answer is D. Theophylline serum levels are increased by conditions that decrease theophylline elimination. Smoking increases the rate of theophylline elimination by increasing the rate of metabolism, resulting in a reduced serum theophylline level. Pneumonia, ciprofloxacin, cor pulmonale, and heart failure decrease the rate of theophylline elimination, resulting in an increased serum theophylline level.

67. The answer is B (III). Atenolol is a β-adrenergic blocking agent, which is a relatively cardioselective agent. Even though this agent is β-1 selective and would be a preferred β-blocker over a nonselective agent (such as propranolol), it should be used cautiously at higher doses because of increased risk of acute bronchospasm. No β-adrenergic blocking agent is entirely safe in an asthmatic patient such as Mr. Torres—spironolactone, a potassium-sparing diuretic, and irbesartan, an ARB, can be prescribed for patients with asthma because they do not affect the respiratory system.

68. The answer is E. Routine monitoring parameters for simvastatin would, of course, include obtaining a lipid panel to determine efficacy of the agent in reducing total and LDL cholesterol. Baseline liver function tests (ALT and AST) should be obtained and every 4 to 6 weeks after initiating therapy for the first 15 months of therapy.

69. The answer is C. Irbesartan is a member of a large class of agents referred to as angiotensin II receptor antagonists, which decrease the conversion of angiotensin I to angiotensin II. This results in a reduction in the release of aldosterone as well as a reduction in the powerful vasoconstrictor effects of angiotensin II.

70. The answer is D. All of the agents listed are calcium-channel blockers and have been used successfully in the treatment of hypertension. However, within the calcium-channel blockers, there are three different chemical groups; amlodipine, nifedipine, felodipine, and isradipine are referred to as dihydropyridine derivatives, which do not slow impulses within the atrioventricular (AV) node. Verapamil, a nondihydropyridine derivative, has been shown to effectively slow impulses within the AV node and has been used in the treatment of tachyarrhythmias, angina pectoris, and hypertension.

71. The answer is A. According to the recommendations of the JNC-7 (a multidisciplinary, national collaborative group), drug therapy is usually initiated with a thiazide diuretic in patients with stage I hypertension not associated with any of the compelling indications. However, additional recommendations include alternative therapy with ACE inhibitors, ARBs, β-adrenergic receptor blockers, or calcium-channel blockers for patients who are unable to tolerate a thiazide diuretic or who do not respond appropriately to them. Spironolactone is a potassium-sparing diuretic that antagonizes aldosterone receptors within the distal convoluted tubule and has minor diuretic effects. Doxazosin is a peripherally acting α-adrenergic blocker that demonstrated potentially negative clinical effects in the Antihypertensive and Lipid-Lowering Treatment to Prevent Heart Attack Trial (ALLHAT) study. Hydralazine is a vasodilator that directly dilates peripheral arteries to reduce blood pressure. Clonidine is a centrally acting antihypertensive that stimulates α_2-adrenergic receptors to decrease sympathetic outflow to lower blood pressure. None of these agents is considered an alternative to thiazide diuretics as initial therapy for stage I hypertension.

72. The answer is E (I, II, and III). In most patients, the cause of Parkinson disease is unknown (idiopathic); however, a small percentage of cases are secondary, and many of these cases are curable. Secondary parkinsonism may be caused by drugs such as dopamine antagonists (phenothiazine, butyrophenones such as haloperidol, reserpine), poisoning by chemicals such as carbon monoxide and heavy metals (such as manganese and mercury), infectious diseases such as viral encephalitis and syphilis, and other causes (arteriosclerosis, degenerative diseases of the central nervous system, and various metabolic disorders).

73. The answer is B (III). Diphenhydramine is an antihistaminic agent that has some mild anticholinergic effects and is used for symptomatic relief of mild tremor. Amantadine is a dopaminergic agent. Trihexyphenidyl is an anticholinergic agent. Treatment of Parkinson disease usually involves the use of antihistaminic drugs, anticholinergic agents, and dopaminergic agents. Owing to its adverse reaction within the central nervous system, diphenhydramine should be used with caution in the elderly.

74. The answer is C. Trihexyphenidyl is an anticholinergic agent used in the treatment of Parkinson disease; the daily dosage range is 6 to 10 mg orally. However, when patients are started on trihexyphenidyl, they are usually titrated upward from an initial 1 mg dose up to 2 mg and increasing the dose 2 mg every 3 to 5 days, as tolerated up to a maximal dose of 15 mg per day.

75. The answer is C (I and II). Entacapone, a catechol-*O*-methyltransferase (COMT) inhibitor, works by delaying the metabolism of levodopa and, therefore, prolonging its availability. It is thus indicated as an adjunctive treatment to levodopa in patients who suffer from a wearing-off effect.

76. The answer is A. Caution is needed when introducing anticholinergics in this patient who has narrow-angle glaucoma. Anticholinergic agents may aggravate certain other underlying conditions and, therefore, should also be used with caution in patients with obstructions of the GI or genitourinary tracts or severe cardiac disease. Side effects usually include dry mouth, blurred vision, constipation, urinary retention, and tachycardia. Central nervous system side effects may include hallucinations, ataxia, mental slowing, confusion, and memory impairment.

77. The answer is E (I, II, and III). Levodopa is capable of causing adverse drug reactions within the GI, cardiovascular, and musculoskeletal systems. Additional organ systems with associated adverse reactions include the central nervous system (confusion, memory changes, depression, hallucinations, and psychosis) and the hematologic system (hemolytic anemia, leukopenia, and agranulocytosis).

78. The answer is B (III). Anticholinergic agents should be given one drug at a time. Several agents are available for therapy, and they all appear to be equally effective. One of the principles of drug therapy is that if a patient does not respond to an agent in one class, try another class. The exception includes the use of dopamine agonists, such as bromocriptine; patients who do not respond to one of the agents may not respond to another.

79. The answer is D. Of the drugs listed, only amantadine has dopaminergic properties. Although the full extent of its mechanism of action is not known, amantadine stimulates the presynaptic release of dopamine and has demonstrated benefit in Parkinson disease. Available dopaminergic agents and their mechanisms include levodopa, which exogenously replenishes striatal dopamine; bromocriptine, which directly stimulates dopamine receptors; selegiline and rasagiline, which selectively inhibits monoamine oxidase type B and selectively prevents the breakdown of dopamine in the brain; pramipexole and ropinirole, which are considered nonergot dopamine agents; rotigotine, which stimulates dopamine receptors; and tolcapone and entacapone, referred to as COMT inhibitors, which delay the breakdown of dopamine in the brain. Pergolide, another dopaminergic agent, was recently removed from the U.S. market.

80. The answer is A. Levodopa must be converted to dopamine, and this conversion must occur centrally, for therapeutic effect. Because dopamine does not readily cross the blood–brain barrier, it is important that only minimal amounts of levodopa be converted to dopamine peripherally. The enzyme for this metabolic reaction is dopa decarboxylase, for which pyridoxine (vitamin B_6) is a coenzyme. Exogenous pyridoxine can, therefore, increase the peripheral metabolism of levodopa, making less dopamine available centrally for the desired effect.

81. The answer is A (I). Carbidopa inhibits the peripheral decarboxylation of levodopa to dopamine. Carbidopa does not cross the blood–brain barrier, therefore making more levodopa available for transport to the brain. This situation minimizes the risk of peripheral side effects and may lower the required dose of levodopa by approximately 75%.

82. The answer is B. The on–off phenomenon refers to swings in drug response to levodopa or dopamine agonists. Loss of drug effectiveness is characteristic of off periods. Bromocriptine, a dopamine agonist, has been shown to be effective in patients who have responded poorly to levodopa or who have experienced a severe on–off phenomenon. It is often used as an adjunct to levodopa therapy.

83. The answer is B (III). Significance is generally determined by using an analysis of variance. A probability of $P < .05$ indicates a statistically significant difference (i.e., one that is not the result of chance alone). Thus, the high-fat breakfast treatment had a longer T_{max} and a lower C_{max}, indicating a delay in absorption. The slower rate of systemic drug absorption may have been caused by a delay in stomach emptying time owing to the ingestion of fat.

84. The answer is D. Mechlorethamine (Mustargen) is nitrogen mustard, which serves as an alkylating agent. Chlorambucil (Leukeran), busulfan (Myleran), and melphalan (Alkeran) are all considered water-soluble compounds that alkylate (alkylating agents) DNA. Doxorubicin (Adriamycin) is an example of a tetracyclic amino sugar-linked antibiotic.

85. The answer is A. Dospan is an erosion-core tablet that employs insoluble plastics, hydrophilic polymers, or fatty compounds to create a matrix device. The slowly dissolving tablet releases the majority of a dose after the primary dose is released from the tablet coating. OROS is an osmotic delivery system. The transdermal drug delivery system (TDDS) is designed to support the passage of drug substances from the skin surface. Pennkinetic is an ion-exchange resin. The hydrodynamically balanced system (HBS) represents a hydrocolloid system.

86. The answer is C. Moxifloxacin, levofloxacin, ciprofloxacin, and gemifloxacin are all quinolone derivatives. Clarithromycin is a macrolide antibiotic claimed to be slightly more active than erythromycin against select gram-positive bacteria.

87. The answer is E (I, II, and III). Immunosuppressive agents are administered to prevent graft rejection after renal transplantation. Azathioprine interferes with DNA and RNA synthesis so that it may reduce cell-mediated and humoral immune responses. Basiliximab is a chimeric monoclonal antibody that binds to block the interleukin 2 receptor on the surface of activated T lymphocytes, thus preventing T-lymphocyte activation and acute rejection. Cyclosporine inhibits T-cell activation in the early stage of immune response to foreign antigen such as a graft.

88. The answer is A (I). Lisinopril represents the class of drugs referred to as ACE inhibitors, which have been shown to provide a beneficial effect when given in the post-MI stage to reduce morbidity and mortality from the MI and prevent left ventricular dysfunction. The Survival and Ventricular Enlargement (SAVE) trial was the first major study to show the direct benefits of ACE inhibitors in post-MI patients. In Mr. Melvin's case, the order for lisinopril was written on the day of his heart attack and the dose was slowly titrated upward to prevent untoward hypotensive effects of the drug. Studies have shown that ACE inhibitors have a beneficial effect in certain patient populations (diabetes mellitus) in the prevention of renal nephropathy, but Mr. Melvin is not receiving lisinopril for this reason. In addition, ACE inhibitors do have a blood pressure–lowering effect, and although Mr. Melvin may have received the drug for high blood pressure, he most likely received the drug for prevention of left ventricular dysfunction after the acute myocardial infarction.

89. The answer is A. The Cockcroft and Gault equation is a common method for estimating creatinine clearance. This equation is based on the serum creatinine concentration and patient characteristics, including age, weight, and gender. Fick's law describes drug diffusion by passive transport from a region of high drug concentration to a region of lower drug concentration. The law of mass action describes the rate of a chemical reaction in terms of the concentrations of the reactants. The Henderson–Hasselbalch equation describes the relationship among pK_a, pH, and the extent of ionization of a weak acid or a weak base. The Noyes–Whitney equation describes the rate of dissolution of a solid drug.

90. The answer is C (I and II). The patient is experiencing symptoms suggesting heart failure, which may occur as a consequence of the acute coronary syndrome (MI) or of the patient receiving too much of the β-blocker metoprolol, or a combination of the two. Lisinopril, an ACE inhibitor, was initiated in this patient to reduce cardiac consequences. In this setting, the physician opted to cut back on the metoprolol dose with the hope of reducing the β-blocking side effects while still providing the drug, which has shown to be beneficial post-MI. In addition, the dose of lisinopril was increased to try to maximize its contributions to the patient's treatment.

91. The answer is C (I and II). TNKase, tPA, and rPA are all three equally effective thrombolytic therapies used to dissolve a clot in patients presenting with a STEMI. It should ideally be administered within 12 hours of MI symptom onset. Thrombolytics are contraindicated in patients at increased risk of intracranial hemorrhage. Thrombolytic agents are not used in the management of NSTEMI.

92. The answer is B (III). β-Adrenergic blockers have been shown to be effective in the acute management of MI patients in the prevention of sudden cardiac death owing to acute MI. They are also indicated in the treatment of angina pectoris, hypertension, and tachyarrhythmias along with numerous other drug-specific indications. However, the acute administration of a β-blocker (primarily atenolol and metoprolol) has become an important part of the treatment of acute MI. Whichever agent is used, usually a series of IV administrations of the drug are given over a short period of time, and then the patient is converted to oral medication daily thereafter. The parameters that need to be evaluated in these patients include blood pressure (if too low, the patient cannot receive a β-blocker), heart rate (if too low, the patient cannot receive a β-blocker), and pulmonary/left ventricular function (although indicated in the treatment of heart failure, patients must be monitored carefully when receiving β-blocker therapy).

93. The answer is D. Monitoring parameters for heparin include the aPTT (measure of anticoagulation effect), hemoglobin and hematocrit (potential bleeding), serum potassium (heparin suppresses aldosterone synthesis), and platelets (heparin my cause thrombocytopenia). Heparin will not affect the neutrophil count.

94. The answer is E. Amiodarone has an extremely long half-life—up to 50 days. The therapeutic effect of amiodarone may be delayed for weeks after oral therapy begins, and adverse reactions may persist after therapy ends.

95. The answer is C (I and II). Propranolol is a β-adrenergic blocking agent that helps reduce some manifestations of hyperthyroidism (e.g., tachycardia, sweating, tremor). In addition to providing symptomatic relief, propranolol inhibits the conversion of thyroxine (T_4) to triiodothyronine (T_3) in high doses.

96. The answer is C (I and II). There are numerous causes for ARF, which is a sudden, potentially reversible interruption of kidney function, resulting in the retention of nitrogenous waste products in body fluids. ARF is classified according to its cause. In prerenal ARF, impaired renal perfusion occurs as a result of dehydration, hemorrhage, vomiting, urinary losses from excessive diuresis, decreased cardiac output owing to heart failure, or severe hypotension. Intrarenal ARF reflects structural kidney damage owing to nephrotoxins

such as aminoglycosides, severe hypotension, malignant hypertension, and radiation. Postrenal ARF occurs because of obstruction of urine flow along the urinary tract as a result of uric acid crystals, thrombi, bladder obstruction, etc. Mr. Rones has a history of heart failure and hypertension, which are both capable of causing ARF. Hyperkalemia does not cause ARF, but rather ARF is associated with hyperkalemia, which might be considered a medical emergency.

97. The answer is E. Mr. Rones has reported allergies to sulfonamides and penicillin, so he should not be given any of the medications. Penicillin V potassium (V-Cillin-K) is a penicillin. Although the pharmacist may not know the exact nature of the reported allergy, a conversation with the physician would answer the question of whether an allergy exists. Trimethoprim-sulfamethoxazole (Bactrim, Septra) and hydrochlorothiazide are both sulfonamide derivatives; again, the pharmacist may not know the exact nature of the reported allergy, but a follow-up conversation with the physician should take place before filling either of these prescriptions for the patient.

98. The answer is E (I, II, and III). Slow-K is a potassium supplement used to prevent hypokalemia. However, Mr. Rones is diagnosed as having hyperkalemia, probably secondary to ARF, and he should not receive the prescription. In addition, moexipril, an ACE inhibitor, is contraindicated in hyperkalemia owing to its potassium-retaining properties. Sudafed (pseudoephedrine HCl) is an indirect-acting sympathomimetic that stimulates receptors, resulting in the release of adrenergic amines; it must be used with great caution in this hypertensive patient. The pharmacist should contact the physician before dispensing either of these prescriptions to determine whether the physician does indeed want to use them.

99. The answer is A (I). Mr. Rones has heart failure as a compelling indication, which would suggest the use of diuretics, ACE inhibitors (ramipril), ARBs (candesartan), β-adrenergic blockers (atenolol), or an aldosterone antagonist such as spironolactone. However, because of the presence of hyperkalemia in this patient, ramipril and candesartan should be avoided if possible.

100. The answer is C. Situations that favor the development of hypokalemia—use of non–potassium-sparing diuretics, failure to administer potassium supplements, administration of agents that decrease serum potassium (Kayexalate, sodium polystyrene sulfonate)—have been reported to be able to cause digoxin toxicity because of the development of hypokalemia. Phenytoin and lidocaine have both been shown to be effective in the treatment of digoxin toxicity–induced arrhythmias. Digoxin is primarily eliminated in the active form via the kidney, but when renal function decreases, as in advancing age, the elimination of the drug is decreased.

Monitoring for renal function can help prevent the development of digoxin toxicity.

101. The answer is D (II and III). Felodipine and isradipine are referred to as second-generation dihydropyridine derivatives, similar in action to nifedipine, which make up the class of calcium-channel blockers. Ramipril and enalapril are two examples of ACE inhibitors. Losartan is an example of the class of drugs referred to as angiotensin II receptor antagonists; and atenolol, carvedilol, and propranolol are examples of the β-adrenergic receptor antagonist class of drugs.

102. The answer is E. Patients such as Mr. Rones who have renal failure lose their ability to eliminate potassium from the kidney, and consequently elevations in serum potassium should be expected. Situations that favor the reabsorption of potassium by the kidney (administration of potassium supplements, use of potassium-sparing diuretics [spironolactone, ACE inhibitors, ARBs]) should be avoided. However, hyperkalemia can be treated by the removal of potassium by the body (dialysis), potassium-removing resin (sodium polystyrene sulfonate), pharmacologic antagonists (calcium chloride or gluconate), and shifting potassium intracellularly (regular insulin with dextrose).

103. The answer is E (I, II, and III). Verapamil (Isoptin) and atenolol (Tenormin) are representatives of the calcium-channel blocker and β-adrenergic blocker groups and, as such, possess negative inotropic and negative chronotropic effects. Patients should be advised to check their heart rates and report any symptoms that represent side effects from the negative inotropic effects of these agents. This helps prevent the development of signs of heart failure.

104. The answer is B. Facts and Comparisons eAnswers provides regular updates on available products along with dosage forms, indications, adverse drug reactions, and other information on products available in the United States. Newly released agents are not immediately described in the AHFS, but they do appear in supplements shortly after their release. Of the resources listed, Facts and Comparisons eAnswers likely offers the greatest benefit. *Merck Index, Trissel's, Hansten's,* and the *PDR* do not provide comprehensive updates on availability throughout the year, so they would not provide much help on a newly released product. *Trissel's* focuses on injectable drug products; *Hansten's,* on drug interactions.

105. The answer is D. Digoxin (Lanoxin) had previously been widely considered the mainstay in the treatment of heart failure. However, its use, particularly in chronic heart failure, has become somewhat controversial, and recent guidelines have limited its use to the short-term management of acute symptoms. Current recommendations favor the use of ACE inhibitors as primary therapy, with the addition of a diuretic if accompanied by shortness of breath, and the use of β-adrenergic blockers. Digoxin does possess two pharmacologic effects that reflect its concentration within the body. With lower total body stores (8 to 12 mg/kg), digoxin exerts a positive inotropic effect on the myocardium: an increase in cardiac output and renal blood flow and a decrease in cardiac filling pressure, venous and capillary pressures, heart size, and fluid volume. With higher total body stores (15 to 18 mg/kg), digoxin produces negative chronotropic effects—a reduction in electrical impulse conduction from the sinoatrial node throughout the atria into the atrioventricular node.

106. The answer is E. It takes four to five half-lives, with no loading doses given, for a patient to reach steady-state serum digoxin concentrations. For an anephric patient, who has a terminal half-life of 3.5 to 4.5 days, 15 to 20 days would be required to reach a steady state. If the patient is in acute heart failure, the treatment of choice is rapid loading of enough digoxin to obtain total body stores of 8 to 12 mg/kg over a 12-hour period, followed by daily maintenance doses. The patient who has normal renal function needs 6 to 8 days of daily maintenance doses to reach steady state, if loading doses are not given.

107. The answer is E. Acebutolol (Sectral) is a long-acting, relatively cardioselective agent that may be beneficial in patients who have lung disease and need to receive fewer doses per day to increase compliance. All β-adrenergic blockers have the potential to cause bronchospasm in patients with suspected lung disease, but the cardioselective agents may provide benefit in lower doses. Carvedilol (Coreg) lacks cardioselectivity and is available as an extended-release product. Esmolol (Brevibloc) is available only in intravenous form and has a very short half-life of approximately 9 minutes. Nadolol (Corgard) is a long-acting agent without cardioselective properties. Propranolol (Inderal LA) would offer no more cardioselective properties than those of Inderal.

108. The answer is A (I). Isosorbide dinitrate (Isordil) and other nitrates have been shown to reduce pulmonary congestion and increase cardiac output by reducing preload and perhaps afterload. Nitrates generally cause venous dilation, with a resultant increase in venous pooling and a reduction in venous return and preload. The combination of nitrates with hydralazine (arteriole dilator) has been shown to reduce morbidity and mortality in patients with heart failure. However, the combination should not be used as initial therapy over ACE inhibitors but should be considered in patients who are intolerant of ACE inhibitors. Dopamine and dobutamine are inotropic agents, and current guidelines provide a Class III recommendation ("conditions for which there is evidence and/or general agreement that a procedure/therapy is not useful/effective and in some cases may be harmful"). In addition, current guidelines provide a Class

IIb recommendation for the use of continuous intravenous infusion of a positive inotropic agent for palliation of heart failure symptoms ("conditions for which there is conflicting evidence and/or a divergence of opinion about the usefulness/efficacy of performing the procedure/therapy and that the usefulness/efficacy is less well established by evidence/opinion").

109. The answer is B. *Martindale: The Complete Drug Reference* is one resource that may be used to identify a drug manufactured in a foreign country. Other resources for identifying drugs manufactured in a foreign country include *Index Nominum, Lexi-Drugs International Online (Lexicomp Online)*, and the *USP Dictionary of United States Adopted Names (USAN) and International Drug Names*. *Facts and Comparisons, Trissel's Stability of Compounded Formulations*, and *AHFS* do not contain this type of information.

110. The answer is A. Peritoneal dialysis is not practical for drugs that are highly bound to plasma or tissue proteins, are nonpolar or lipid soluble, or have a large volume of distribution. Drugs that are polar and have a small apparent volume of distribution tend to have a larger concentration in plasma and highly perfused tissues. These polar drugs are more easily dialyzed in the case of drug intoxication.

111. The answer is E (I, II, and III). An important potential problem with the use of herbal medications is the inability to retrieve up-to-date information on many substances currently available through various vendors. Previously, the FDA's Center for Food Safety and Applied Nutrition created the "Special Nutritional Adverse Event Monitoring System" Web site for dietary supplements. Unfortunately, that site was not updated after 1999 and is currently no longer available. Before the site's removal, the center developed an extensive list of supplements considered unsafe by the FDA because of reported damage to various organ systems.

112. The answer is B. Iron is available in different oral forms as ferrous gluconate, ferrous sulfate, and ferrous fumarate. Each form has a different iron content. Ferrous gluconate contains 12% elemental iron, ferrous sulfate 20%, and ferrous fumarate 33%.

113. The answer is C. In extemporaneous compounding, various methods may be used to reduce the particle size of a drug, including levigation, pulverization by intervention, spatulation, and trituration. Geometric dilution is a method of mixing a small amount of a drug with a large amount of powder in a geometric progression so that the final powder mixture is homogeneous. Pulverization by intervention uses the addition of nonsolvent.

114. The answer is E. The total dose is 2.5 mg/kg/hr = 1200 mg. At a strength of 5 mg/L, each 50-mL vial contains 250 mg. The number of vials needed for this patient can be calculated by dividing the total dose (1200 mg) by the amount of antibiotic per vial (250 mg) to get 4.8 vials (five vials).

115. The answer is B. For most drugs with poor aqueous solubility, the dissolution rate (the rate at which the drug is solubilized) is the rate-limiting step for systemic drug absorption. Disintegration is the fragmentation of a solid dosage form into smaller pieces.

116. The answer is A (I). Atazanavir, indinavir, and nelfinavir are referred to as examples of protease inhibitors and are used in the treatment of HIV infection in combination with other groups of antiretroviral agents. Abacavir, lamivudine, and stavudine are examples of nucleoside reverse transcriptase inhibitors and are used in combination with protease inhibitors in the treatment of HIV. Delavirdine, efavirenz, and nevirapine are examples of nonnucleoside reverse transcriptase inhibitors and are used in the treatment of HIV as well.

117. The answer is A (I). The rate of dissolution of a weak acid drug is directly influenced by the surface area of the solid particles, the water in oil partition coefficient, and the concentration gradient between the drug concentrations in the stagnant layer and the bulk phase of the solvent. An increase in the pH of the medium will make the medium more alkaline, and the weak acid will convert to the ionized species, becoming more water soluble. Increasing the particle size decreases the effective surface area of the solid drug. Increasing the viscosity of the medium slows the diffusion of drug molecules into the solvent.

118. The answer is E (I, II, and III). All three of these statements are correct. The further classifications of bipolar disorder relate to the type and frequency of hypomanic, manic, and depressive episodes. Mood stabilizers—lithium, valproic acid, and carbamazepine—have historically been the mainstays of therapy.

119. The answer is A. Although the mechanism of action for lithium remains virtually unknown, this agent remains the therapy of choice for the acute and maintenance treatment of mania and hypomania. Membrane stabilization, inhibition of norepinephrine release, accelerated norepinephrine metabolism, increased presynaptic reuptake of norepinephrine and serotonin, and decreased receptor sensitivity appear to be therapeutic properties of lithium.

120. The answer is D. Equivalent weight (Li_2CO_3) = molecular weight/valence = 73.89/2 = 36.945. Thus, 1 milliequivalents (mEq) drug = 36.945 mg. The number of mEq contained in 300 mg of Li_2CO_3 = mg drug/equivalent weight (mg) = 300/36.945 = 8.12 mEq.

121. The answer is E (I, II, and III). Lithium therapy is monitored effectively by periodic determinations of serum lithium levels. Lithium has a narrow therapeutic index, with a therapeutic range of 0.5 to 1.2 mEq/L. A variety of factors can affect serum lithium levels; important among these are the time between the last dose and the taking of the blood sample and the concomitant drug therapy (e.g., thiazide diuretics may increase serum lithium levels; extra sodium in the diet may decrease lithium levels [note the salt-restricted diet in order]). If the patient were acutely manic on admission, it might indicate that he was not taking his lithium medication as prescribed. Patients presenting with acute mania generally require levels in the higher end of the therapeutic range.

122. The answer is A (I). The minimum, or trough, serum drug concentration is the most appropriate of the three; it is always lowest just before the administration of the next dose. The best time to monitor serum lithium levels is 12 hours after the last dose—that is, just before the first dose of the day. The exact times for the peak drug concentration and the average drug concentration are uncertain for any individual patient. The drawing of a sample to obtain a "peak" serum level uses an approximate time for maximum absorption of the drug. The average serum drug concentration cannot be obtained directly but is approximated by dividing the area under the curve (AUC) dosing interval by the time (T) of the dosage interval.

123. The answer is E (I, II, and III). The lithium level, which was ordered on admission returned at 0.9 mEq/L and the physician opted to add a second agent rather than reevaluate the lithium level from admission. Guidelines suggest that bipolar patients unable to respond to lithium should consider adding an antipsychotic such as olanzapine. Baseline laboratory tests for olanzapine include blood glucose, a lipid profile, height and weight, and EKG for those with cardiovascular risk factors.

124. The answer is D. Lithium is eliminated renally by glomerular filtration and competes with sodium for reabsorption in the renal tubules. Thiazide diuretics interfere with sodium reabsorption and, therefore, may favor lithium reabsorption, leading to elevated lithium levels. If the hydrochlorothiazide is being used to "treat" the prehypertension, it should be discontinued now until the patient's manic episode is stabilized. Blood pressure monitoring would need to be continued to determine if drug therapy is even needed at all. If an antihypertensive agent is indicated, alternatives could be introduced, which would not interfere with sodium/lithium elimination.

125. The answer is D. Lithium can cause a leukocytosis (elevated WBC count) as an early-onset adverse effect. The other agents do not cause this effect.

126. The answer is C (I and II). Antidepressants such as the tricyclic antidepressants (amitriptyline, nortriptyline, and protriptyline), have not been shown to offer any benefit over other mood stabilizers currently used in the treatment of bipolar disorders.

127. The answer is D. Chlorpromazine is a traditional (first-generation) antipsychotic agent. The others listed are considered atypical (second-generation) antipsychotics.

128. The answer is A.

129. The answer is C. Loading dose = 200 mg/m^2 × 0.89 m^2 = 178 mg.

130. The answer is D. Furosemide is a loop diuretic that acts principally at the ascending limb of the loop of Henle, where it inhibits the cotransport of sodium and chloride from the luminal filtrate. Loop diuretics increase the excretion of water, sodium, and chloride.

131. The answer is C (I and II). Topical OTC nasal decongestants are sympathomimetic amines and include, among others, phenylephrine (e.g., Neo-Synephrine) and oxymetazoline (e.g., Afrin). Pseudoephedrine is an oral decongestant and is not available as a topical nasal decongestant.

132. The answer is C (I and II). The JNC-7 recommendations include thiazide-type diuretics (hydrochlorothiazide), either alone or in combination with one other agent (e.g., ACE inhibitor, ARB, β-adrenergic receptor blocker, or calcium-channel blocker), for first-line treatment of stage I hypertension, if there are no indications for another type of drug. Tenormin (atenolol), a β-blocker, would therefore be considered as a potential first-line agent. Catapres (clonidine) is an α$_2$-adrenergic agonist and is not part of this first-line list.

133. The answer is E (I, II, and III). Tardive dyskinesia is characterized by a mixture of orofacial dyskinesia, tics, chorea, and athetosis. Signs and symptoms usually appear while patients are receiving first-generation antipsychotic agents. Recommendations for avoiding the onset of tardive dyskinesia include using antipsychotic agents only when clearly indicated, keeping the daily dose as low as possible and for as short a duration as possible, monitoring patients closely for signs and symptoms of tardive dyskinesia, and using atypical antipsychotics as first-line agents (which have little or no propensity to cause tardive dyskinesia). Also, chronic use of anticholinergic agents is not recommended because these agents may increase the risk of tardive dyskinesia.

134. The answer is A (I). Parnate (tranylcypromine) is a monoamine oxidase (MAO) inhibitor. Serious adverse drug reactions have been reported in patients receiving MAO inhibitors with opioid drugs. These serious interactions (hypotension, hyperpyrexia, coma) have occurred in patients receiving MAO inhibitors with meperidine (Demerol) but have not been reported to occur with morphine. Meperidine should be considered contraindicated in patients receiving MAO inhibitors. NSAIDs, a group that includes ketorolac, do not produce adverse interactions with MAO inhibitors. If a narcotic is necessary, morphine may be used cautiously, although waiting 14 days between the onset of morphine therapy and the discontinuation of MAO inhibitor therapy would be judicious.

135. The answer is D. Ondansetron (Zofran® is a selective 5-HT$_3$-receptor antagonist, blocking serotonin both peripherally on vagal nerve terminals and centrally at the chemoreceptor trigger zone for chemotherapy-induced and special postoperative cases of nausea and vomiting. Bupropion (Zyban) is available for use as an aid in smoking cessation. Sertraline (Zoloft) is a selective inhibitor of serotonin reuptake and an agent prescribed for the treatment of depression. Linezolid (Zyvox) is used in the treatment of resistant gram-positive bacterial infections such as vancomycin-resistant enterococcus and methicillin-resistant *Staphylococcus aureus*. Simvastatin (Zocor) is a β-hydroxy-β-methylglutaryl-coenzyme A (HMG-CoA) reductase inhibitor used in the treatment of hypercholesterolemia.

136. The answer is A. Aripiprazole (Abilify) is an atypical antipsychotic approved for the treatment of schizophrenia. Rabeprazole (Aciphex) is a PPI commonly used for GERD and peptic ulcer disease. Butoconazole (Gynazole-1) is an antifungal approved for use in the treatment of vulvovaginal candidiasis. Clotrimazole is an antifungal agent used in the treatment of susceptible fungal infections.

137. The answer is B. Vitamin D increases the absorption of calcium. Thiamine (vitamin B$_6$), ascorbic acid (vitamin C), vitamin E, and pantothenic acid are other vitamins.

138. The answer is A (I). Moxifloxacin is one of the currently available quinolones that is considered a respiratory agent, which can be used in the treatment of community acquired pneumonia. Ciprofloxacin is a quinolone, but not considered an alternative for respiratory infections. Doxycycline is tetracycline antibiotic, which has been used in the treatment of mild-to-moderate infections, acne vulgaris, periodontitis, pelvic inflammatory disease, and most recently anthrax.

139. The answer is C (I and II). According to the guidelines established by the American College of Rheumatology, patients are diagnosed as having rheumatoid arthritis if they have satisfied at least four of the following seven criteria, with the first four continuing for at least 6 weeks: (1) morning stiffness; (2) arthritis in three or more joint areas; (3) arthritis of wrist, hand, or finger joints; (4) symmetric arthritis; (5) subcutaneous nodules (rheumatoid nodules); (6) abnormal serum rheumatoid factor; and (7) radiologic changes with erosion or bone decalcification of involved joints.

140. The answer is B (III). Hydroxychloroquine (Plaquenil) is a disease-modifying antirheumatic drug (DMARD); its therapeutic benefit may take up to 6 months to develop. Hydroxychloroquine is given in dosages of 400 to 600 mg/day and has been associated with severe and sometimes irreversible adverse effects on the eyes, skin, central nervous system, and bone marrow. Because the drug may have severe effects on the eyes, an ophthalmologist should check visual acuity every 3 to 6 months, and therapy should be discontinued at the first signs of retinal toxicity.

141. The answer is A. Clopidogrel bisulfate (Plavix) is an antiplatelet drug indicated for the reduction of atherosclerotic events (MI, stroke, and vascular death) in patients with atherosclerosis documented by recent stroke, recent MI, or established peripheral arterial disease. Several agents are collectively referred to as DMARDs, including the commonly used hydroxychloroquine (Plaquenil), sulfasalazine (Azulfidine), methotrexate (Rheumatrex), penicillamine (Cuprimine), and gold salts (Myochrysine). Like hydroxychloroquine (Plaquenil), they are added to first-line therapy to slow or delay progression of the disabling symptoms and effects of rheumatoid arthritis.

142. The answer is E (I, II, and III). Celecoxib (Celebrex) represents a class of NSAIDs referred to as cyclooxygenase 2 (COX-2) receptor inhibitors. It is believed to offer a potential benefit over traditional NSAIDs by reducing the gastrointestinal consequences associated with use of these agents. Naproxen (Naprosyn) is an NSAID that is also used in the treatment of rheumatoid arthritis. Nabumetone, another NSAID agent, is believed to have a greater specificity for the COX-2 receptor than the COX-1 receptor; it has also been used in the symptomatic control of rheumatoid arthritis. Each agent could be a suitable alternative for ibuprofen, and celecoxib in particular might reduce the GI side effects associated with the other NSAIDs.

143. The answer is E (I, II, and III). All of the trade and generic names match.

144. The answer is E (I, II, and III). The onset of most of the DMARDs is prolonged; therefore, anti-inflammatory drugs are usually given concurrently as a bridge until therapeutic effects of the DMARD occur. The American College of Rheumatology recommends that DMARD therapy be initiated within 3 months of diagnosis, despite good control with NSAIDs. The lowest effective dose should be used to minimize adverse effects.

145. The answer is B. Patients with rheumatoid arthritis often have a normocytic, normochromic anemia, often referred to as an anemia of chronic disease. In fact, anemia has been reported to occur in as many as 60% of all rheumatoid arthritis, only surpassed in occurrence by joint symptoms. This anemia does not respond to drug therapy (i.e., iron therapy). Sometimes, this may produce a diagnostic dilemma because patients on NSAIDs may develop gastric irritation with chronic blood loss, which would lead to iron deficiency anemia. Other blood tests can help differentiate these two types of anemia—for example, serum iron to iron binding capacity and mean corpuscular volume (usually decreased in iron deficiency).

146. The answer is B (III). Arthrotec is a combination of an NSAID (diclofenac sodium) and misoprostol. Misoprostol is a synthetic prostaglandin E_1 analog with mucosal protective properties and is given to patients at risk for developing NSAID-induced gastric or duodenal ulcers. Ms. Trombley is 40 years of age and is, therefore, at risk for NSAID-induced peptic ulcer disease. Diarrhea may be a side effect from misoprostol, but this medication would not be used to treat constipation. This combination is not a DMARD.

147. The answer is E (I, II, and III). The patient had been started on hydroxychloroquine in February, and with dose increases and an apparent lack of response into June, it was becoming apparent that the patient was not responding, and a change in therapy was needed. However, the decision to introduce the TNF-inhibitor, etanercept (Enbrel) needed to be held off until the active UTI was resolved. When the time came to initiate etanercept therapy, methotrexate was added as well with the intention of adding a therapeutic benefit, as described in the literature.

148. The answer is B. Etanercept (Enbrel) is a DMARD used to delay the progression of the disease. It binds to TNF-α and -β, inhibiting the inflammatory response mediated by immune cells. It is indicated as monotherapy or in conjunction with methotrexate. It is given by subcutaneous injection. It is not a COX-2 inhibitor.

149. The answer is C. Appropriate treatment measures are listed in choices A, B, D, and E. All bedrooms (where the concentration of pinworm eggs is likely to be the greatest) should be vacuumed—not swept—to remove the eggs.

150. The answer is C. Tinea infections are superficial fungal dermatophyte infections of the skin. These infections are usually named based on the area of the skin involved: tinea cruris (groin), tinea capitis (head), tinea pedis (feet), tinea corporis (body), and tinea unguium (nails). Sally has tinea pedis.

151. The answer is D. The antiseptic agent hexylresorcinol is not considered safe and effective for the treatment of tinea infections. The other four agents are all considered safe and effective for treating tinea pedis.

152. The answer is A. Diphenhydramine and doxylamine are two ethanolamine antihistamines, generally considered the most sedating class of antihistamines. Brompheniramine, chlorpheniramine, dexbrompheniramine, and pheniramine are part of the alkylamine class of antihistamines, which are among the least sedating of the first-generation antihistamines. Thonzylamine, is not available for use in the U.S. market but is an ethylenediamine antihistamine; this class is between the other two classes in terms of sedation effects. Loratadine is a second-generation nonsedating antihistamine that recently was moved to OTC status.

153. The answer is B. The second-generation nonsedating antihistamine, loratadine (e.g., Claritin), is available OTC. This patient's specific symptoms are related to histamine effects, so an antihistamine is warranted. Given his occupation, the pharmacist would not want to give this patient a sedating antihistamine, such as diphenhydramine. Even though loratadine is considered a nonsedating antihistamine, a small percentage of patients experience somnolence (8%) and fatigue (4%). Mr. Conway should certainly see how this agent affects him before he attempts to drive. He does not have nasal congestion, so the decongestant (pseudoephedrine) is not warranted at this time.

154. The answer is A. Nonsalicylate NSAIDs (ibuprofen, naproxen) are the most effective OTC agents for primary dysmenorrhea. Aspirin and acetaminophen are generally less effective. Ketoprofen had been available, previously without a prescription, however, now does requires one so you would need to contact her physician in order to obtain such a prescription. Ketoprofen is the correct answer here because it should be used only in patients 16 years of age and older.

155. The answer is C (I and II). Pyrethrins with piperonyl butoxide (synergized pyrethrins) and permethrin are the two safe and effective OTC agents used to treat head lice. Patients should be warned to use these as directed because there is a growing trend of lice resistance to these products. Lindane is available only by prescription and has generally fallen into disfavor.

156. The answer is C. Novolin is a trade name for human insulin that is a fixed-dose mixture of 70% NPH (intermediate action) and 30% regular insulin (short action).

157. The answer is E (I, II, and III). The elevated BUN and SCr would likely indicate that she has some renal impairment. The WBC count is elevated and could be caused by the presence of a bacterial infection. The presence of nitrites in the urine most commonly indicates the presence of gram-negative bacteria. Since Ms. Urmeister's urinalysis did not reveal any nitrites, the likely bacterial cause of her suspected UTI is a gram-positive pathogen such as *Enterococcus*. Based on the presence of leukocytes and leukocyte esterase in her urinalysis, her WBC count, and her symptoms one can confirm the diagnosis of a UTI.

158. The answer is C. Amoxicillin would be the most appropriate therapy choice for the treatment of the UTI based on the patient's current medication regimen, renal function, and likely causative organism. Sulfamethoxazole/trimethoprim would not be the best option due to the major interaction with her concomitant warfarin (Coumadin) therapy (increases INR, increases risk of bleeding). Nitrofurantoin would not be the best option due to the patient's renal function and CrCl of < 60 mL/min, at which point its use is contraindicated. Ciprofloxacin would not be an option because of her allergy to this medication. Metronidazole is not indicated for the treatment of a bacterial UTI.

159. The answer is E. Warfarin has two main mechanisms of action. It works to inhibit the production of the vitamin K–dependent clotting factors II, VII, IX, and X and the production of the anticoagulant proteins C and S. Heparin produces its anticoagulant effect by increasing the activity of antithrombin III. Dabigatran is a direct thrombin inhibitor.

160. The answer is A. Routine monitoring parameters for warfarin include prothrombin time, INR, hematocrit, and stool guaiac. Serum ketones would be used to diagnose and monitor a patient with diabetic ketoacidosis.

161. The answer is B. The patient does not have an indication for omeprazole or any information that warrants its use. Simvastatin is being used to treat the patient's hyperlipidemia, metoprolol is being used to control the patient's atrial fibrillation, and docusate is a stool softener to treat her hard stools.

162. The answer is D. The CHADS(2) score is used to assess the risk of stroke in a patient with atrial fibrillation. Components of the CHADS(2) score are diagnosed heart failure, hypertension (treated or untreated), age ≥ 75 years, diabetes, and prior ischemic stroke, TIA, or thromboembolism. Renal function is not one of the items used to calculate this score.

163. The answer is A. Dofetilide is a potassium channel blocker antiarrhythmic. All of the other pairs are matched correctly.

164. The answer is B. The following are significant major adverse effects of amiodarone: pulmonary toxicity (which may present as pulmonary fibrosis), hypothyroidism, corneal microdeposits, and hepatotoxicity. *Hypo*tension is a major concern, not *hyper*tension.

165. The answer is B. Morphine sulfate is a narcotic analgesic with venous pooling properties that reduces preload. Preload reduction decreases the oxygen demand placed on the heart. For this reason, along with its ability to alleviate pain and reduce anxiety (anxiety and pain also increase oxygen demand), morphine is frequently used in the myocardial infarction patient.

166. The answer is C. NicoDerm CQ patch contains nicotine (not nitroglycerin) and has been shown to be effective in helping patients stop smoking. Nitroglycerin patches are available in several brands (e.g., Nitro-Dur). All of the other generic names match with a trade name.

167. The answer is C (I and II). Isosorbide dinitrate (Isordil) is used in both angina pectoris and heart failure. The development of angina pectoris centers around the balance between oxygen demand and oxygen supply to the myocardium. When the demand for oxygen exceeds the supply of oxygen, an angina attack occurs. Isosorbide dinitrate, like other nitrates, is a venous dilator resulting in reduced oxygen demand by the heart through a decrease in (venous return) preload. Isosorbide works in the heart failure patient by reducing venous return of blood to the heart, therefore, again, decreasing preload with a resultant decrease in fluid for the heart to pump. Clinical studies have demonstrated that the combination of isosorbide dinitrate with the arteriole dilator hydralazine has reduced mortality and morbidity in heart failure patients. Heart failure is a potential consequence of an acute MI, and angina pectoris is a common underlying problem in many patients who have had an MI.

168. The answer is A. Reteplase (Retavase) is a thrombolytic and has been shown to be effective during the first several hours after a STEMI. However, for an NSTEMI there is no evidence to support the use of a thrombolytic. Metoprolol, like other β-adrenergic blockers administered shortly after an acute MI, has been shown to be effective in reducing mortality and morbidity. Aspirin in the dose of 162 to 325 mg should be given as soon as possible after the event. Patients with ongoing NSTEMI or ischemic discomfort should receive sublingual nitroglycerin. Morphine is used to treat myocardial pain and discomfort and causes venous pooling, reduces preload, cardiac workload, and oxygen consumption.

169. The answer is B. Sudafed (Pseudoephedrine), a sympathomimetic amine, has central nervous system (CNS) stimulating properties and is the most likely agent to cause sleep disruption. Metamucil (psyllium) as a bulk laxative is not absorbed. Flonase (fluticasone) would be very unlikely. Benadryl (diphenhydramine) is one of the OTC agents used to treat insomnia and would more likely cause drowsiness. CNS stimulation from regular doses of aspirin is highly unlikely.

170. The answer is E. Middle ear infection (otitis media) and external ear infection (swimmer's ear or otitis externa) require prescription antibiotics to treat. Water-clogged ears can be treated with an OTC product containing isopropyl alcohol and anhydrous glycerin. Impacted cerumen can be treated with carbamide peroxide.

171. The answer is A. Oxymetazoline has a duration of action of 12 hours and should be used no more than twice daily. The other topical nasal decongestants listed are administered every 6 hours (naphazoline), every 4 hours (phenylephrine, ephedrine), or every 8 to 10 hours (xylometazoline).

172. The answer is B. The SPF is the minimal erythema dose (MED) of sunscreen-protected skin divided by the MED of unprotected skin. An SPF of 15 means that, if the sunscreen is applied properly, the user can stay out in the sun about 15 times longer to get a minimal redness reaction compared to being in the sun with unprotected skin (i.e., with no sunscreen application): 15 × 10 minutes = 150 minutes = 2.5 hours.

173. The answer is A. If the patient misses a dose of Rogaine (minoxidil), he should just continue with the next dose. One should not make up missed doses. The other items noted are appropriate counseling points to cover.

174. The answer is C. Benzoyl peroxide, sulfur, salicylic acid, and sulfur plus resorcinol are all considered safe and effective agents for the treatment of acne. Triclosan is an antibacterial agent with antigingivitis and antiplaque activity in the oral cavity and no proven efficacy against acne.

175. The answer is D. Nonprescription treatment of acne is restricted to mild noninflammatory acne. It is clear that this young lady has more significant inflammatory acne (including mild scarring). She has apparently had only a modest response to the OTC agents, and she needs to be referred to a physician for additional prescription therapy. The other noted suggested treatments are all OTC agents indicated for noninflammatory acne.

176. The answer is D. This agent (benzoyl peroxide) is generally considered the nonprescription drug of choice for the treatment of acne. It does have the twofold mechanism of action described in selection D. The other selections are incorrect.

177. The answer is C. If topical nasal decongestants are used for more often than 3 to 5 days, rhinitis medicamentosa (rebound congestion) may occur in the nasal passages. Thus, the patient ends up experiencing as a side effect what he sought to treat in the first place. For the common cold, a 3- to 5-day use of a topical nasal decongestant should be all that is needed.

178. The answer is D (II and III). Coreg CR is an extended-release form of carvedilol, a β-adrenergic blocking agent. Many of the currently available extended-release dosage forms cannot be cut or crushed because that would disrupt the integrity of the delivery system and would have the potential to provide active drug for more rapid absorption, thus causing toxicity.

179. The answer is D (II and III). First-order reactions are characterized by an exponential change in the drug amount or concentration with time, and these changes produce a straight line when plotted on a semilog graph. The half-life for a first-order reaction is a constant.

180. The answer is D (II and III). FluMist is an inhaled influenza vaccine preparation approved for ages 2 to 49.

181. The answer is A. Calcium is available for oral administration in a salt form of lactate, gluconate, phosphate, and carbonate; it is not available for oral administration in a salt form of chloride. Dosage regimens should be individualized because of differences in calcium content of the various salts.

182. The answer is C. Osteoporosis, hyperglycemia, fluid retention, and cataracts are long-term complications of therapy with steroids, including prednisone. Steroids generally increase the white blood cell count, therefore, leukopenia is incorrect.

183. The answer is C. Cidofovir (Vistide) is an antiviral agent used to treat cytomegalovirus replication by selective inhibition of DNA synthesis. It is not a protease inhibitor and is not indicated for treatment of HIV infection. Saquinavir (Invirase), ritonavir (Norvir), atazanavir (Reyataz), and indinavir (Crixivan) are protease inhibitors used to treat HIV infection.

184. The answer is A (I). A pyrogen test is a fever test in rabbits or an in vitro test using the limulus (horseshoe crab). A positive test shows the presence of fever-producing substances (pyrogens) in a sterile product; these substances may be dead microorganisms or extraneous proteins.

185. The answer is A (I). Increases in BUN and SCr generally indicate renal impairment. Levels of LDH, AST, and ALT rise with liver dysfunction and indicate liver damage.

186. The answer is D. Nausea and vomiting are common adverse reactions to chemotherapy. Common antiemetic agents include ondansetron (Zofran), metoclopramide (Reglan), aprepitant (Emend), and dronabinol (Marinol). Cimetidine (Tagamet) has no value as an antiemetic.

187. The answer is A. Laboratory findings in ARF may include hyperuricemia, hyperkalemia, hypocalcemia, and metabolic acidosis. In acute renal failure, phosphate excretion decreases, causing *hyper*phosphatemia, not *hypo*phosphatemia.

188. The answer is E. Iodine is a trace element essential to the synthesis of thyroxine (T$_4$) and triiodothyronine (T$_3$). Iodine also is needed for physical and mental development and metabolism. Iodine deficiency can cause cretinism in children and infants.

189. The answer is D. The use of a folic acid supplement in a pregnant woman can prevent neural tube defects in the baby.

190. The answer is C. Bentoquatam (Ivy-Block) is an organoclay that should be applied at least 15 minutes before poison ivy plant exposure and then every 4 hours for continued protection. Because the oleoresin (urushiol) can rapidly penetrate the skin, it should be washed off soon after exposure (within 10 minutes is ideal). Obviously, learning how to identify the poison ivy plant and avoiding it would be the best ways of preventing the dermatitis.

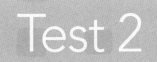

Use the patient profile below to answer questions 1 to 11.

PATIENT RECORD (INSTITUTION/NURSING HOME)

Patient Name: Shirley Curtis
Address: 8179 Vadith Ct.

Age: 62	Height: 5′7″
Sex: F	Race: African American Weight: 118 lb

Allergies: Penicillin: local hives
Social History: 20 pack-year history

DIAGNOSIS

Primary	(1)	Acute psychotic episode
	(2)	Schizophrenia × 10 years
Secondary	(1)	Hypertension controlled with medications

LAB/DIAGNOSTIC TESTS

	Date	Test
(1)	8/14	Basic metabolic panel ordered with following key results: Na 140 mEq/L; K 4.7 mEq/L; Cl 95 mEq/L; CO$_2$ 25 mEq/L; BUN 11 mg/dL; Cr 1.0 mg/dL; Hb 12.5 g/dL; HCT 39%; blood pressure 150/90 mm Hg; HR 95; RR 16; T 37.5

MEDICATION ORDERS (Including Parenteral Solutions)

	Date	Drug and Strength	Route	Sig
(1)	8/14	Haloperidol decanoate 50 mg	IM	stat
(2)	8/14	Haloperidol 5 mg	IM	q4h prn agitation
(3)	8/15	Benazepril 20 mg	po	i qd
(4)	8/16	Diphenhydramine 50 mg	po	stat
(5)	8/17	Risperidone 4 mg	po	i qd
(6)	9/17	Risperidone 4 mg	po	i bid

ADDITIONAL ORDERS

	Date	Comments
(1)	8/14	Admit to security ward—chart notes previous positive response to haloperidol per last hospitalization.
(2)	8/14	May restrain.

| (3) | 8/17 | DC haloperidol. |
| (4) | 8/30 | Discharge patient on risperidone with follow-up visit in 30 days. |

DIETARY CONSIDERATIONS (Enteral and Parenteral)

	Date	Comments
(1)	None	

PHARMACIST NOTES AND OTHER PATIENT INFORMATION

	Date	Comments
(1)	8/14	Smoker 2 packs/day for 10 years.
(2)	8/14	Positive family history for schizophrenia (mother).
(3)	8/14	Positive family history for alcoholism (father).
(4)	8/14	Medication history: includes haloperidol; may be compliance problem.
(5)	8/14	Contacted physician upon receipt of initial haloperidol order, in order to suggest a change based on current patient symptoms.

1. Ms. Curtis is hospitalized for an acute psychotic episode of her schizophrenia. The most common symptoms of schizophrenia are

   A. hallucinations and delusions.
   B. poor attention and apathy.
   C. insomnia and amotivation.
   D. combativeness and thought disorder.
   E. disorganized speech and asocial behavior.

2. The patient profile indicates that Ms. Curtis responded to haloperidol therapy the last time she was hospitalized for an acute psychotic episode. Antipsychotic therapy for this patient can be assessed by monitoring the target symptom of

   A. delusions.
   B. withdrawal.
   C. asocial behavior.
   D. apathy.
   E. poor judgment.

3. Extrapyramidal side effects can occur with all of the typical antipsychotics, especially high-potency ones like haloperidol. All of the following are extrapyramidal side effects *except*

   A. akathisia.
   B. tardive dyskinesia.
   C. acute dystonia.
   D. pseudoparkinsonism.
   E. neuroleptic malignant syndrome.

4. On 8/14, a note by the pharmacist focused on the need to contact the physician regarding the haloperidol order that was initially written for Ms. Curtis, on admission. Which of the following explains the purpose for the phone call?

   I. Incorrect dose ordered for the haloperidol for an acute psychosis patient.
   II. Incorrect form of haloperidol ordered for an acute psychosis patient.
   III. Incorrect route of administration ordered for an acute psychosis patient.

   A. I only
   B. III only
   C. I and II
   D. II and III
   E. I, II, and III

5. Within 48 hours of initiating haloperidol, the patient experiences uncontrolled and involuntary neck twisting and a fixed upward gaze. The treatment of choice in this patient would be

   A. immediate haloperidol dose reduction by one-half.
   B. immediate oral administration of bromocriptine 5 mg.
   C. immediate intramuscular (IM) administration of diazepam 5 mg.
   D. immediate IM administration of diphenhydramine 50 mg.
   E. immediate change to an alternative antipsychotic agent, such as thioridazine.

6. In the medical record provided by Ms. Curtis' primary care provider, the physician recorded that at one patient visit "the patient was having difficulty keeping her legs and feet still." This movement abnormality most likely represented

   A. a dystonic reaction, which may be treated with oral diazepam.
   B. akathisia, which should respond to a dosage reduction in her haloperidol.
   C. drug-induced parkinsonism, which may respond to oral bromocriptine.
   D. a warning sign of reduced seizure threshold; low-dose antiseizure therapy should be initiated.
   E. tardive dyskinesia; the antipsychotic dose should be lowered.

7. During a discussion with Ms. Curtis about her compliance with haloperidol therapy, the patient states that she did not like taking oral haloperidol because it made her "stiff." This apparent pseudoparkinsonism reaction *can* be treated by

   I. changing her therapy to an atypical antipsychotic agent (SGA).
   II. decreasing the dose of the haloperidol.
   III. adding an anticholinergic agent.

   A. I only
   B. III only
   C. I and II
   D. II and III
   E. I, II, and III

8. Ms. Curtis was switched to risperidone, a second-generation antipsychotic, and discharged on this agent. In addition to this agent, all of the following are atypical antipsychotics *except*

   A. aripiprazole.
   B. olanzapine.
   C. ziprasidone.
   D. thioridazine.
   E. quetiapine.

9. Ms. Curtis might be a candidate for a long-acting IM formulation of antipsychotic given the fact that she apparently had some compliance problems in the past. Which of the following agents are used as such?

   I. haloperidol decanoate
   II. fluphenazine decanoate
   III. long-acting risperidone

   A. I only
   B. III only
   C. I and II
   D. II and III
   E. I, II, and III

10. Second-generation antipsychotic agents (SGAs) would be preferred over first-generation agents (FGAs) because they

   I. have increased efficacy for negative symptoms (apathy, asocial behavior, etc.) compared to typical antipsychotics.
   II. have been associated with less extrapyramidal symptoms (EPSs).
   III. have been shown to be much more effective on positive symptoms (hallucinations, delusions, etc.) than the FGAs.

   A. I only
   B. III only
   C. I and II
   D. II and III
   E. I, II, and III

11. Clozapine (Clozaril) is an SGA that is reserved for use in patients who are refractory to treatment with other antipsychotics. Treatment plans for patients receiving this agent should include routine monitoring for

   A. renal failure.
   B. agranulocytosis.
   C. hair loss.
   D. severe diarrhea.
   E. excessive sodium loss.

End of this patient profile; continue with the examination.

12. When counseling a parent with a 3-year-old on the administration of otic drops to his child, the pharmacist should instruct the parent to pull the ear

   A. backward and upward.
   B. backward and downward.
   C. 90 degrees outward.
   D. straight forward.
   E. none of the above.

13. Which of the following agents is the only U.S. Food and Drug Administration (FDA)-approved nonprescription cerumen-softening agent?

   A. carbamide peroxide
   B. mineral oil
   C. hydrogen peroxide
   D. sweet oil
   E. glycerin

14. Which of the following would be considered the *most important* counseling point for a patient taking mineral oil as a laxative?

A. Remain in an upright position while taking this agent.
B. Take with food.
C. It may interfere with the absorption of water-soluble vitamins.
D. An adult can take up to 3 oz as a dose.
E. Do not take if fluid compromised.

15. An older gentleman complains that his hemorrhoids are bothering him again. He has not had problems with them in quite some time. He is concerned because he has noticed that this time around he has had some bleeding into the toilet bowl. What product would you recommend to this elderly gentleman?

A. Anusol suppositories
B. Tucks pads
C. Preparation H ointment
D. hydrocortisone ointment
E. none; he should be referred to a physician

16. A middle-aged woman explains that she has recently developed hemorrhoids and she wants something to stop the itching. Upon checking her profile in the computer, you find out that she is currently taking atenolol 20 mg/day for her hypertension and Lipitor 40 mg/day for her hyperlipidemia. Which of the following would *not* be appropriate for this woman?

A. Anusol HC-1
B. Tucks pads (witch hazel, glycerin)
C. Anusol ointment
D. Preparation H cream
E. hydrocortisone 1% cream

Use the information below to answer questions 17 to 19.

A 49-year-old woman has recently been diagnosed with rheumatoid arthritis. Celebrex (celecoxib) was initially prescribed for her condition. She was eventually prescribed Enbrel (etanercept) and a course of prednisone 5 mg/day was prescribed at the same time.

17. Which of the following apply to the drug celecoxib in the treatment of rheumatoid arthritis?

   I. This agent works by inhibiting prostaglandin synthesis by decreasing activity of the enzyme cyclooxygenase 2 (COX-2), which results in decreased formation of prostaglandin precursors.
   II. It does not alter the course of rheumatoid arthritis, nor does it prevent joint destruction.
   III. It may cause serious skin reactions.

   A. I only
   B. III only
   C. I and II
   D. II and III
   E. I, II, and III

18. The reason why prednisone is being used in this patient is best described by which of the following?

   I. as "bridge" therapy to allow the Enbrel to fully take effect
   II. to alter the course of the disease
   III. to minimize the side effects of nonsteroidal anti-inflammatory drugs (NSAIDs)

   A. I only
   B. III only
   C. I and II
   D. II and III
   E. I, II, and III

19. All of the following apply to the use of Enbrel (etanercept) in this patient *except* which one?

   A. This agent is used as one of a number of disease-modifying antirheumatic drugs (DMARDs).
   B. It is believed now that agents like Enbrel should be initiated in the rheumatoid arthritis patient within the first 3 months despite good control with NSAIDs.
   C. Inflammatory markers for the disease (e.g., erythrocyte sedimentation rate [ESR]) are reduced significantly by DMARDs (e.g., Enbrel) but not NSAIDs.
   D. It binds to tumor necrosis factor α (TNF-α) and β, inhibiting the inflammatory response mediated by immune cells.
   E. There is no exception; all of the above apply to the use of Enbrel in this patient.

End of this patient profile; continue with the examination.

20. When recommending an appropriate sun protectant for patients, it is important to recommend a product that protects against both ultraviolet A (UVA) and ultraviolet B (UVB) radiation wavelengths. Which agent or combination of agents would provide such protection?

   I. titanium dioxide
   II. ecamsule, octocrylene, and avobenzone
   III. homosalate and padimate O

   A. I only
   B. III only
   C. I and II
   D. II and III
   E. I, II, and III

Use the patient profile below to answer questions 21 to 31.

MEDICATION PROFILE (COMMUNITY)

Patient Name: Mary Smith
Address: 14 Francis St.

Age: 62   Height: 5'2″
Sex: F   Race: Caucasian   Weight: 110 lb
Allergies: Penicillin

DIAGNOSIS

Primary   (1)   Breast cancer
Secondary   (1)   Chemotherapy-induced nausea and vomiting

MEDICATION RECORD (Prescription and OTC)

	Date	Rx No.	Physician	Drug and Strength	Quan	Sig	Refills
(1)	5/31	432525	Golub	Dexamethasone 4 mg	8	2 tabs po at 10 P.M. on 5/31 then 2 tabs × 3 days daily beginning at least 1 hour before chemotherapy on 6/1	5
(2)	6/1	432576	Golub	Taxotere 100 mg IV	1	administer in clinic	0
(3)	6/1	432577	Golub	Adriamycin 75 mg IV	1	IV push × 2 min	0
(4)	6/1	432578	Golub	Cytoxan 750 mg IV	1	IV push × 2 min	0
(5)	6/1	432580	Golub	Compazine 10 mg	10	i q4h prn nausea, po	1
(6)	6/1	432581	Golub	Ativan 1 mg	10	i q4h prn nausea	1
(7)	6/1	432582	Golub	Compazine suppositories 25 mg	6	i q6h prn PR	1
(8)	6/1	432583	Golub	Emend Tri-Pack	1	125 mg po 60 min before chemotherapy on 6/1 then 80 mg po daily on 6/2 and 6/3	5
(9)	6/1	432584	Golub	Ondansetron 8 mg	2	2 tabs 60 min before chemotherapy on 6/1	5
(10)	6/2	432585	Golub	Neulasta 6 mg SC	1	6 mg SQ on 6/2	5

PHARMACIST NOTES AND OTHER PATIENT INFORMATION

	Date	Comments
(1)	6/1	Weight 50 kg; body surface area 1.5 m².
(2)	6/1	Treatment plan: TAC every 21 days for 6 cycles.
(3)	6/1	Return to clinic 6/21 for CBC and IV chemotherapy.
(4)	6/1	Docetaxel 75 mg/m²; doxorubicin 50 mg/m²; cyclophosphamide 500 mg/m².
(5)	6/1	Neulasta 6 mg SC on day 2 of each cycle of chemotherapy.
(6)	6/1	Patient has implanted port for chemotherapy administration.
(7)	6/1	Note: to begin Arimidex 1 mg orally daily after chemotherapy and radiation therapy completed.

21. Ms. Smith was placed on the TAC (Taxotere-Adriamycin-Cytoxan) regimen for her breast cancer. All of the following statements about combination cancer chemotherapy regimens are true *except* which one?

    A. Combination cancer chemotherapy regimens are used to improve survival and response outcomes for cancer treatment.
    B. Drugs in combination generally should have the same mechanisms of action.
    C. The drugs act during different cell cycle phases.
    D. The drugs should be associated with different adverse effects.
    E. Cell cycle–specific agents may be given with cell cycle–nonspecific agents.

22. Ms. Smith is receiving cyclophosphamide as one of her chemotherapeutic agents. Cyclophosphamide is classified as:

    A. an alkylating agent.
    B. an antimetabolite.
    C. a natural alkaloid.
    D. a hormonal agent.
    E. a platinum derivative.

23. Which chemotherapy agent(s) is/are associated with a low (10% to 30%) incidence of nausea and vomiting?

    I. doxorubicin
    II. cyclophosphamide
    III. docetaxel

    A. I only
    B. III only
    C. I and II
    D. II and III
    E. I, II, and III

24. Dexamethasone is administered before and after TAC chemotherapy to prevent

    I. fluid retention which may result in pulmonary edema.
    II. chemotherapy-induced nausea and vomiting.
    III. anaphylaxis to the vehicle used to make the docetaxel soluble.

    A. I only
    B. III only
    C. I and II
    D. II and III
    E. I, II, and III

25. Which of the following is/are (a) vesicant chemotherapy agent(s)?

    A. Cyclophosphamide
    B. Docetaxel
    C. Doxorubicin
    D. Both A and B
    E. Both B and C

26. What brand name product should be dispensed for ondansetron?

    A. Aloxi
    B. Zofran
    C. Kytril
    D. Emetrol
    E. Anzemet

27. Ms. Smith will begin taking anastrozole (Arimidex) to block the effects of estrogen following completion of chemotherapy and radiation therapy. Which of the following drugs is *not* used as an antiestrogen agent in the treatment of breast cancer?

    A. Clomiphene (Clomid)
    B. Tamoxifen (Nolvadex)
    C. Letrozole (Femara)
    D. Fulvestrant (Faslodex)
    E. Toremifene (Fareston)

28. Which of the following statements is/are correct regarding Ms. Smith's antiemetic regimen?

    I. Chemotherapy-induced nausea and vomiting is best treated with as needed antiemetics such as prochlorperazine (Compazine) given after nausea and vomiting starts.
    II. Aprepitant (Emend) is added to ondansetron therapy to prevent anticipatory nausea and vomiting.
    III. The combination of dexamethasone, aprepitant, and ondansetron is the standard regimen used with chemotherapy that includes doxorubicin and cyclophosphamide.

    A. I only
    B. III only
    C. I and II
    D. II and III
    E. I, II, and III

29. Ms. Smith develops a *Staphylococcus aureus* infection at her implanted port site. Because of her history, she is hospitalized for treatment and evaluation. Based on Ms. Smith's profile, which antibiotic(s) would be (a) reasonable therapy choice(s)?

    I. vancomycin
    II. dicloxacillin
    III. Unasyn

    A. I only
    B. III only
    C. I and II
    D. II and III
    E. I, II, and III

30. The microbiology laboratory reports Ms. Smith's cultures reveal the *S. aureus* to be vancomycin and methicillin resistant. Which of the following is the best choice for therapy given this information?

    A. linezolid
    B. Rocephin
    C. Vancocin
    D. meropenem
    E. Cedax

31. Pegfilgrastim is used to

    I. reduce the risk of anemia and certain cancers of the blood.
    II. maintain cell membrane integrity, reduce cellular aging, and inhibit melanoma cell growth.
    III. reduce the risk of neutropenia, which can be life-threatening.

    A. I only
    B. III only
    C. I and II
    D. II and III
    E. I, II, and III

End of this patient profile; continue with the examination.

32. In the geriatric patient, drugs with anticholinergic activity can increase the risk of cognitive impairment by up to 50%. All of the following agents have anticholinergic activity to be avoided in this patient population *except*

    A. Detrol LA
    B. Tylenol PM
    C. amitriptyline
    D. sertraline
    E. diphenhydramine

Use the information below to answer questions 33 and 34.

Hydrophilic ointment *USP* has the following formula:
Methylparaben 0.25 g
Propylparaben 0.15 g
Sodium lauryl sulfate 10 g
Propylene glycol 120 g
Stearyl alcohol 250 g
White petrolatum 370 g
Purified water to make approximately 1000 g

33. How much stearyl alcohol is needed to make 30 g of hydrophilic ointment?

   A. 0.3 g
   B. 1.2 g
   C. 3.7 g
   D. 7.5 g
   E. 8.3 g

34. Hydrophilic ointment is generally classified as:

   A. a hydrocarbon base.
   B. an absorption base.
   C. a water-removable base.
   D. a water-soluble base.
   E. a water-insoluble base.

End of this section; continue with the examination.

35. Which of the following sleep medications does *not* act on the benzodiazepine receptor?

   A. eszopiclone
   B. zaleplon
   C. zolpidem
   D. ramelteon
   E. triazolam

36. What patient counseling information should be provided when a patient is prescribed montelukast?

   A. Montelukast should be taken 1 hour before or 2 hours after a meal.
   B. It is first-line therapy for acute bronchospasm.
   C. It works the same way as Spiriva.
   D. Worsened allergic rhinitis symptoms may be noted.
   E. If it is prescribed for asthma, the drug should be taken in the evening.

37. Which product is most likely to induce hypokalemia in an otherwise normal hypertensive patient?

   A. Dyazide
   B. Vasotec
   C. Aldactazide
   D. hydrochlorothiazide
   E. eplerenone

38. All of the following are potential advantages of low-molecular-weight heparin (LMWH) over unfractionated heparin *except* which one?

   A. increased plasma half-life
   B. lower incidence of heparin-induced thrombocytopenia
   C. less risk of osteoporosis
   D. uses the same monitoring process as for heparin (activated partial thromboplastin time [aPTT])
   E. more predictable dose response

39. All of the following oral tablet strengths are available for lisinopril *except*:

   A. 2.5 mg.
   B. 5.0 mg.
   C. 10.0 mg.
   D. 25.0 mg.
   E. 40.0 mg.

40. All of the following agents are FDA-approved bisphosphonates for the prevention and treatment of osteoporosis *except*:

   A. zoledronic acid.
   B. raloxifene.
   C. ibandronate.
   D. alendronate.
   E. risedronate.

41. All of the following are fat soluble vitamins *except*:

    A. vitamin C.
    B. vitamin D.
    C. vitamin K.
    D. vitamin A.
    E. vitamin E.

42. According to the Henderson–Hasselbalch equation, $pH = pK_a + \log([base]/[salt])$. When pK_a equals 9 and the ratio of the nonionized species to the ionized species is 10:1, the pH equals:

    A. 8.
    B. 9.
    C. 10.
    D. 11.
    E. 12.

43. Which substance should be used in a case of overdosage with methotrexate?

    A. brewer's yeast
    B. leucovorin
    C. *para*-aminobenzoic acid
    D. sulfisoxazole
    E. trimethoprim

44. All of the following would be possible appropriate treatment options for *Clostridium difficile* infection *except*:

    A. loperamide.
    B. vancomycin.
    C. metronidazole.
    D. rifaximin.
    E. fidaxomicin.

Use the patient profile below to answer questions 45 to 59.

MEDICATION PROFILE (COMMUNITY)

Patient Name: Robert Trombone
Address: 6150 Ellis Ln.

Age: 62   Height: 5'6"

Sex: M   Race: White   Weight: 186 lb

Allergies: No known allergies

DIAGNOSIS

Primary   (1)   Hypertension
               (2)   Gouty arthritis
               (3)   Obesity

MEDICATION RECORD (Prescription and OTC)

	Date	Rx No.	Physician	Drug and Strength	Quan	Sig	Refills
(1)	11/21	15776	Mason	Hydrochlorothiazide 50.0 mg	30	i qd	5
(2)	11/21			Commit lozenges 2.0 mg	72	as directed	
(3)	12/4	15998	Mason	Phentermine 30.0 mg	30	i qd A.M.	0
(4)	1/7	16578	Mason	Naproxen 250.0 mg	20	3 stat, then i tid	2
(5)	1/7	16579	Mason	Benazepril 20.0 mg	30	i qd	6
(6)	1/12			Acetaminophen 500.0 mg	100	i–ii prn	
(7)	6/22	20967	Mason	Colchicine 0.6 mg	60	i bid	2
(8)	7/30	21366	Mason	Allopurinol 300.0 mg	30	i qd	6

PHARMACIST NOTES AND OTHER PATIENT INFORMATION

	Date	Comments
(1)	1/6	Patient called and stated that he has severe pain and swelling in his right big toe that awakened him last night; referred him to his physician for evaluation.
(2)	1/7	Patient states that his MD told him that his serum uric acid was 11.5 mg/dL.
(3)	1/7	DC hydrochlorothiazide.
(4)	1/12	Patient brought aspirin to counter for purchase; advised to use acetaminophen instead.

45. Based on Mr. Trombone's height and weight, he has a BMI of ~ 30. Which of the following statements apply to his situation?

   I. BMI stands for basal metabolic index.
   II. His BMI value meets the definition of obesity.
   III. Gradual weight loss would likely lower his serum uric acid.

   A. I only
   B. III only
   C. I and II
   D. II and III
   E. I, II, and III

46. Phentermine should be used cautiously in this patient because

   I. he has gout.
   II. his BMI is not high enough.
   III. he has elevated blood pressure.

   A. I only
   B. III only
   C. I and II
   D. II and III
   E. I, II, and III

47. Although he is waiting to see if his phentermine prescription can be filled, Mr. Trombone asks, "Is there any safe and effective over-the-counter medication that I can take to treat my obesity?" You reply, "The FDA has ruled that

    I. Orlistat has moved from prescription to over-the-counter (OTC) status and can be used."
    II. pseudoephedrine has taken the place of phenylpropanolamine as a safe and effective agent."
    III. benzocaine is effective."

    A. I only
    B. III only
    C. I and II
    D. II and III
    E. I, II, and III

48. Based on the information noted for 1/6 and 1/7, it appears that Mr. Trombone is suffering from an acute attack of gout. Which of the following *best* describes the usual pattern of the arthritis in gout?

    A. Morning stiffness for 1 hour.
    B. Periods of acute attacks with intense pain that completely resolve.
    C. Arthritis most commonly in the metacarpophalangeal and proximal interphalangeal joints of the hands.
    D. Gradual building of pain over a few days, then a sudden burst of intense pain that typically occurs in the late afternoon.
    E. Acute inflammation of two or more joints in a symmetrical pattern.

49. The Commit lozenges were recommended for Mr. Trombone for what purpose?

    I. to help treat his apparent sore throat
    II. as a treatment for an apparent cough
    III. as an aid to help him stop smoking

    A. I only
    B. III only
    C. I and II
    D. II and III
    E. I, II, and III

50. All of the following statements concerning Mr. Trombone's acute gouty arthritis attack are correct *except* which one?

    A. Corticosteroids should never be used to treat these attacks.
    B. A good response to colchicine therapy may help confirm the diagnosis of gouty arthritis, but some other forms of arthritis may respond to this agent.
    C. The first attack of gouty arthritis usually involves only one joint; when this is the first metatarsophalangeal joint of the foot, it is termed *podagra*.
    D. The patient will likely have an elevated serum uric acid level.
    E. Attacks most typically occur during the middle of the night.

51. Why did the pharmacist advise Mr. Trombone against taking the occasional aspirin for his headache?

    I. In low doses, aspirin can cause retention of uric acid in the body.
    II. Milligram per milligram acetaminophen is much more effective than aspirin for pain from episodic tension-type headaches.
    III. His increased risk for Reye syndrome.

    A. I only
    B. III only
    C. I and II
    D. II and III
    E. I, II, and III

52. All of the following statements concerning gout or uric acid excretion apply to Mr. Trombone *except* which one?

    A. As a man, Mr. Trombone is much more likely to develop gout compared to a woman.
    B. Most of Mr. Trombone's body uric acid is excreted through the gastrointestinal (GI) tract.
    C. Foods high in purine content may increase his serum uric acid level.
    D. If he were to take colchicine, it would have no effect on his serum uric acid level.
    E. Naproxen is a good choice over colchicine to treat his acute attack of gout because diarrhea secondary to colchicine therapy is common.

53. Mr. Trombone obtains refills on his naproxen for two additional episodes of gouty arthritis. Which of the following would be appropriate considerations in this patient?

    I. With his three attacks, Mr. Trombone is a candidate for uric acid–lowering therapy.

    II. Small daily doses of oral colchicine would likely benefit this patient by helping prevent additional attacks of acute gouty arthritis, especially if uric acid–lowering therapy is begun.

    III. It would be useful to consider switching him to another antihypertensive, as the current agent may be contributing to his hyperuricemia.

    A. I only
    B. III only
    C. I and II
    D. II and III
    E. I, II, and III

54. Which of the following apply to the allopurinol (Zyloprim) prescription for Mr. Trombone?

    I. This drug is known as a xanthine oxidase inhibitor.

    II. He can take this just once daily because of the long half-life of the metabolite.

    III. He must drink plenty of fluids to prevent uric acid crystallization in the urine after starting this drug.

    A. I only
    B. III only
    C. I and II
    D. II and III
    E. I, II, and III

55. Cheryl Trombone, Robert's wife, comes into the pharmacy and asks you to recommend a vaginal product for her yeast infection. Which of the following would apply to Mrs. Trombone?

    I. To use the OTC agents for this condition, she must have had at least one previous episode of vaginal candidiasis that was medically diagnosed.

    II. The OTC vaginal candidiasis products come in 1-, 3-, and 7-day treatment regimens.

    III. The characteristic symptoms of this condition are a vaginal discharge that is described as "cottage cheese–like" with no offensive odor, dysuria, or vulvar or vaginal redness.

    A. I only
    B. III only
    C. I and II
    D. II and III
    E. I, II, and III

56. One of Mr. Trombone's children, Megan (age 14), developed diarrhea. Which of the following agents are now considered by the FDA to be safe and effective OTC antidiarrheal agents?

    I. attapulgite
    II. kaolin
    III. bismuth subsalicylate

    A. I only
    B. III only
    C. I and II
    D. II and III
    E. I, II, and III

57. You decide to recommend Pepto Bismol Original Liquid for the treatment of Megan's diarrhea. Which of the following apply to this agent?

    I. This product contains bismuth subsalicylate.

    II. This product should not be given to a teenager who has chickenpox.

    III. Harmless black-stained stools may occur with the administration of this product.

    A. I only
    B. III only
    C. I and II
    D. II and III
    E. I, II, and III

58. A further inquiry into the possible reason for Megan's diarrhea reveals that she seems to get it most often after eating ice cream or other dairy products. You decide against recommending Pepto Bismol in favor of another product called Lactaid Original Caplets. Which of the following can be stated about her condition and your product recommendation?

   I. She probably has lactose intolerance.
   II. Lactaid Original contains lactase, which would be the appropriate agent for treating her.
   III. The diarrhea is caused by the calcium in the dairy products.

   A. I only
   B. III only
   C. I and II
   D. II and III
   E. I, II, and III

59. Ryan (age 13) and Greg (age 15), Mr. Trombone's other children, are planning to go to the beach with some friends. Mr. Trombone's family has fair skin, and Mr. Trombone wants to make sure that his sons are protected from the sun. Which of the following would apply to the use of sunscreens for these two teens?

   I. A product with a sun protection factor (SPF) of 30 or 30+ would provide maximal protection against sunburn.
   II. An adequate amount should be applied, and then it should be reapplied frequently because of loss of sunscreen from sweating or swimming.
   III. The SPF indicates protection against both UVA and UVB radiation.

   A. I only
   B. III only
   C. I and II
   D. II and III
   E. I, II, and III

Use the patient profile below to answer questions 60 to 69.

MEDICATION PROFILE (COMMUNITY)

Patient Name: Marilyn Fox
Address: 48 Worthy Rd.
Age: 22   Height: 5′5″
Sex: F   Race: White   Weight: 125 lb
Allergies: No known allergies

DIAGNOSIS

Primary   (1)   Pelvic inflammatory disease
             (2)   Anemia
             (3)   Vaginal candidiasis
Secondary   (1)   None

MEDICATION RECORD (Prescription and OTC)

	Date	Rx No.	Physician	Drug and Strength	Quan	Sig	Refills
(1)	9/3	617583	Tacs	Cefoxitin 2g	1	2 g IM × 1	0
(2)	9/3	617584	Tacs	Probenecid 500 mg	2	2 tabs stat	0
(3)	9/3	617585	Tacs	Tetracycline 500 mg	28	i q6h × 14 d	0
(4)	9/3	617586	Tacs	Tylenol with Codeine No. 3	20	i q4h prn	1
(5)	9/3			Feosol	100	i bid	
(6)	9/7	617843	Greene	Doxycycline 100 mg	30	i bid × 14 d	0
(7)	9/7	617967	Greene	Diflucan 150 mg	1	150 mg po × 1	0
(8)	10/1	618103	Greene	Triphasil	28	i qd	12

PHARMACIST NOTES AND OTHER PATIENT INFORMATION

	Date	Comments
(1)	9/7	DC tetracycline because of GI intolerance; change to doxycycline with food (doxycycline is current CDC recommendation for PID, not tetracycline).

60. Ms. Fox has purchased some Feosol. All of the following statements about iron supplementation are correct *except* which one?

    A. Iron can cause dark discoloration of the stool.
    B. Taking iron with food can decrease absorption.
    C. The usual dose of elemental iron is 200 mg/day in divided doses.
    D. Ferrous gluconate has the highest percentage of elemental iron of all the oral iron salts.
    E. Non–enteric-coated preparations of iron supplements are preferred over enteric-coated products.

61. Ms. Fox's anemia is apparently the result of an iron deficiency. Which of the following would apply to this type of an anemia before treatment with iron supplementation?

    I. One would likely note a microcytic hypochromic blood smear.
    II. The serum hemoglobin (Hb) and the mean cell volume (MCV) would be low.
    III. The serum total iron-binding capacity (TIBC) would usually be high.

    A. I only
    B. III only
    C. I and II
    D. II and III
    E. I, II, and III

62. Which products in Ms. Fox's profile may interact adversely with Feosol?

    I. Rocephin
    II. codeine
    III. tetracycline

    A. I only
    B. III only
    C. I and II
    D. II and III
    E. I, II, and III

63. Ms. Fox's initial diagnosis is pelvic inflammatory disease (PID). Which of the following statements apply to this condition?

    I. PID is usually caused by the organisms *Neisseria gonorrhoeae* and *Chlamydia trachomatis.*
    II. An acceptable outpatient drug regimen for empiric treatment of this condition is cefoxitin and doxycycline.
    III. The initial administration of cefoxitin IM is a rational one.

    A. I only
    B. III only
    C. I and II
    D. II and III
    E. I, II, and III

64. Why did Ms. Fox receive the Probenecid?

    I. She must have gout.
    II. Her serum uric acid level must be elevated.
    III. To prolong the serum levels of the cefoxitin.

    A. I only
    B. III only
    C. I and II
    D. II and III
    E. I, II, and III

65. Which of the following drugs from Ms. Fox's profile is most likely responsible for her yeast infection (vaginal candidiasis)?

    A. tetracycline
    B. Feosol
    C. Triphasil-28
    D. Tylenol with Codeine No. 3
    E. None of the above is likely responsible.

66. All of the following statements about doxycycline are correct *except* which one?

    A. It is active against many gram-positive and gram-negative organisms, *Rickettsia, Mycoplasma,* and *Chlamydia.*
    B. It is mainly excreted in the feces.
    C. Its absorption is increased with concurrent use of antacids and milk.
    D. It commonly causes GI distress.
    E. It may produce phototoxic reactions if the patient is exposed to sunlight.

67. Which of the following would most accurately describe the antibacterial activity of tetracycline antibiotics?

    I. They are mainly bacteriostatic at normal serum concentrations.
    II. They interfere with protein synthesis by binding to the 30S and possibly the 50S ribosomal subunit(s).
    III. They may cause alterations in the bacterial cytoplasmic membrane.

    A. I only
    B. III only
    C. I and II
    D. II and III
    E. I, II, and III

68. The selection of Diflucan to treat Ms. Fox's vulvovaginal candidiasis (VVC) is appropriate because

    I. it is less messy than vaginal creams.

    II. it is the only oral antifungal agent currently approved by the FDA for the treatment of VVC.

    III. it promotes patient compliance.

    A. I only

    B. III only

    C. I and II

    D. II and III

    E. I, II, and III

69. Based on Ms. Fox's profile, she has had only one occurrence of vulvovaginal candidiasis. Which of the following apply to recurrent vulvovaginal candidiasis?

    I. It would be diagnosed if she experienced at least four such infections in a 12-month period.

    II. If this is her diagnosis, she should not try to self-treat with any of the nonprescription products.

    III. Vaginal cultures should be obtained to confirm diagnosis and identify unusual species.

    A. I only

    B. III only

    C. I and II

    D. II and III

    E. I, II, and III

End of this patient profile; continue with the examination.

70. Which of the following would be used to treat antibiotic-associated *C. difficile* colitis?

    I. clindamycin

    II. fidaxomicin

    III. vancomycin

    A. I only

    B. III only

    C. I and II

    D. II and III

    E. I, II, and III

71. Which drug is a substituted imidazole for treating many systemic fungal infections and is an effective systemic agent when taken orally?

    A. butoconazole

    B. clotrimazole

    C. ketoconazole

    D. miconazole

    E. nystatin

Use the patient profile below to answer questions 72 to 83.

MEDICATION PROFILE (COMMUNITY)

Patient Name: Chanda Tanis
Address: 68 Ferris Dr.
Age: 36   Height: 5′4″
Sex: F   Race: African American   Weight: 110 lb
Allergies: Amitriptyline: local rash; phenobarbital: Stevens–Johnson syndrome

DIAGNOSIS

Primary	(1)	Epilepsy
	(2)	Mild hypertension
Secondary	(1)	Gastroesophageal reflux disease

MEDICATION RECORD (Prescription and OTC)

	Date	Rx No.	Physician	Drug and Strength	Quan	Sig	Refills
(1)	1/5	11238	Dunbar	Phenytoin 100 mg	100	iii caps q A.M.	6
(2)	1/5	11239	Dunbar	Divalproex 250 mg	200	ii tabs qid	6
(3)	1/5	11240	Dunbar	Carbamazepine 200 mg	60	i tab bid	6
(4)	1/30	11473	Huang	Folic acid 1 mg	100	i qd	2
(5)	1/30			Multivitamins	100	i qd	
(6)	1/30			Ibuprofen 200 mg	30	ii prn	
(7)	2/14	12372	Huang	Atacand HCT 16/12.5	30	i qd	3
(8)	2/14	12373	Huang	Ranitidine 150 mg	60	i bid	6

PHARMACIST NOTES AND OTHER PATIENT INFORMATION

	Date	Comments
(1)	1/10	Phenytoin level 16 μg/mL.
(2)	2/4	Nystagmus observed at routine visit.
(3)	2/4	Contacted Dr. Dunbar regarding prescription concern.

72. Which drugs should be avoided by this patient?

  I.   phenytoin
  II. primidone
  III. carbamazepine

  A. I only
  B. III only
  C. I and II
  D. II and III
  E. I, II, and III

73. Ms. Tanis has had difficulty swallowing various tablets and capsules. Which medications should she avoid crushing before administration?

  I.   carbamazepine (Tegretol)
  II. divalproex sodium (Depakote ER)
  III. folic acid

  A. I only
  B. III only
  C. I and II
  D. II and III
  E. I, II, and III

74. Which of the following are common side effects associated with phenytoin therapy?

    I. gingival hyperplasia
    II. megaloblastic anemia
    III. Stevens–Johnson syndrome

    A. I only
    B. III only
    C. I and II
    D. II and III
    E. I, II, and III

75. Therapeutic serum levels of phenytoin are generally considered to be in the range of

    A. 2 to 10 μg/mL.
    B. 10 to 20 μg/mL.
    C. 15 to 35 μg/mL.
    D. 20 to 40 μg/mL.
    E. 45 to 65 μg/mL.

76. Which of the following poses potential for drug–drug interactions with phenytoin?

    I. Depakote
    II. folic acid
    III. Tegretol

    A. I only
    B. III only
    C. I and II
    D. II and III
    E. I, II, and III

77. Good oral hygiene is especially important for reducing adverse reactions related to

    I. phenytoin.
    II. divalproex sodium.
    III. carbamazepine.

    A. I only
    B. III only
    C. I and II
    D. II and III
    E. I, II, and III

78. The serum level of carbamazepine (Tegretol) is unaffected by

    A. erythromycin ethylsuccinate (EES).
    B. Ery-Tab.
    C. amoxicillin.
    D. isoniazid.
    E. fluconazole (Diflucan).

79. Which drug is most likely responsible for Ms. Tanis' nystagmus?

    A. Dilantin
    B. Depakote
    C. Tegretol
    D. folic acid
    E. Advil

80. Dilantin is available as

    I. a capsule.
    II. a tablet.
    III. an ampule.

    A. I only
    B. III only
    C. I and II
    D. II and III
    E. I, II, and III

81. In addition to hydrochlorothiazide 12.5 mg, Atacand HCT 16/12.5 contains

    A. ramipril 5.0 mg.
    B. amlodipine 5.0 mg.
    C. candesartan 16.0 mg.
    D. quinapral 5.0 mg.
    E. captopril 12.5 mg.

82. The most commonly reported dose-related side effects associated with carbamazepine are

    A. rash, renal failure, and decreased white blood cells.
    B. diplopia, nausea, and ataxia.
    C. liver toxicity, pulmonary fibrosis, and autoimmune disorders.
    D. angina, urticaria, and vomiting.
    E. headache, rash, and prolonged blood clotting.

83. True comparisons of Advil to Tylenol include which statements?

    I. Tylenol has less anti-inflammatory activity than does Advil.
    II. Tylenol is contraindicated in children because they are susceptible to Reye syndrome.
    III. Tylenol irritates the GI tract more than does Advil.

    A. I only
    B. III only
    C. I and II
    D. II and III
    E. I, II, and III

End of this patient profile; continue with the examination.

84. The brand name for fosphenytoin is

    A. Dilantin
    B. Cerebyx
    C. Valium
    D. Lamictal
    E. Topamax

85. What type of drug interaction is taking place when reduced blood levels of tetracycline result from taking the drug concurrently with a calcium-containing antacid?

    A. synergism
    B. complexation
    C. chemical antagonism
    D. electrostatic interaction
    E. enzyme inhibition

86. Which of the following adverse drug reactions has been reported with the use of quinupristin/dalfopristin (Synercid)?

    A. photosensitivity
    B. infusion site pain, erythema, or itching
    C. neutropenia
    D. cardiomyopathy
    E. renal failure

87. Naloxone is used in combination with Talwin Nx to

    I. decrease the first-pass effects of pentazocine when administered orally.
    II. produce additive analgesic effects with pentazocine when administered orally.
    III. provide narcotic antagonist activity when administered intravenously.

    A. I only
    B. III only
    C. I and II
    D. II and III
    E. I, II, and III

88. If co-trimoxazole oral suspension contains 40 mg trimethoprim and 200 mg sulfamethoxazole per 5 mL, how many milliliters of suspension are required to provide a dose equivalent to one Bactrim DS tablet?

    A. 5 mL
    B. 10 mL
    C. 15 mL
    D. 20 mL
    E. 25 mL

89. Which of the following medications are classified as sustained-release theophylline products?

    I. Elixophyllin
    II. Uniphyl
    III. Theo-24

    A. I only
    B. III only
    C. I and II
    D. II and III
    E. I, II, and III

90. Based on a patient's malnutrition and symptoms such as fatigue, weight loss, and paresthesias, the physician suspects pernicious anemia. Which test is the most likely to diagnose this condition?

    A. Schilling test
    B. hematocrit
    C. hemoglobin
    D. serum folate
    E. Schlichter test

91. Which forms are available for potassium chloride?

    I. oral solution
    II. powder in a packet
    III. liquid

    A. I only
    B. III only
    C. I and II
    D. II and III
    E. I, II, and III

92. What is the side effect most commonly associated with doxazosin?

    A. hyperkalemia
    B. postural hypotension
    C. cough
    D. taste disturbances
    E. angioedema

93. All of the following statements are true of Prilosec OTC *except* which one?

    A. It is available as a 20-mg dose.
    B. It is available as a purple capsule.
    C. It is indicated for treatment of frequent heartburn.
    D. The patient should not take it > 14 days without a physician's direction.
    E. The patient should not repeat a 14-day course more often than every 4 months, unless directed by a physician.

94. Which of the following is the proper treatment for syphilis?

 A. ceftriaxone 1g IM once
 B. metronidazole 500 mg three times a day for 10 days
 C. azithromycin 1 g by mouth once
 D. benzathine penicillin 2.4 million units once
 E. tetracycline 500 mg four times a day for 14 days

95. Potassium supplementation is contraindicated in patients using

 A. chlorthalidone.
 B. hydrochlorothiazide (HCTZ).
 C. furosemide.
 D. triamterene.
 E. ethacrynic acid.

96. To determine the absolute bioavailability of a new controlled-release dosage form of quinidine gluconate, the extent of quinidine bioavailability after the new dosage form should be compared with

 I. the area under the curve (AUC) after an intravenous (IV) bolus dose of quinidine gluconate.
 II. the AUC after a reference standard controlled-release form of quinidine gluconate.
 III. the AUC after an oral solution of quinidine gluconate.

 A. I only
 B. III only
 C. I and II
 D. II and III
 E. I, II, and III

97. Which of the following is contraindicated in a patient with a history of anaphylaxis related to sulfamethoxazole/trimethoprim (Septra) administration?

 A. carbamazepine
 B. Depakote
 C. Dilantin
 D. acetazolamide
 E. ethosuximide

Use the patient profile below to answer questions 98 to 104.

PATIENT RECORD (INSTITUTION/NURSING HOME)

Patient Name: Grace Wiley
Address: 5768 So. 24th Street
Age: 35   Height: 5′9″
Sex: F   Race: Caucasian   Weight: 126 lb
Allergies: No known allergies

DIAGNOSIS

Primary   (1)   Bleeding duodenal ulcer
             (2)   Hypotension
Secondary   (1)   None

LAB/DIAGNOSTIC TESTS

	Date	Test
(1)	6/22	Hb 9 g/dL; HCT 30%; Na 126 mEq/L; K 3.4 mEq/L; Cl 90 mEq/L; CO_2 content 24 mEq; BUN 25 mg/dL; Cr 0.8 mg/dL; guaiac positive

MEDICATION ORDERS (Including Parenteral Solutions)

	Date	Drug and Strength	Route	Sig
(1)	6/22	D5/0.45% NaCl 1000 mL	IV	125 mL/hr
(2)	6/22	Ranitidine 50 mg	IV	q6h
(3)	6/23	Esomeprazole 40 mg	per NG tube	qd × 10 days
(4)	6/23	Clarithromycin Suspension	per NG tube	500 mg bid × 10 days
(5)	6/23	Amoxicillin Suspension	per NG tube	1 g bid × 10 days

ADDITIONAL ORDERS

	Date	Comments
(1)	6/22	Endoscopy stat.
(2)	6/22	Insert NG tube.
(3)	6/22	Check *Helicobacter pylori* status.
(4)	6/25	Patient discharged from the hospital.

DIETARY CONSIDERATIONS (Enteral and Parenteral)

	Date	Comments
(1)	None	

PHARMACIST NOTES AND OTHER PATIENT INFORMATION

	Date	Comments
(1)	6/22	Patient has 10 pack-years history of smoking.
(2)	6/22	Patient has recently completed a course of ibuprofen for sports injury.
(3)	6/23	Open Nexium capsule, administer esomeprazole beads in 50 mL water via NG tube.
(4)	6/23	Patient *H. pylori* positive.
(5)	6/23	Discontinue ranitidine.

98. As noted in Ms. Wiley's patient profile, she was tested for *H. pylori*. Which of the following statements is/are true regarding *H. pylori*?

  I. It is present in the majority of patients with duodenal ulcer.
  II. *H. pylori* eradication can cure peptic ulcer disease and reduce ulcer recurrence.
  III. An active duodenal ulcer is best managed with a combination of antisecretory therapy plus appropriate antibiotic(s).

  A. I only
  B. III only
  C. I and II
  D. II and III
  E. I, II, and III

99. In the admission interview, the pharmacist records that the patient has recently completed a regimen of ibuprofen. This information is significant in the patient's history because

  I. ibuprofen may cause ulcers even in *H. pylori*–negative individuals.
  II. ibuprofen may injure the gastric mucosa directly.
  III. ibuprofen inhibits synthesis of prostaglandins, thereby compromising the mucosal-protective effect of these substances.

  A. I only
  B. III only
  C. I and II
  D. II and III
  E. I, II, and III

100. If Ms. Wiley were allergic to penicillin, what anti-infective agent should be substituted for the amoxicillin?

  A. azithromycin
  B. cefaclor
  C. clindamycin
  D. metronidazole
  E. vancomycin

101. As noted in the profile, Ms. Wiley received ranitidine. The elimination half-life for ranitidine is approximately 2 hours. What percentage of this drug would be eliminated from the body 4 hours after an intravenous (IV) bolus dose?

  A. 12.5%
  B. 25.0%
  C. 50.0%
  D. 75.0%
  E. 87.5%

102. Ms. Wiley received ranitidine. Of the following H_2 antagonists, which one is a particular concern because it interacts with a large number of other medications?

  A. ranitidine
  B. cimetidine
  C. nizatidine
  D. famotidine

103. All of the following reduce acid secretion by inhibiting the proton pump of the parietal cell *except*:

  A. lansoprazole.
  B. posaconazole.
  C. pantoprazole.
  D. esomeprazole.
  E. omeprazole.

104. After leaving the hospital, the patient is given prescriptions for Nexium, amoxicillin, and Biaxin to complete the *H. pylori* eradication regimen. You should counsel the patient regarding all of the following *except* which one?

  A. Continue Nexium 40 mg for a total of 10 days.
  B. Clarithromycin can be taken with food to minimize GI side effects.
  C. Taste disturbances are common with Biaxin.
  D. Complete a full 10 days of antibiotic/antisecretory therapy for optimal eradication results.
  E. Refrigerate Biaxin suspension.

End of this patient profile; continue with the examination.

105. All of the following are true regarding bismuth subsalicylate preparations *except*:

  A. may turn the tongue black.
  B. may turn the stool black.
  C. is effective in the treatment of acute diarrhea.
  D. may increase the risk of developing Lyme disease.
  E. may cause salicylate toxicity when administered with aspirin.

106. Which statement concerning the drug misoprostol is true?

  A. It is effective for protecting patients from NSAID-induced gastric ulcer.
  B. It frequently produces dose-related diarrhea.
  C. It is contraindicated in women who are pregnant.
  D. It is a prostaglandin.
  E. Concomitant use with magnesium antacids increases the likelihood for constipation.

Use the information below to answer questions 107 and 108.

Hydrocortisone acetate 10 mg
Bismuth subgallate 1.75%
Bismuth resorcinol compound 1.20%
Benzoyl benzoate 1.20%
Peruvian balsam 1.80%
Zinc oxide 11.00%
Suppository base qs ad 2 g

107. The most appropriate suppository base in this preparation is

   A. glycerin.
   B. glycerinated gelatin.
   C. polyethylene glycol.
   D. theobroma oil.
   E. surfactant base.

108. How many milligrams of Peruvian balsam are needed to prepare 12 suppositories?

   A. 180
   B. 216
   C. 288
   D. 420
   E. 432

109. Which of the following requires that patients be screened for tuberculosis infection before initiation of therapy?

   A. celecoxib
   B. infliximab
   C. sulfasalazine
   D. captopril
   E. omeprazole

110. A patient comes into your pharmacy with complaints of "jock itch." He says he's been putting a topical cream on it for the past 10 days to help the itching, but the rash seems to be "spreading." What is the most likely content of this topical cream?

   A. miconazole
   B. terbinafine
   C. hydrocortisone
   D. clotrimazole
   E. tolnaftate

111. Which medication may result in a "disulfiram-like reaction" when taken with alcohol?

   A. tetracycline
   B. metronidazole
   C. amoxicillin
   D. clindamycin
   E. azithromycin

112. Which medications may discolor urine, sweat, and other body fluids and should be discussed as part of patient counseling?

   A. rifampin
   B. lisinopril
   C. hydrochlorothiazide
   D. clarithromycin
   E. propranolol

113. Which of the following medications has the adverse effect of worsening renal function?

   I. cisplatin
   II. foscarnet
   III. amphotericin B

   A. I only
   B. III only
   C. I and II
   D. II and III
   E. I, II, and III

114. Which of the following conditions may predispose a patient to toxicity from a highly protein-bound drug?

   I. hypoalbuminemia
   II. hepatic disease
   III. malnutrition

   A. I only
   B. III only
   C. I and II
   D. II and III
   E. I, II, and III

115. What is the primary reason for selecting an antacid containing both an aluminum salt and a magnesium salt as opposed to a single-ingredient antacid?

   A. lower cost
   B. a balance of untoward effects such as constipation and diarrhea
   C. minimal potential for concomitant drug interactions
   D. better palatability
   E. decreased frequency of administration

116. For which of the following antibiotics should the patient's creatinine phosphokinase (CPK) be monitored?

   A. amoxicillin
   B. daptomycin
   C. azithromycin
   D. linezolid
   E. clindamycin

Use the patient profile below to answer questions 117 to 128.

PATIENT RECORD (INSTITUTION/NURSING HOME)

Patient Name: Robert Smith
Address: Sharon View Nursing Home, 98 Colling Rd.
Age: 81   Height: 5′8″
Sex: M   Race: White   Weight: 175 lb
Allergies: No known allergies

DIAGNOSIS

Primary	(1)	Pneumonia
	(2)	Asthma
Secondary	(1)	Alzheimer disease
	(2)	Hypercholesterolemia
	(3)	Hypertension

LAB/DIAGNOSTIC TESTS

	Date	Test
(1)	10/2	Total cholesterol 242 mg/dL
(2)	10/14	WBC 9.2×10^3/mm^3; Cr 1.4 mg/dL

MEDICATION ORDERS (Including Parenteral Solutions)

	Date	Drug and Strength	Route	Sig
(1)	10/1	Advair Diskus	inhalation	ii puffs bid
(2)	10/1	Zafirlukast 20 mg	po	i bid
(3)	10/1	Rosuvastatin 20 mg	po	qd
(4)	10/1	Felodipine 5 mg	po	qd
(5)	10/12	Terbutaline 5 mg	po	i tab tid
(6)	10/15	Cefuroxime 1.5 g	IV	q8h
(7)	10/21	Amoxil 500 mg	po	q8h
(8)	10/22	Ciprofloxacin 750 mg	po	bid
(9)	10/22	Theo-24 300 mg	po	iii qd A.M.

ADDITIONAL ORDERS

	Date	Comments
(1)	10/15	Encourage fluids.
(2)	10/15	Rinse mouth with water after Advair dosing.

DIETARY CONSIDERATIONS (Enteral and Parenteral)

	Date	Comments
(1)	10/1	Low-fat diet.

PHARMACIST NOTES AND OTHER PATIENT INFORMATION

	Date	Comments
(1)	10/14	Fever to 102.4°F.
(2)	10/18	Temperature 98.6°F.
(3)	10/22	DC Amoxil because rash occurred.

117. What is the generic name for Accolate?

   A. metaproterenol
   B. albuterol
   C. ipratropium bromide
   D. zafirlukast
   E. cromolyn sodium

118. Which drug is most likely to cause tremor?

   A. Atrovent
   B. terbutaline
   C. Maxipime
   D. nicotinic acid
   E. Amoxil

119. Which statements concerning cefuroxime are true?

   I. It is a first-generation cephalosporin.
   II. It may produce a disulfiram-type reaction if this patient receives alcohol-containing products concurrently.
   III. It is commonly used in patients with community-acquired pneumonia.

   A. I only
   B. III only
   C. I and II
   D. II and III
   E. I, II, and III

120. Which of the following should *not* be used to provide acute relief of bronchospasm?

   A. albuterol
   B. pirbuterol
   C. Atrovent
   D. bitolterol
   E. Proventil

121. All of the following statements concerning amoxicillin are true *except* which one?

   A. It has an antimicrobial spectrum of activity similar to that of ampicillin.
   B. It is appropriately dosed every 6 hours.
   C. It may cause a generalized erythematous, maculopapular rash in addition to urticarial hypersensitivity.
   D. It produces diarrhea less frequently than does ampicillin.
   E. It is contraindicated in patients with a history of hypersensitivity to cyclacillin.

122. Which agents should Mr. Smith avoid?

   I. ampicillin
   II. ciprofloxacin
   III. erythromycin

   A. I only
   B. III only
   C. I and II
   D. II and III
   E. I, II, and III

123. When using an inhaler a patient should

   A. wait 5 minutes between puffs.
   B. rinse mouth with water between puffs.
   C. check peak flow readings before and after puffs.
   D. wait 1 minute between puffs.
   E. lie down for 10 minutes after dose has been administered.

124. Which agents are suitable for this patient's infection?

   I. cinoxacin
   II. norfloxacin
   III. ofloxacin

   A. I only
   B. III only
   C. I and II
   D. II and III
   E. I, II, and III

125. Which statements concerning fever are true?

    I. When treating a fever, either acetaminophen or aspirin would be acceptable antipyretic therapy.
    II. Fever is a useful assessment tool; treat only if the fever is dangerously high or the patient experiences chills.
    III. Fever should be treated aggressively; antipyretic therapy should begin on day 1 of antibiotic therapy.

    A. I only
    B. III only
    C. I and II
    D. II and III
    E. I, II, and III

126. Which drugs require that serum levels be measured and recorded in the patient's medication profile?

    I. theophylline
    II. cefuroxime
    III. terbutaline

    A. I only
    B. III only
    C. I and II
    D. II and III
    E. I, II, and III

127. Crestor is available as tablets in all of the following strengths *except*

    A. 5 mg.
    B. 10 mg.
    C. 20 mg.
    D. 40 mg.
    E. 80 mg.

128. The physician would like the patient to use a generic drug product equivalent to Uniphyl. For a generic drug product to be bioequivalent

    I. both the generic and the brand name drug products must be pharmaceutical equivalents.
    II. both the generic and brand name drug products must have the same bioavailability.
    III. both the generic and brand name drug products must have the same excipients.

    A. I only
    B. III only
    C. I and II
    D. II and III
    E. I, II, and III

End of this patient profile; continue with the examination.

129. Which of the following are thought to shorten the activity of theophylline?

    I. smoking
    II. phenobarbital
    III. cimetidine

    A. I only
    B. III only
    C. I and II
    D. II and III
    E. I, II, and III

130. Procrit is used in chronic renal failure to treat

    A. peripheral neuropathy.
    B. anemia.
    C. hyperphosphatemia.
    D. metabolic alkalosis.
    E. hyperuricemia.

131. The most common adverse effect of raloxifene is

    A. irregular uterine bleeding.
    B. rash and allergic reactions.
    C. hot flashes and leg cramps.
    D. nausea and GI upset.
    E. breast tenderness.

132. Emulsifying agents can be described as

    I. compounds that lower interfacial tension.
    II. molecules that contain a hydrophobic and a hydrophilic functional group.
    III. compounds that have surfactant properties.

    A. I only
    B. III only
    C. I and II
    D. II and III
    E. I, II, and III

133. Amitiza is indicated for treatment of

    A. acute diarrhea.
    B. migraine headache.
    C. chronic idiopathic constipation.
    D. gastroesophageal reflux disease (GERD).
    E. insomnia.

134. Which agents interfere with folic acid metabolism?

    I. trimethoprim
    II. methotrexate
    III. pyrimethamine

    A. I only
    B. III only
    C. I and II
    D. II and III
    E. I, II, and III

135. In the preparation shown here, salicylic acid is used for which property?

Salicylic acid 13.9%

Zinc chloride 2.7%

Flexible collodion base qs ad 30 mL

    A. analgesic
    B. antipyretic
    C. astringent
    D. keratolytic
    E. rubefacient

136. All of the following agents represent an approved OTC treatment for acne vulgaris *except*

    A. PROPA pH.
    B. Liquimat.
    C. Rezamid.
    D. Carmol-HC.
    E. Loroxide.

137. Which statements about type 1, or insulin-dependent, diabetes mellitus are true?

    I. The disease is more common in obese patients > 40 years of age.
    II. The cause of the disease is decreased insulin secretion and peripheral tissue insensitivity to insulin.
    III. Increased serum glucose levels can cause ketoacidosis in these patients.

    A. I only
    B. III only
    C. I and II
    D. II and III
    E. I, II, and III

138. Which type of hormone is represented in the structure here?

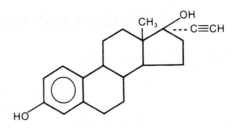

    A. androgen
    B. estrogen
    C. glucocorticoid
    D. mineralocorticoid
    E. progestin

139. All of the following situations are thought to contribute to the development of Parkinson disease *except*

    A. dopamine deficiency.
    B. norepinephrine deficiency.
    C. γ-aminobutyric acid (GABA) deficiency.
    D. acetylcholine deficiency.
    E. serotonin deficiency.

140. Which of the following statements is correct regarding paliperidone?

    A. It is a prodrug that is converted to risperidone following administration.
    B. It is classified as a dopamine agonist.
    C. The paliperidone extended-release tablet formulation should be administered with a laxative to ensure a predictable transit time through the GI tract.
    D. It should not be used concurrently with medications that prolong the QT interval.
    E. Unlike risperidone, paliperidone is not expected to elevate prolactin levels.

Use the patient profile below to answer questions 141 to 149.

PATIENT RECORD (INSTITUTION/NURSING HOME)

Patient Name: Heather Finegan
Address: 2325 Prospect Blvd.
Age: 52   Height: 5′6″
Sex: F   Race: Caucasian   Weight: 158 lb
Allergies: Penicillin: local rash

DIAGNOSIS

Primary   (1)   Acute pneumonia
             (2)   Chronic obstructive pulmonary disease
Secondary   (1)   History of recurrent pneumonia

LAB/DIAGNOSTIC TESTS

	Date	Test
(1)	2/28	Chest x-ray (bilateral lower lobe infiltrate)
(2)	2/28	WBC 18,000/mm^3; differential: segs 80%, bands 10%
(3)	2/28	Na 140.0 mEq/L; K 4.0 mEq/L; Cl 96.0 mEq/L; Bicarb 24.0 mEq/L; BUN 32.0 mg/dL; Cr 1.4 mg/dL; glucose 124.0 mg/dL; albumin 2.5 g/dL
(4)	2/28	Arterial blood gases: pH 7.4, P_{O_2} 70 mm Hg, P_{CO_2} 45 mm Hg, O_2 saturation 90%
(5)	2/28	Temp 102°F (oral); sputum c and s; theophylline level stat = 7.5 μg/mL

MEDICATION ORDERS (Including Parenteral Solutions)

	Date	Drug and Strength	Route	Sig
(1)	2/28	Aminophylline 250 mg	IVPB	stat
(2)	2/28	Aminophylline infusion	IV drip	40 mg/hr
(3)	2/28	Acetaminophen 650 mg	po or rectal	q4h prn
(4)	2/28	Ceftazidime 1 g	IVPB	q8h
(5)	2/28	Gentamicin 140 mg	IVPB	stat
(6)	2/28	Gentamicin 100 mg	IVPB	q12h
(7)	2/28	Albuterol 5% neb soln	inhalation	q4h prn

ADDITIONAL ORDERS

	Date	Comments
(1)	3/1	Gentamicin peak and trough after third dose.
(2)	3/1	Theophylline level (steady state).
(3)	3/2	Cimetidine 300 mg IVPB q8h.
(4)	3/4	Theophylline level.

DIETARY CONSIDERATIONS (Enteral and Parenteral)

	Date	Comments
(1)		
(2)		

PHARMACIST NOTES AND OTHER PATIENT INFORMATION

Date	Comments
(1)	Check influenza vaccination status.

141. Based on a volume of distribution of 0.5 L/kg theophylline in Ms. Finegan, the IV bolus dose of aminophylline would be expected to achieve an initial *total* theophylline serum concentration of

A. 3.2 μg/mL.
B. 6.9 μg/mL.
C. 10.7 μg/mL.
D. 13.1 μg/mL.
E. 14.4 μg/mL.

142. After IV bolus administration, theophylline follows the pharmacokinetics of a two-compartment model. Drugs that exhibit the characteristics of two-compartment pharmacokinetics have

I. an initial rapid distribution followed by a slower elimination phase.
II. a rapid distribution and equilibration into highly perfused tissues (central compartment) followed by a slower distribution and equilibration into the peripheral tissues (tissue compartment).
III. a plasma drug concentration that is the sum of two first-order processes.

A. I only
B. III only
C. I and II
D. II and III
E. I, II, and III

143. Results of the theophylline level on 3/1 indicate a serum level of 14.0 μg/mL. Without any change in the theophylline infusion and without any interruption in therapy, the theophylline level on 3/4 was reported as 17.5 μg/mL. Which statement most likely represents the reason for this increase?

A. The blood drawn for the theophylline level was not timed at steady state.
B. The blood taken for the theophylline level was drawn from the same arm in which theophylline was infusing.
C. The presence of ceftazidime in the blood sample caused a falsely elevated theophylline level.
D. The coadministration of cimetidine competitively blocked the metabolism of theophylline, resulting in a decreased elimination of theophylline.
E. The patient had a larger than usual volume of distribution for theophylline.

144. After the third dose of gentamicin, levels of the drug were reported as follows:

Peak—drawn half hour after ending a half-hour infusion, was 6.2 μg/mL.

Trough—drawn half hour before the next dose, was 1.2 μg/mL.

Gentamicin follows first-order elimination kinetics. Which statements concerning gentamicin pharmacokinetics are correct?

I. The elimination rate constant cannot be calculated.
II. If C_{max} is 7.2 μg/mL, the volume of distribution can be calculated as 16.6 L (0.23 L/kg).
III. The elimination half-life can be calculated as 4.65 hours.

A. I only
B. III only
C. I and II
D. II and III
E. I, II, and III

145. The culture and sensitivity report for the sputum specimen indicates the following minimum inhibitory concentrations (MICs):

ceftazidime < 8.0 $\mu g/mL$; piperacillin < 8.0 $\mu g/mL$; gentamicin $= 4.0$ $\mu g/mL$; tobramycin < 0.5 $\mu g/mL$ ciprofloxacin $= 8.0$ $\mu g/mL$

Based on these results, a rational therapeutic decision would be to

A. continue existing regimens without change.
B. continue ceftazidime only.
C. continue gentamicin; change ceftazidime to piperacillin.
D. change gentamicin to tobramycin; continue ceftazidime.
E. change ceftazidime to piperacillin; discontinue gentamicin.

146. Ms. Finegan has reported a penicillin allergy. The incidence of cephalosporin–penicillin cross-hypersensitivity is reported to be approximately

A. 0%.
B. 10%.
C. 25%.
D. 75%.
E. 95%.

147. Ms. Finegan has been stabilized on an IV infusion of aminophylline equivalent to 16 mg theophylline per hour. The physician would like to convert her to an oral controlled-release theophylline product such as Theo-24 or something comparable. Which dosage of Theo-24 would the pharmacist recommend for initial therapy?

A. 200 mg q24h
B. 300 mg q24h
C. 400 mg q24h
D. 500 mg q24h
E. 600 mg q24h

148. Which statements about converting Ms. Finegan from IV to oral sustained-release theophylline therapy are true?

I. Considering the theophylline infusion rate of 40 mg/hr, conversion to a sustained-release product at 300 mg q8h is appropriate.
II. Oral theophylline drug products produce more variable drug concentrations compared to an IV drug infusion.
III. Subsequent theophylline levels should be determined when no doses have been missed in the preceding 48 hours, and the sample should be drawn 3 to 7 hours after the last dose.

A. I only
B. III only
C. I and II
D. II and III
E. I, II, and III

149. The patient would like to receive a generic equivalent of Theo-24. In the process of selecting a generic theophylline product, the pharmacist obtains the following information on the generic theophylline product from the pharmaceutical manufacturer:

Thirty-six healthy subjects (26 men and 10 women) received either a single oral dose of 300 mg theophylline in controlled-release tablet form or an equal daily dose of 100 mg theophylline elixir given tid. A two-way crossover design was used for this study. In this study, no significant difference was observed in the AUC (0 to 24 hours) for serum theophylline concentrations from the tablet compared with the elixir dosage forms. A graph of the plasma drug concentrations versus time was included.

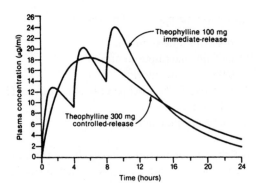

From this study, the pharmacist concludes that the

   I. theophylline tablet demonstrates controlled-release characteristics compared with those of the theophylline elixir.
  II. extent of theophylline bioavailability from both the tablet and the elixir is the same.
 III. theophylline elixir is bioequivalent to the theophylline tablet.

  A. I only
  B. III only
  C. I and II
  D. II and III
  E. I, II, and III

End of this patient profile; continue with the examination.

150. Influenza vaccine use in chronic obstructive pulmonary disease (COPD) patients

  A. has no demonstrated benefit.
  B. is recommended for asthma but not COPD.
  C. is recommended annually, usually in the fall, for COPD patients.
  D. is too risky for COPD patients owing to drug interaction potential.
  E. is effective for 5 years after immunization; no need for more frequent administration.

151. Ingredients with antitussive action that may be found in OTC cough preparations include

   I. dextromethorphan.
  II. diphenhydramine.
 III. dihydrocodeinone.

  A. I only
  B. III only
  C. I and II
  D. II and III
  E. I, II, and III

152. Which of the following statements about antithyroid agents are true?

    I. Propylthiouracil (PTU) and methimazole may help attain remission through direct interference with thyroid hormone synthesis.
    II. PTU or methimazole may be used preoperatively to establish and maintain a euthyroid state until definitive surgery can be performed.
    III. PTU has been associated with serious blood dyscrasias such as agranulocytosis.

    A. I only
    B. III only
    C. I and II
    D. II and III
    E. I, II, and III

153. The belladonna alkaloids are

    I. vincristine.
    II. vinblastine.
    III. atropine.

    A. I only
    B. III only
    C. I and II
    D. II and III
    E. I, II, and III

154. Spiriva may aggravate

    A. narrow-angle glaucoma.
    B. asthma.
    C. COPD.
    D. irritable bowel syndrome.
    E. excessive salivation.

155. Which statements describe potential problems with drug substances packaged in ampules?

    I. Ampules are made of glass, which can break on opening or during transport.
    II. Drug substances packaged in ampules must be filtered to prevent broken particles of glass from being infused.
    III. Once the ampule is broken open, it must be used; therefore, it cannot be a multiple-dose product.

    A. I only
    B. III only
    C. I and II
    D. II and III
    E. I, II, and III

156. The hypotonic parenteral product is

    A. normal saline solution.
    B. half-normal saline solution.
    C. 0.9% sodium chloride.
    D. dextrose 40.0% total parenteral nutrition (TPN) solution.
    E. 3.0% sodium chloride solution.

157. Which infusion methods allow reliable administration of a medication with a narrow therapeutic index?

    I. continuous IV infusion
    II. intermittent IV infusion
    III. IV bolus with intermittent infusion

    A. I only
    B. III only
    C. I and II
    D. II and III
    E. I, II, and III

Use the patient profile below to answer questions 158 to 166.

PATIENT RECORD (INSTITUTION/NURSING HOME)

Patient Name: John Stevens
Address: Shady Grove Nursing Home
Age: 81   Height: 5′9″
Sex: M   Race: African American   Weight: 150 lb
Allergies: No known allergies

DIAGNOSIS

Primary   (1)   Chronic renal failure
              (2)   Dementia
Secondary   (1)   Anemia

LAB/DIAGNOSTIC TESTS

	Date	Test
(1)	5/4	BUN 75.0 mg/dL; Cr 6.0 mg/dL; K 7.5 mEq/L; HCT 24%; Hb 7.8 g/dL; phosphate 7.6 mg/dL
(2)	5/7	K 7.5 mEq/L

MEDICATION ORDERS (Including Parenteral Solutions)

	Date	Drug and Strength	Route	Sig
(1)	5/4	Mylanta 30 mL	po	prn
(2)	5/4	Kayexalate 30 g	po	qid prn
(3)	5/4	Calcitriol 1 mg	po	i qd
(4)	5/4	Calcium carbonate 1 g	po	ii qid
(5)	5/4	Colace 100 mg	po	bid
(6)	5/7	Haloperidol 1 mg	po	bid
(7)	5/9	Amphojel 30 mL	po	qid pc
(8)	5/9	Ferrous sulfate 300 mg	po	qid pc

ADDITIONAL ORDERS

	Date	Comments
(1)	None	

DIETARY CONSIDERATIONS (Enteral and Parenteral)

	Date	Comments
(1)	5/4	Protein-restricted diet.

PHARMACIST NOTES AND OTHER PATIENT INFORMATION

	Date	Comments
(1)	5/9	DC Mylanta.

158. Which mechanism describes how Amphojel achieves its therapeutic effect in Mr. Stevens?

    A. potassium binding
    B. phosphate binding
    C. acid neutralizing
    D. base neutralizing
    E. ion exchange

159. Kayexalate achieves its therapeutic effect by acting as an exchange resin. Which ion is exchanged with sodium?

    A. potassium
    B. phosphorus
    C. calcium
    D. nitrogen
    E. magnesium

160. Which type of anemia is most likely to occur in chronic renal failure?

    A. normochromic, normocytic
    B. hypochromic, normocytic
    C. hypochromic, microcytic
    D. normochromic, macrocytic
    E. hypochromic, macrocytic

161. Which medications would need a dosage reduction in renal failure?

    I. haloperidol
    II. digoxin
    III. tobramycin

    A. I only
    B. III only
    C. I and II
    D. II and III
    E. I, II, and III

162. Calcitriol is the same substance as

    A. calcium carbonate.
    B. calcium gluconate.
    C. 1,25-dihydroxycholecalciferol.
    D. calcium leucovorin.
    E. dihydrotachysterol.

163. Which drugs in Mr. Stevens' therapeutic regimen are likely to cause constipation?

    I. Amphojel
    II. Kayexalate
    III. calcitriol

    A. I only
    B. III only
    C. I and II
    D. II and III
    E. I, II, and III

164. Life-threatening cardiac arrhythmias owing to hyperkalemia should be treated with

    I. calcium chloride or calcium gluconate intravenously.
    II. loop diuretics to rapidly eliminate potassium.
    III. sodium polystyrene sulfonate.

    A. I only
    B. III only
    C. I and II
    D. II and III
    E. I, II, and III

165. Which adverse effect of haloperidol is most likely to occur in Mr. Stevens?

    A. neuroleptic malignant syndrome
    B. extrapyramidal symptoms
    C. urinary retention
    D. cardiovascular effects
    E. decreased seizure threshold

166. When Mr. Stevens complained of GI discomfort, the physician prescribed cimetidine. The nurse should be alerted that cimetidine interacts with

    I. Amphojel.
    II. Colace.
    III. ferrous sulfate.

    A. I only
    B. III only
    C. I and II
    D. II and III
    E. I, II, and III

Use the patient profile below to answer questions 167 to 176.

PATIENT RECORD (INSTITUTION/NURSING HOME)

Patient Name: Mina Peterson
Address: 1422 Arlington St.
Age: 31   Height: 5′6″
Sex: F   Race: White   Weight: 130 lb
Allergies: Penicillin: rash

DIAGNOSIS

Primary	(1)	Acute nonlymphocytic leukemia
Secondary	(1)	Drug-induced congestive heart failure

LAB/DIAGNOSTIC TESTS

	Date	Test
(1)	None	

MEDICATION ORDERS (Including Parenteral Solutions)

	Date	Drug and Strength	Route	Sig
(1)	3/5	Cytarabine 200 mg/m^2	IV	qd × 7 days
(2)	3/5	Daunorubicin 45 mg/m^2	IV	qd × 3 days
(3)	3/6	Lorazepam 1 mg	IV	30 min prechemotherapy
(4)	3/6	Dolasetron 1.8 mg/kg	IV	30 min prechemotherapy
(5)	3/6	Dexamethasone 20 mg	IV	30 min prechemotherapy
(6)	3/6	Ortho-Novum 1/50	po	i qd
(7)	3/7	Nystatin Suspension	po	5 mL swish and swallow
(8)	3/7	Cetacaine Spray	to throat	prn
(9)	3/7	Colace 100 mg	po	i tid
(10)	3/7	Gentamicin 100 mL in D$_5$W	IV	i tid

ADDITIONAL ORDERS

	Date	Comments
(1)	3/7	Serum creatinine before gentamicin dosing.

DIETARY CONSIDERATIONS (Enteral and Parenteral)

	Date	Comments
(1)	None	

PHARMACIST NOTES AND OTHER PATIENT INFORMATION

	Date	Comments
(1)	3/5	Patient has had three previous courses of chemotherapy.
(2)	3/5	Family requests antidepressant therapy be reinstituted (previously received SSRI); patient asks for OTC ranitidine.

167. Which drug in Ms. Peterson's profile is most likely to cause congestive heart failure?

    A. cytarabine
    B. metoclopramide
    C. dexamethasone
    D. lorazepam
    E. daunorubicin

168. The most likely complications seen with Ms. Peterson's chemotherapy include

    I. renal failure.
    II. peripheral neuropathy.
    III. alopecia.

    A. I only
    B. III only
    C. I and II
    D. II and III
    E. I, II, and III

169. When the second dose of chemotherapy is administered, extravasation occurs. Management of this condition includes all of the following measures *except*

    A. leaving the needle in place.
    B. administering potassium chloride.
    C. applying ice.
    D. administering a corticosteroid.
    E. injecting sodium bicarbonate.

170. The probable reason for administration of Ortho-Novum 1/50 in this patient is

    A. birth control.
    B. estrogen stimulation of white blood cell production.
    C. discontinuation of menstrual bleeding.
    D. progestin stimulation of white blood cell production.
    E. chemotherapy for acute nonlymphocytic leukemia.

171. Approximately 10 days after chemotherapy, the cells most commonly affected include

    I. granulocytes.
    II. platelets.
    III. erythrocytes.

    A. I only
    B. III only
    C. I and II
    D. II and III
    E. I, II, and III

172. In preparing Ms. Peterson's chemotherapy, the pharmacist should take all of the following precautions *except*

    A. a horizontal laminar flow hood.
    B. a surgical gown.
    C. latex gloves.
    D. negative-pressure technique for vials.
    E. syringes with Luer-Lock fittings.

173. A patient who is taking an antihypertensive medication

    A. should avoid the serotonin and norepinephrine reuptake inhibitor (SNRI) venlafaxine.
    B. can safely take a tricyclic antidepressant.
    C. should reduce the dosage of antihypertensive when initiating antidepressant therapy.
    D. should not take any antidepressant medication.
    E. can take duloxetine without risk of increased blood pressure.

174. Ms. Peterson develops a hospital-acquired pneumonia and requires an antibiotic. Which drug should be administered with caution to this patient?

    A. clindamycin
    B. tetracycline
    C. vancomycin
    D. ceftazidime
    E. tobramycin

175. Gentamicin is also ordered for Ms. Peterson's infection. The major toxicities of gentamicin include

    I. hepatotoxicity.
    II. neurotoxicity.
    III. nephrotoxicity.

    A. I only
    B. III only
    C. I and II
    D. II and III
    E. I, II, and III

176. The FDA-recommended dose of ranitidine to treat GERD is

    A. 75 mg.
    B. 150 mg twice a day.
    C. 300 mg at bedtime.
    D. 150 mg four times a day.
    E. 300 mg four times a day.

End of this patient profile; continue with the examination.

177. Which sign or symptom reflects a vitamin K deficiency?

   A. dementia
   B. bleeding
   C. depression
   D. dermatitis
   E. diarrhea

178. Body surface area (BSA) is used in calculating chemotherapy doses because

   A. it is an indicator of tumor cell mass.
   B. it correlates with cardiac output.
   C. it correlates with GI transit time.
   D. the National Cancer Institute requires that it be used.
   E. the FDA requires that it be used.

179. Aspirin in high doses has been shown to extend the activity of methenamine in the treatment of urinary tract infections. What mechanism is responsible for this drug interaction?

   A. Urinary alkalinization reduces methenamine elimination.
   B. Urinary acidification reduces methenamine elimination.
   C. Urinary alkalinization promotes methenamine elimination.
   D. Urinary acidification promotes methenamine elimination.
   E. Acidification of the gastric contents decreases methenamine absorption.

180. Mary Jones presents with a prescription for boceprevir. Which of the following in the patient's profile of medications are contraindicated with concomitant therapy?

   A. aspirin
   B. carbamazepine
   C. ibuprofen
   D. metoprolol
   E. hydrocortisone cream

181. Which of the following narcotics has the longest duration of effect?

   A. methadone
   B. controlled-release morphine
   C. levorphanol
   D. transdermal fentanyl
   E. dihydromorphone

182. What is the principal ingredient in Burow's solution?

   A. acetic acid
   B. aluminum acetate
   C. boric acid
   D. sodium hypochlorite
   E. aluminum hydroxide

183. Which therapeutic agents have been developed from recombinant DNA technology?

   I. Activase
   II. Neupogen
   III. Epogen

   A. I only
   B. III only
   C. I and II
   D. II and III
   E. I, II, and III

184. Effects of the GI anticholinergic agent propantheline include

   I. dry mouth, blurred vision, and urinary retention.
   II. increased secretions, diarrhea, and pupillary constriction.
   III. acceleration of gastric emptying time.

   A. I only
   B. III only
   C. I and II
   D. II and III
   E. I, II, and III

185. Coumadin should be given with caution to patients in end-stage liver disease because

   I. Coumadin binding to albumin decreases.
   II. plasma albumin concentrations decrease.
   III. prothrombin clotting time increases.

   A. I only
   B. III only
   C. I and II
   D. II and III
   E. I, II, and III

186. A woman has a prescription for 32 mEq KCl by mouth. The pharmacy has 600-mg KCl controlled-release tablets. How many tablets does she need to take each day to provide this dose (molecular weight of KCl is 74.5)?

   A. 2 tablets
   B. 3 tablets
   C. 4 tablets
   D. 5 tablets
   E. 6 tablets

Use the information below to answer questions 187 and 188.

A woman brings the following prescription to the pharmacy after visiting her oncologist:
Carafate 1 g   8 tablets
Sorbitol 70% 40 mL
Vari-Flavors 2 packets
Water qs ad   120 mL
Sig: swish and expectorate 10 mL q4h

187. What is the percentage of sucralfate in the final suspension?

A. 1.0%
B. 6.7%
C. 12.4%
D. 8.0%
E. 15.0%

188. How much sucralfate is in 10 mL of this product?

A. 1.0 g
B. 500.0 mg
C. 66.7 mg
D. 0.667 g
E. 6.7 g

End of this patient profile; continue with the examination.

189. Passive diffusion of a drug molecule across a cell membrane depends on the

I. lipid solubility of the drug.
II. extent of ionization of the drug.
III. concentration difference on either side of the cell membrane.

A. I only
B. III only
C. I and II
D. II and III
E. I, II, and III

190. Which type of laxative includes the agent psyllium?

A. stimulant
B. bulk-forming
C. emollient
D. saline
E. lubricant

Test 2 Answers and Explanations

1. The answer is A. All of the symptom pairs listed are possible symptoms of schizophrenia. The most common are hallucinations (perception disturbances in sensory experiences of the environment) and delusions (incorrect or false beliefs).

2. The answer is A. Treatment of schizophrenia is primarily symptomatic. Target symptoms of schizophrenia have been categorized as "positive" and "negative" and may be used as a guide in evaluation of therapy. Positive symptoms (e.g., hallucinations, delusions, combativeness, insomnia) as compared to negative symptoms (e.g., poor judgment, apathy, asocial behavior, withdrawal, flat affect).

3. The answer is E. Neuroleptic malignant syndrome is an uncommon, but potentially fatal adverse effect of antipsychotics and other drugs which have antidopaminergic activity; although it has also been associated with drugs void of antidopaminergic activity. Signs and symptoms include fever, rigidity, altered mental status, unstable blood pressure, tachycardia, elevated creatine kinase levels, and an increased white blood cell count. Treatment includes supportive care and the use of bromocriptine and/or dantrolene.

4. The answer is C (I and II). The patient is admitted to the hospital in an acute psychotic state, and the decision is made to initiate therapy with haloperidol. Haloperidol is available in several forms; the initial order for haloperidol decanoate 50 mg IM represents the treatment of a chronic psychotic patient, which is administered on a monthly basis, once a patient has been stabilized. It is not intended for the acute management of psychosis. Instead, the patient should have received an order for haloperidol lactate, where doses of 2 to 10 mg IM or IV are given every 4 to 8 hours at the initiation of therapy for acutely agitated patients.

5. The answer is D. An acute dystonic reaction is characterized by involuntary tonic contractions of skeletal muscles of virtually any striated muscle group. The greatest period of risk for such a reaction usually is within the first 24 to 48 hours of initiating an antipsychotic agent; 95% of dystonic reactions have occurred within 96 hours of antipsychotic initiation or dosage increase. Ms. Curtis is experiencing torticollis (muscle spasm of the neck causing the head to be twisted to the side) and oculogyric crisis (a spasm of the eye muscles causing one or both eyes to become fixed in an upward gaze). The reaction is treated initially with an anticholinergic agent such as diphenhydramine or benztropine, given intramuscularly or intravenously. Relief is usually seen within 15 to 20 minutes. The antipsychotic may be continued along with a short course of anticholinergic agent. Alternative agents include the benzodiazepines diazepam and lorazepam.

6. The answer is B. Akathisia is a subjective experience of motor restlessness, and patients usually complain of an inability to sit still. This adverse symptom occurs in 20% to 40% of patients receiving high-potency first-generation agents (FGAs). Onset of akathisia occurs within the first few weeks or months of therapy, and treatment may include dosage reduction, lipophilic β-blockers, benzodiazepines, or anticholinergic agents.

7. The answer is E (I, II, and III). All three approaches would be useful in helping this patient. Given the option of using equally effective second-generation antipsychotic agents, with which these reactions are rare, and the previously noted reactions that Ms. Curtis has experienced with the haloperidol, it seems prudent that the best option would be to discontinue the haloperidol and switch her to a second-generation agent.

8. The answer is D. Thioridazine (Mellaril) is a first-generation antipsychotic. The other agents—aripiprazole (Abilify), olanzapine (Zyprexa), ziprasidone (Geodon), and quetiapine (Seroquel)—are all second-generation agents.

9. The answer is E (I, II and III). Haloperidol decanoate is given IM every 3 to 4 weeks. Fluphenazine decanoate is administered every 2 to 3 weeks. Long-acting risperidone is administered IM every 2 weeks and was the first of the second-generation agents to be available in this dosage form.

10. The answer is C (I and II). With the exception of clozapine, all antipsychotics (FGAs and SGAs) are thought to have similar efficacy for positive symptoms. Clozapine has demonstrated efficacy for treatment-refractory schizophrenia.

11. The answer is B. Agranulocytosis, defined as a granulocyte count $< 500/mm^3$, occurs in association with clozapine use at a cumulative incidence at 1 year of approximately 1.3%. This reaction could prove fatal if it is not detected early and therapy is not interrupted. Patients should have a white blood cell (WBC) count before therapy begins and a clear plan for frequent (weekly), routine WBC assessment throughout therapy.

12. The answer is B. The objective is to straighten the ear canal so that the drops are easily instilled. In a child, this is accomplished by pulling the ear backward and downward.

In an adult patient, the ear canal is straightened by pulling it backward and upward.

13. The answer is A. Carbamide peroxide is effective in softening, loosening, and helping remove cerumen from the ear canal. Although the other agents have been used in practice for years, there are no data to support their efficacy above carbamide peroxide in anhydrous glycerin. Sweet oil is another name for olive oil.

14. The answer is A. Mineral oil (liquid petrolatum) is the only OTC lubricant laxative available. It may rarely be recommended in situations in which a soft stool is warranted, to avoid the patient from straining. In most of these cases, a stool softener would be preferable (e.g., docusate sodium). Lipid pneumonia may result if the patient takes this medication while lying down. It should not be given to bedridden patients or before bedtime for ambulatory patients. It should be taken on an empty stomach because taking it with meals will delay gastric emptying. Although the clinical effect is uncertain, mineral oil may decrease the absorption of fat-soluble vitamins A, D, E, and K. The usual dose is 15 to 45 mL (1 to 3 tablespoons). Patients will not lose fluid with this lubricant laxative as they would with a saline laxative.

15. The answer is E. Symptoms of hemorrhoids such as burning, discomfort, irritation, inflammation, itching, pain, and swelling can all be treated safely and effectively with various OTC agents. Patients with bleeding, seepage, prolapse, thrombosis, and severe pain should be referred to a physician to rule out a cause other than a hemorrhoid.

16. The answer is D. All of the agents would be effective for treating itching from hemorrhoids. Anusol HC-1 contains hydrocortisone, and Anusol ointment contains pramoxine (OTC topical anesthetic). Preparation H cream contains phenylephrine in addition to shark liver oil, petrolatum, and glycerin. Because drugs absorbed in the anal area go directly into the systemic circulation, this agent might increase the blood pressure in this patient. An appropriate warning label against its use in hypertensive patients is on the product.

17. The answer is E (I, II, and III). Celecoxib (Celebrex) is a COX-2 inhibitor used for pain and inflammation of rheumatoid arthritis. These agents do not alter the course of the disease, nor do they prevent joint destruction. Warnings concerning postmarketing reports of serious skin reactions and hypersensitivity reactions in patients receiving this drug were issued in November 2002. Patients experiencing a rash while receiving this medication are advised to discontinue the drug immediately.

18. The answer is A (I). Low-dose systemic corticosteroids can work well either orally or parenterally for anti-inflammatory and immunosuppressant activity. They do not alter the course of the disease, but they are often used to bridge therapy as patients are started on disease-modifying antirheumatic drugs (DMARDs). Corticosteroids will not counteract the side effects of the NSAIDs.

19. The answer is E. All of the statements (A through D) apply to the use of Enbrel.

20. The answer is C (I and II). Titanium dioxide is a physical sunscreen agent that blocks ultraviolet radiation over both the UVA and UVB spectrum (actually over the entire solar spectrum). Ecamsule (Mexoryl SX) helps protect against short UVA rays whereas avobenzone (Parsol 1789) helps protect against long UVA rays, and octocrylene helps protect against UVB rays. These three sunscreen agents are combined into a product (Anthelios Sx) which provides both UVA and UVB protection. Homosalate and padimate O block only UVB radiation.

21. The answer is B. Combination cancer chemotherapy regimens are used to improve survival and response outcomes for cancer treatment, and usually involve two or more agents. Drugs given in combination generally should have different mechanisms of action, should act during different cell cycle phases, should have known activity as single agents, and should be associated with different adverse effects. Cell cycle–specific drugs may be given in combination with cell cycle–nonspecific agents.

22. The answer is A. Cyclophosphamide is an alkylating agent. These agents affix an alkyl group to cellular DNA, causing cross-linking of DNA strands, which triggers cell death. Cell cycle–nonspecific agents kill nondividing as well as dividing cells.

23. The answer is B (III). Only docetaxel is associated with a low incidence of nausea and vomiting. Both cyclophosphamide and doxorubicin are associated with moderate incidences of nausea and vomiting (31% to 90%), which are caused largely by stimulation of the chemoreceptor trigger zone in the brain.

24. The answer is C (I and II). Docetaxel (Taxotere) may cause fluid retention leading to pulmonary edema. Dexamethasone is administered to help prevent this effect. Dexamethasone is also an adjuvant antiemetic for prevention of nausea and vomiting due to the doxorubicin-cyclophosphamide components of TAC chemotherapy. Premedication with dexamethasone and H_1 and H_2 antagonists is required for paclitaxel (Taxol) to prevent potential hypersensitivity reactions.

25. The answer is E. Both doxorubicin and docetaxel are considered to be vesicants. Vesicants cause extreme irritation and may cause tissue necrosis if they extravasate or leak from blood vessels into surrounding tissues. Placement of implanted infusion ports decreases the risk of extravasation but does not eliminate the risk.

26. The answer is B. Ondansetron is the generic name for Zofran. The brand names for the other products are Aloxi (palonosetron), Kytril (granisetron), Emetrol (phosphorated carbohydrate solution), and Anzemet (dolasetron).

27. The answer is A. Clomiphene (Clomid) is an ovulation stimulant and a selective estrogen receptor modulator (SERM) that is not used in the treatment of breast cancer. All of the other agents listed may be used as adjuvant hormonal therapy for breast cancer.

28. The answer is B (III only). Chemotherapy-induced nausea and vomiting is best controlled by preventing it with an appropriate antiemetic regimen. Nausea and vomiting, common occurrences with many chemotherapeutic drugs, result from stimulation of the brain's CTZ. Some patients experience anticipatory nausea and vomiting before getting chemotherapy and this is best managed through the use of a benzodiazepine (such as lorazepam) prior to treatment. Severe nausea and vomiting may reduce patient tolerance to treatment regimens. Effective use of antiemetic drug regimens is an important adjunct to successful chemotherapy.

29. The answer is A (I only). Although all three drugs are reliable antistaphylococcal therapy, Ms. Smith's history of penicillin allergy is a contraindication for the use of penicillin derivatives such as dicloxacillin and Unasyn (ampicillin and sulbactam). Vancomycin (Vancocin) is not a penicillin derivative and is a valuable alternative for penicillin-sensitive patients. It has excellent activity against *S. aureus* (including most methicillin-resistant strains).

30. The answer is A. Linezolid (Zyvox) is effective treatment for vancomycin-resistant *S. aureus*. Vancocin is a brand of vancomycin, to which the organism has demonstrated resistance. Rocephin, meropenem, and Cedax (ceftibuten) are generally ineffective for vancomycin-resistant *S. aureus*.

31. The answer is B (III only). Pegfilgrastim (Neulasta) is used to reduce the risks of neutropenic complications in patients with cancer who are receiving myelosuppressive chemotherapy. Potential benefits include a decreased incidence of febrile neutropenia, hospitalization, and antibiotic treatment.

32. The answer is D. Sertraline (Zoloft) is a selective serotonin reuptake inhibitor (SSRI) without anticholinergic properties. The other four agents have significant anticholinergic effects: Tolterodine (Detrol LA), Tylenol PM (acetaminophen with diphenhydramine), amitriptyline, and diphenhydramine which could result in cognitive impairment in the elderly.

33. The answer is D. *250 g/1000 g = X g stearyl* alcohol/ 30 g total

$$X = 7.5 \text{ g stearyl alcohol}$$

34. The answer is C. The *USP* lists four general classes of ointments that are used as vehicles: (1) hydrocarbon bases, represented by white petrolatum and white ointment; (2) absorption bases, represented by hydrophilic petrolatum and cold cream; (3) water-removable bases, represented by hydrophilic ointment; and (4) water-soluble bases, represented by polyethylene glycol ointment. Ophthalmic ointments are listed separately by the *USP* as ointments for application to the eye.

35. The answer is D. Ramelteon (Rozerem) is the first agent that acts on the melatonin system, binding to the melatonin 1 and melatonin 2 receptors in the brain. Eszopiclone (Lunesta), zaleplon (Sonata), and zolpidem (Ambien) are benzodiazepine agonists that bind to the γ-aminobutyric acid 1 (GABA-1) receptor and the benzodiazepine receptor, but they are not benzodiazepines in structure. Triazolam (Halcion) is structurally a benzodiazepine that binds to the benzodiazepine receptor on the GABA-A receptor complex.

36. The answer is E. Montelukast should be taken in the evening if it is prescribed for asthma. Montelukast may be administered without regard to meal times. It is used to treat symptoms of allergic rhinitis so these should not increase. It is not FDA approved for use in the reversal of acute bronchospasm in asthma. Montelukast is a leukotriene antagonist whereas Spiriva (tiotropium) is an anticholinergic agent.

37. The answer is D. Hydrochlorothiazide by itself causes hypokalemia. Triamterene-hydrochlorothiazide (Dyazide), and spironolactone-hydrochlorothiazide (Aldactazide) obviously contain the thiazide diuretic hydrochlorothiazide (HCTZ), which can cause hypokalemia. However, Dyazide and Aldactazide contain a potassium-sparing diuretic, which helps prevent potassium losses. Enalapril (Vasotec) is an angiotensin-converting enzyme inhibitor that inhibits potassium loss from the kidney by inhibiting angiotensin effects. Eplerenone is a selective aldosterone blocker which can cause the serum potassium to increase.

38. The answer is D. LMWHs (tinzaparin, dalteparin, enoxaparin) can be given without anticoagulation monitoring because they have a more predictable dose-response relationship. LMWHs have longer half-lives than unfractionated heparin and can be administered subcutaneously with greater bioavailability. LMWHs are also associated with a lower risk of adverse effects typical of heparin, such as thrombocytopenia and osteoporosis.

39. The answer is D. Lisinopril tablets are available as 2.5-, 5.0-, 10.0-, 20.0-, 30.0-, and 40.0-mg tablets.

40. The answer is B. Raloxifene (Evista) is a selective estrogen receptor modulator (SERM). All of the other agents are bisphosphonates: Zoledronic acid (Reclast), Ibandronate (Boniva), Alendronate (Fosamax), and Risedronate (Actonel).

41. The answer is A. Vitamins A, D, K, and E are all fat-soluble vitamins. Vitamin C is a water-soluble vitamin.

42. The answer is C. Substitution in the Henderson–Hasselbalch equation gives pH = 9 + log (10/1) = 9 + 1 = 10. When pH is equal to pK_a, the ratio of nonionized to ionized species is 1. When the pK_a is 1 unit above or below the pH, the ratio of nonionized to ionized species is 10:1 or 1:10, respectively. For weak acid drugs, the reverse is true.

43. The answer is B. Methotrexate (amethopterin, or MTX) is a competitive inhibitor of dihydrofolic acid reductase. Leucovorin (citrovorum factor) is used to neutralize the effects of MTX.

44. The answer is A. Loperamide interferes with peristalsis to slow GI motility which minimizes the excretion of the exotoxins of *C. difficile*. It is contraindicated in patients who have diarrhea caused by pseudomembranous colitis. The other agents are treatment options for *C. difficile*: vancomycin, metronidazole (Flagyl), rifaximin (Xifaxan), and fidaxomicin (Dificid).

45. The answer is D (II and III). BMI stands for body mass index. BMI = [weight (lb)/height (in^2)] $\times$ 703; (186/66^2) $\times$ 703 = 30. It is the most commonly used indicator for obesity. Height and weight charts are available to quickly determine this number. A BMI $\geq$ 30 defines obesity. Gradual weight loss does result in a decrease in serum uric acid.

46. The answer is B (III). Phentermine is structurally similar to amphetamine, but it has less severe central nervous system stimulation. Because it can cause significant increases in blood pressure, its use in hypertensive patients is not advisable. His BMI of 30 justifies the use of pharmacotherapy-facilitated weight loss (a BMI of 27 justifies the use of drug therapy if other risk factors such as hypertension are present); however, another agent without the adverse effect on blood pressure should probably be selected. There is no contraindication to the use of phentermine in a patient with gout.

47. The answer is A (I). In 2007, Orlistat (Alli) became the first weight loss drug officially sanctioned by the U.S. government for OTC use. The sympathomimetic agent phenylpropanolamine and the topical anesthetic benzocaine were originally ruled as safe and effective OTC weight loss drugs. Because of safety issues (hemorrhagic stroke), phenylpropanolamine was removed from the OTC drug market. Pseudo-

ephedrine, an oral decongestant that remains on the market for that indication, has not been shown to be an effective weight loss agent. Because of insufficient evidence of efficacy, the FDA advised manufacturers of benzocaine-containing products to remove these from the market. The manufacturers have complied, so there are no safe and effective OTC weight loss agents on the market.

48. The answer is B. Gouty arthritis attacks occur acutely with complete resolution after a few days. The morning stiffness described in choice A is typical of rheumatoid arthritis. Metacarpophalangeal and proximal interphalangeal joint involvement is classic for rheumatoid arthritis. Gouty arthritis most commonly affects the first metatarsophalangeal joint of the big toe. Gouty arthritis attacks typically occur suddenly in the middle of the night. This scenario matches the pharmacist's note in the profile. Joint inflammation with simultaneous involvement of the same joint areas on both sides of the body may be characteristic of rheumatoid arthritis.

49. The answer is B (III). Commit lozenges contain nicotine polacrilex (the same ingredient as nicotine gum), which is one of the newer dosage forms for nicotine replacement. Patients are instructed to use the 2-mg or 4-mg strength based on the amount of time after awakening when the urge to smoke occurs. Patients who have this urge within 30 minutes should use the 4-mg product.

50. The answer is A. Although not generally given as first-line agents, corticosteroids (e.g., oral prednisone) may be used to treat acute gouty arthritis. NSAIDs and oral colchicine are the usual first-line agents. A positive response to colchicine may help confirm the diagnosis of acute gouty arthritis, but other causes of acute arthritis may respond positively to this agent. Choices C, D, and E are "classic" components of gout. Mr. Trombone's presentation per his phone call to the pharmacy matches the descriptions in choices C and E. The serum uric acid reported in Mr. Trombone's profile (11.5 mg/dL) is elevated.

51. The answer is A (I). Aspirin in low doses ($<$ 2 g/day) inhibits the tubular secretion of uric acid, causing uric acid to be retained. For the treatment of minor pain such as headache, dosages for both aspirin and acetaminophen are essentially the same. Reye syndrome, an acute and potentially fatal illness, occurs with rare exceptions in children $<$ 15 years. Fatty liver with encephalopathy develops with this syndrome. The onset most often follows an influenza or chickenpox infection. The risk for this syndrome increases with salicylate ingestion. Because of Mr. Trombone's age, he is not at risk for this condition.

52. The answer is B. By almost a 10:1 margin, gout affects more males than females. Most (about two-thirds) of the uric acid excreted by the body is through the kidneys, and this is helpful in using drugs such as probenecid, which aids in the excretion of uric acid through the kidneys. High-purine foods (i.e., organ meats) should be avoided because these may increase serum uric acid levels. Colchicine has no effect on serum uric acid levels. Most clinicians now select NSAIDs over colchicine because of the high incidence of diarrhea from colchicine.

53. The answer is E (I, II, and III). Initially, acute gouty arthritis attacks resolve completely, usually with no residual effects. The repeated attacks of gouty arthritis and the fact that his serum uric acid level is elevated would indicate the need for uric acid–lowering therapy. Prophylactic low doses of colchicine (usually 0.5 to 1.0 mg/day) may help prevent acute attacks of gouty arthritis, especially during the initiation of uric acid–lowering therapy. Thiazide diuretics (hydrochlorothiazide) may cause hyperuricemia, and switching this patient to a different antihypertensive agent would be appropriate.

54. The answer is C (I and II). Allopurinol (Zyloprim) is a xanthine oxidase inhibitor that works to prevent uric acid formation from xanthine. The long half-life of the main active metabolite (oxypurinol) permits the drug to be dosed just once daily. Unlike the uricosuric agent (probenecid), which blocks tubular absorption of uric acid resulting in increased amounts of uric acid in the urine, allopurinol actually decreases uric acid formation. Therefore, increased fluid intake is not required as it is with the uricosuric drugs.

55. The answer is E (I, II, and III). To use the OTC agents, a woman must have had this condition once before, must have had it diagnosed by a physician previously, and must experience the same type of symptoms. These agents are available in 1-, 3-, and 7-day regimens. These are all "azole" antifungal agents. The characteristic symptoms are noted in choice III. Other vaginal conditions that are not amenable to OTC treatment will produce symptoms that require medical referral, such as a malodorous discharge and dysuria.

56. The answer is D (II and III). Kaolin by itself (without pectin), bismuth subsalicylate, and loperamide are now considered safe and effective by the FDA for OTC use for diarrhea. Also lactase products are specifically indicated for lactose-intolerant patients. Attapulgite and calcium polycarbophil, which were previously considered safe and effective, were reclassified in April 2003 as Class III agents owing to insufficient effectiveness data. Even though the FDA has granted kaolin monograph status, no single-ingredient kaolin products are currently available in the United States.

57. The answer is E (I, II, and III). Pepto Bismol does contain bismuth subsalicylate. As with other salicylates, these should not be given to children or teenagers with the flu or chickenpox because of the increased risk of Reye syndrome.

A black-stained stool, which is harmless, may occur and should not be confused with melena, which is blood in the stool. Harmless darkening of the tongue can also occur with bismuth subsalicylate use.

58. The answer is C (I and II). Lactose intolerance is relatively common. Disaccharides, like lactose and sucrose, are normally hydrolyzed by lactase. If lactase is not present, these disaccharides may produce an osmotic diarrhea. Products such as Lactaid Original, which contain lactase, can be administered before eating dairy products to relieve this problem. Also, lactose-free milk products can be used in place of regular milk. Calcium, although probably not in the doses present in various dairy products, will eventually cause constipation, not diarrhea.

59. The answer is C (I and II). An SPF of 30 blocks about 97% of UVB radiation and would certainly provide maximal protection against sunburn. Any benefit from using SPFs above 30 would be negligible. All sun-exposed surfaces should be covered liberally and evenly. An average-size adult in a swimsuit would require about 1 oz per application. Perspiration, swimming, and toweling off all contribute to the need for reapplication. The SPF is a measure of only UVB protection. UVA radiation, which is relatively constant throughout the day, is not blocked by sunscreen agents that are limited to the UVB spectrum. The sunscreen agent avobenzone blocks most of the UVA rays.

60. The answer is D. Ferrous sulfate (Feosol) and fumarate have higher percentages of elemental iron than the gluconate salt. Enteric-coated formulations do not dissolve until they enter the small intestine, which causes a reduction in iron absorption. The other statements concerning iron supplementation are correct.

61. The answer is E (I, II, III). Iron-deficiency anemia usually produces a microcytic hypochromic type of anemia. The red blood cells are smaller and lighter in color than normal. The hemoglobin level in the blood will be low. Red blood cell indices such as MCV and the mean cell hemoglobin concentration (MCHC) will both be low, reflecting the microcytic and hypochromic nature of the red cells. Total iron-binding capacity will be high.

62. The answer is B (III). Iron preparations form a chelate with tetracycline, inhibiting its absorption; therefore, iron preparations should not be administered with oral tetracyclines. If a patient needs both types of therapy, the iron product should be administered 3 hours before or 2 hours after the tetracycline to minimize the adverse interaction.

63. The answer is E (I, II, and III). Common organisms that can cause PID include *N. gonorrhoeae* and *C. trachomatis.* Empiric treatment is, therefore, directed toward eradicating these organisms. One of the options for empiric outpatient treatment uses a combination regimen of cefoxitin given intramuscularly once followed by doxycycline given for 14 days.

64. The answer is B (III). The patient does not have any symptoms of gout or any notation of an elevated uric acid level. Benemid (probenecid) could be used for long-term management of those two conditions, but she received only one dose. Probenecid competes with the tubular secretion of β-lactam antibiotics, resulting in prolongation of serum levels. The Centers for Disease Control and Prevention (CDC) recommendations for pelvic inflammatory disease include probenecid as part of the regimen.

65. The answer is A. Tetracycline and other broad-spectrum antibiotics are a common cause for vulvovaginal candidiasis. Estrogen-containing oral contraceptives (e.g., Triphasil-28) might cause this problem, but it was started after the candida infection. The other agents, ferrous sulfate and Tylenol with Codeine, are not associated with the development of this infection.

66. The answer is C. Tetracyclines are broad-spectrum agents effective against gram-negative and gram-positive organisms, spirochetes, *Mycoplasma* and *Chlamydia* organisms, rickettsial species, and certain protozoa. Phototoxic reactions (enhanced sunburn) can develop with exposure to sunlight. Doxycycline has the least binding affinity for calcium ions of any of the tetracyclines, but the net effect is a slight decrease in absorption, not an increase. Unlike other tetracycline derivatives, food and/or antacids do not significantly inhibit absorption of doxycycline. GI distress is a common adverse effect of all tetracyclines; it may be minimized by concurrent administration with food.

67. The answer is E (I, II, and III). Tetracyclines are mainly bacteriostatic, but at high concentrations they can be bactericidal. They inhibit bacterial protein synthesis by binding to the 30S and possibly the 50S ribosomal subunit(s), thus interfering with the transfer of genetic information. They may also inhibit the bacterial cytoplasmic membrane, reducing membrane stability and thus causing bacterial cell lysis.

68. The answer is E (I, II, and III). Single-dose oral fluconazole has been shown to have clinical efficacy as good as or better than topical antifungal products. Because it can be given as a single oral tablet, it is considered cleaner than topical agents, many of which need to be dosed three or more times to reach the efficacy afforded by one oral dose of fluconazole. These factors have led to improved patient compliance.

69. The answer is E (I, II, and III). Patients who experience these recurrent vulvovaginal candidiasis infections may be experiencing a mixed infection or a strain of candidal infection other than *C. albicans*. Vaginal cultures should be obtained to confirm diagnosis and identify unusual species (particularly *Candida glabrata*). These infections might be resistant to standard therapy. All of the statements are correct.

70. The answer is D (II and III). Clindamycin is commonly associated with the development of pseudomembranous colitis or *C. difficile* colitis as a side effect. Vancomycin and metronidazole are the most commonly antibiotics used to treat antibiotic-associated *C. difficile* colitis when discontinuation of the offending antibiotic does not fully resolve the condition. Fidaxomicin (Dificid) is the most recently approved alternative to these agents. Fidaxomicin has been shown to be noninferior with vancomycin with a significantly lower rate of recurrence of *C. difficile*.

71. The answer is C. Ketoconazole is an oral agent effective for treating systemic fungal infections. Butoconazole, clotrimazole, and miconazole are administered topically or vaginally for local infection. Nystatin is a polyene antifungal antibiotic, not a substituted imidazole derivative. It is available for topical and vaginal administration to treat local infections. Nystatin oral tablets are not absorbed and are, therefore, therapeutic only for infections of the GI tract, especially oral and esophageal *Candida* infections.

72. The answer is D (II and III). Phenytoin, primidone, and carbamazepine are all agents indicated for treatment of generalized tonic–clonic seizures. Primidone metabolizes to phenobarbital; therefore, patients who are allergic to phenobarbital should not receive primidone. Carbamazepine is contraindicated in patients with hypersensitivity to tricyclic antidepressants, such as amitriptyline.

73. The answer is C (I and II). Tegretol and Depakote are both slow-release products of carbamazepine and divalproex preparations and should not be crushed. All slow-released products must remain intact to prevent dissolution in the stomach.

74. The answer is E (I, II, and III). Although the mechanism has only been speculated, the impact that phenytoin might have on the metabolism of folic acid is responsible for the development of select anemias (i.e., megaloblastic), as well as the potential development of gingival hyperplasia (an overgrowth of the gums), both of which might be avoided through the supplementation of folic acid. Stevens–Johnson syndrome is an autoimmune and life-threatening skin reaction.

75. The answer is B. The normal therapeutic range for phenytoin serum levels is 10 to 20 μg/mL. Nystagmus, ataxia, and slurred speech have been reported with serum levels of 20 to 30 μg/mL, with coma reported when the level reaches 40 μg/mL.

76. The answer is D (II and III). Folic acid enhances phenytoin clearance, which can result in reduced phenytoin serum levels and loss of efficacy. Carbamazepine (Tegretol) may also enhance phenytoin metabolism and thus reduce plasma phenytoin levels and therapeutic efficacy. Phenytoin has the same effect on carbamazepine.

77. The answer is A (I). Good oral hygiene including gum massage, frequent brushing and flossing, and appropriate dental care may decrease gingival hyperplasia related to phenytoin use.

78. The answer is C. Penicillins such as amoxicillin have not been shown to affect carbamazepine (Tegretol) levels. Erythromycin (EES or Ery-Tab), isoniazid, and fluconazole (Diflucan) all have reportedly increased carbamazepine levels.

79. The answer is A. Nystagmus is an early sign of phenytoin (Dilantin) intoxication. Other reactions common with phenytoin use are confusion, slurred speech, drowsiness, and ataxia. All are dose-related adverse effects involving the central nervous system.

80. The answer is C (I and II). Phenytoin sodium (Dilantin) is available as an extended-release capsule and as a chewable tablet. However, the Dilantin version of the IM/IV version has been discontinued and is only available in the generic form.

81. The answer is C. Atacand 16.0/12.5 contains the angiotensin receptor blocker candesartan 16.0 mg and hydrochlorothiazide (HCTZ) 12.5 mg.

82. The answer is B. Diplopia, nausea, and ataxia are the most common dose-related side effects associated with carbamazepine.

83. The answer is A (I). Acetaminophen (Tylenol) has analgesic and antipyretic activity but very little anti-inflammatory activity. Aspirin, not acetaminophen, is contraindicated in small children with fever caused by a viral infection because they are susceptible to Reye syndrome.

84. The answer is B. The brand name for fosphenytoin is Cerebyx. The generic name for Dilantin is phenytoin, for Valium is diazepam, for Lamictal is lamotrigine, and for Topamax is topiramate.

85. The answer is B. When tetracycline is administered with a calcium-containing antacid, a complex is formed that reduces the absorption of tetracycline. Synergism is an example of potentiation of one drug's interaction with another—for example, any NSAID and opioid, when combined, their combined effect is greater than the addition of each individual effect. Competitive antagonism results when two agents compete for the same receptor site, such as when atropine sulfate competes with acetylcholine for the cholinergic receptor site.

86. The answer is B. Reported adverse drug reactions with quinupristin/dalfopristin (Synercid) are generally mild and infusion-related: pain, erythema, or itching at the infusion site; increases in pulse and diastolic blood pressure; headache, nausea, or vomiting; and diarrhea. Synercid does not alter hematologic or renal indices, but it may increase liver function tests slightly.

87. The answer is B (III). Naloxone, which is a pure opioid antagonist, reverses or prevents the effects of opioids but has no opioid-receptor agonist activity. Naloxone is not absorbed after oral administration; however, after IV administration, it blocks the pharmacologic effects of pentazocine (Talwin), producing withdrawal symptoms in opioid-dependent persons.

88. The answer is D. Bactrim DS contains 160 mg trimethoprim and 800 mg sulfamethoxazole; thus 20 mL of co-trimoxazole suspension would be required to provide an equivalent dose.

89. The answer is D (II and III). Elixophyllin is the brand name for a theophylline elixir preparation. Uniphyl and Theo-24 are theophylline sustained-release preparations.

90. The answer is A. The Schilling test is used to diagnose pernicious anemia, or vitamin B_{12} deficiency. Hematocrit, hemoglobin, and serum folate measurements are not specific for vitamin B_{12} deficiency. The Schlichter test is used in bacterial endocarditis to ensure adequate antibiotic concentration in the blood.

91. The answer is E (I, II, and III). Potassium chloride is available as an oral solution, as a powder, and as a liquid to be given orally as well as a sterile product for IV administration. For ambulatory use, potassium chloride is available as an oral solution or as a powder in a packet to be mixed with water or juice. The injection form is for rapid IV potassium repletion or as an addition to total parenteral nutrition (TPN).

92. The answer is B. Postural hypotension is commonly experienced with α_1-blockers, including doxazosin, because of the direct action on the vasculature.

93. The answer is B. Prilosec OTC is available as salmon-colored tablets; prescription Prilosec 20 mg is available as purple capsules.

94. The answer is D. Benzathine penicillin 2.4 million units once is the preferred therapy for syphilis. All other choices (ceftriaxone, metronidazole, azithromycin, or tetracycline regimens) are inappropriate.

95. The answer is D. Hyperkalemia is a major risk with potassium-sparing diuretics, and potassium supplementation is, therefore, contraindicated. To reduce the risk of hyperkalemia, the patient may use a combination of diuretic products such as Dyazide (triamterene with HCTZ), Aldactazide (spironolactone with HCTZ), or other combinations.

96. The answer is A (I only). Absolute bioavailability is a measurement of the fraction of the dose that is systemically absorbed. To estimate absolute bioavailability, the AUC after the drug product is given orally is compared with the AUC after an IV bolus dose, because only the IV bolus dose is known to be 100% absorbed. Relative bioavailability compares the AUC of one dosage form with that of another dosage form, usually a drug solution or reference drug product given by the same route of administration.

97. The answer is D. Acetazolamide (Diamox) is a carbonic anhydrase inhibitor and a nonbacteriostatic sulfonamide derivative. Sulfamethoxazole/trimethoprim (Septra, Bactrim) is a sulfonamide antibiotic. Therefore, cross-sensitivity may exist between these drugs.

98. The answer is E (I, II, and III). *H. pylori* infection is present in the majority of duodenal ulcer patients. The major benefit to eradication of the infection is prevention of recurrent ulcer disease. Ulcers recur in 50% to 80% of *H. pylori*–positive patients whose duodenal ulcers are healed within 1 year. Eradication prevents recurrence in most patients. Treatment of active duodenal ulcers is best managed with a combination of antisecretory agents to relieve symptoms and heal the ulcer, and appropriate antibiotics to eradicate the infection and prevent recurrence.

99. The answer is E (I, II, and III). NSAIDs such as ibuprofen are inhibitors of prostaglandin synthesis. Although the inhibition is an important mechanism for anti-inflammatory therapy, it also compromises the protective effects that prostaglandins exert on the gastric mucosa. NSAIDs can also injure the gastric mucosa directly by allowing back-diffusion of hydrogen ions into the mucosa. NSAIDs are independent risk factors for peptic ulcer disease and can cause ulcers in *H. pylori*–negative patients. In fact, NSAIDs are the principal cause of ulcers in patients who are not infected.

100. The answer is D. In patients with a penicillin allergy, metronidazole can be substituted for amoxicillin. This therapy is reserved for this particular situation because resistance and decreased efficacy occurs.

101. The answer is D. For any first-order process, 50% of the initial amount of drug is eliminated at the end of the first half-life, and 50% of the remaining amount of drug (i.e., 75% of the original amount) is eliminated at the end of the second half-life. The half-life for ranitidine is about 2 hours; therefore, in 2 hours 50% of the drug is eliminated, and in 4 hours 75% of the drug is eliminated.

102. The answer is B. Cimetidine inhibits a number of cytochrome P450 isoenzymes which results in interactions with a number of other medications. CYP450 drug interactions with ranitidine, famotidine, and nizatidine are uncommon at OTC doses.

103. The answer is B. Lansoprazole, omeprazole, pantoprazole, and esomeprazole are proton pump inhibitors. Posaconazole is a broad-spectrum antifungal agent.

104. The answer is E. Biaxin (clarithromycin) suspension should be stored at room temperature and should not be refrigerated as it forms a gel. It should be shaken well before use. An appropriate advice for the patient should include recommendations to take the complete 10 days of antibiotics required for eradication, together with Nexium 40 mg daily. Finally, administration of clarithromycin with food may minimize GI complaints.

105. The answer is D. Adolescents and children who have or are recovering from influenza or chicken pox and take salicylates are at risk for Reye syndrome (not Lyme disease). Bismuth compounds discolor the stool and tongue to be black; this may alarm patients because black stools may also be a sign of blood (GI bleeding). Large doses of bismuth subsalicylate in combination with aspirin may cause salicylate toxicity. It is indicated for the treatment of acute diarrhea.

106. The answer is E. If misoprostol is given with magnesium-containing antacids, it may increase the risk of diarrhea (not constipation). Misoprostol is approved to protect patients from NSAID-induced gastric ulcers. Misoprostol is a synthetic prostaglandin that appears to suppress gastric acid secretion and may provide a mucosal protective effect. It is used in patients taking NSAID therapy to counter the undesired effect that these compounds exert on prostaglandin activity in the parietal cell of the gastric mucosa. Misoprostol is contraindicated in pregnant women because it may induce spontaneous uterine contractions.

107. The answer is D. Theobroma oil (cocoa butter) is a mixed triglyceride suppository base that melts at 34° to 35°C. Its emollient and nonirritating characteristics allow its use as a base for hemorrhoidal suppositories. Glycerinated gelatin suppositories are used as vaginal suppositories for the local application of antibacterial agents. Glycerin or soap suppositories contain sodium stearate, which is used for its laxative effect. Polyethylene glycol bases are water-miscible suppository bases used with various drugs for systemic absorption.

108. The answer is E. The amount of Peruvian balsam in one suppository (2 g) is equal to 0.018 × 2000 mg; therefore, for 12 suppositories

0.018 × (2000 mg/suppository) × 12 suppositories = 432 mg.

109. The answer is B. Infliximab prescribing information contains a warning that tuberculosis (frequently disseminated or extrapulmonary at clinical presentation) and other infections have been observed in patients receiving the drug. It is recommended that patients be evaluated for latent tuberculosis with a tuberculin skin test and that therapy of latent tuberculosis be initiated before therapy with infliximab. The other agents listed do not have this warning.

110. The answer is C. Topical miconazole, terbinafine, clotrimazole, and tolnaftate cream are all indicated for the treatment of tinea cruris fungal infections (jock itch) and, depending on the agent, are administered for 1 to 2 weeks. Because the patient describes the rash as spreading, it could likely be because of using hydrocortisone which would relieve the itching but not treat the underlying infection.

111. The answer is B. Patients receiving metronidazole may experience a disulfiram-type reaction if they consume alcohol concurrently with the drug. This reaction has not been noted in patients receiving the other agents.

112. The answer is A. Rifampin colors urine, sweat, tears, saliva, and feces orange-red. The other agents noted have not produced this effect.

113. The answer is E (I, II, and III). Cisplatin, foscarnet, and amphotericin B can decrease renal function. Renal function tests should, therefore, be monitored in patients receiving these drugs.

114. The answer is E (I, II, and III). Drugs that are highly bound to albumin will have higher concentrations of free drug circulating in the blood if albumin levels are reduced. Hypoalbuminemia, liver (hepatic) disease, and malnutrition are several of the more common conditions that result in decreased albumin levels, which necessitate alterations in dosage in highly albumin-bound drugs.

115. The answer is B. Antacids, which act to neutralize gastric acids, are available primarily as magnesium, aluminum, calcium, or sodium salts. A product that is a combination of magnesium and aluminum salts permits a lower dosage of each compound. In addition, with such a combination, the constipating effect of the aluminum salt counteracts the laxative effect of the magnesium salt, thereby minimizing the consequences of each compound.

116. The answer is B. CPK baseline levels should be obtained and CPK levels should be monitored at a minimum of weekly when the patient is on daptomycin therapy. This does not apply to the other antibiotics listed.

117. The answer is D. The generic name for Accolate is zafirlukast. It is a leukotriene receptor antagonist used for the prophylaxis and treatment of asthma.

118. The answer is B. Tremor is often the dose-limiting side effect related to terbutaline use. Tremor also has been reported to occur with other sympathomimetic drugs.

119. The answer is B (III). Cefuroxime (Ceftin, Kefurox, Zinacef) is a second-generation cephalosporin. Alcohol consumption can result in a disulfiram-type reaction in patients receiving cefamandole (or the third-generation agents moxalactam and cefoperazone), but this does not occur with cefuroxime. Cefuroxime often is prescribed as an alternative to ampicillin (as is cefamandole) to treat community-acquired pneumonia and is administered in a dosage of 2.25 to 4.50 g per day, which is divided and given every 8 hours. All cephalosporins should be used cautiously in penicillin-allergic patients.

120. The answer is C. Atrovent (ipratropium) should not be used for symptom relief or for exacerbations of bronchospasm. The onset of action is within 15 minutes, and the agent is useful mainly for maintenance regimens in patients with COPD and some patients with asthma. The other agents listed have more rapid onsets (within 5 minutes) and are useful to relieve acute bronchospasm.

121. The answer is B. Amoxicillin has a spectrum of antimicrobial activity similar to that of ampicillin. It has a longer half-life, which allows less frequent dosing (250 to 500 mg every 8 hours, as opposed to ampicillin, which is given in a dosage of 250 mg to 2 g every 4 to 6 hours). Both drugs may produce an erythematous, maculopapular rash not seen with other penicillins. Amoxicillin has more complete oral absorption than ampicillin—a characteristic that may explain the lower frequency of diarrhea as a side effect. It is contraindicated in patients with a history of hypersensitivity to other penicillins.

122. The answer is A (I). With this patient's recent history of rash caused by amoxicillin, ampicillin should be avoided because an erythematous, maculopapular rash or an urticarial hypersensitivity is seen with other penicillins. Ciprofloxacin and erythromycin are both reasonable alternatives in terms of the potential interaction of these agents with theophylline (Slo-Phyllin).

123. The answer is D. For optimal dose retention, patients should be instructed to wait 1 minute between each puff. Longer waits between puffs are unnecessary and may contribute to nonadherence to the prescribed regimen. Patients using steroid inhalers, especially, should be instructed to rinse well after completing their dosing. If the immediate response to an inhaled β-agonist needs to be documented, patients should wait until all of their puffs have been administered before checking their peak flows. Lying down is unnecessary following administration of inhaled agents.

124. The answer is B (III). Only ofloxacin (Floxin) is suitable for systemic infections such as pneumonia. Cinoxacin was previously approved only for urinary tract infections, but was recently discontinued in the United States. Norfloxacin is indicated for only urinary tract infections.

125. The answer is C (I and II). Fever is an important monitoring parameter in infectious diseases; however, administration of antipyretics masks fever. Subsidence of a fever (defervescence) usually indicates a favorable response to therapy. Fever should be treated only if the patient has chills or if the fever is dangerously high. If needed, acetaminophen or aspirin is acceptable. Because fever sometimes stems from noninfectious conditions that do not respond to antibiotics (e.g., metabolic disorders, drug reactions, and neoplasms), fever should not be treated with anti-infective agents unless infection has been identified as the cause.

126. The answer is A (I). Of the medications that this patient is receiving, only theophylline levels are commonly measured. These tests are available through commercial clinical laboratories.

127. The answer is E. Crestor is currently available as 5-, 10-, 20-, and 40-mg tablets. There is currently no 80-mg tablet.

128. The answer is C (I and II). Bioequivalent drug products must contain the same active ingredient in the same chemical form and in the same amount (i.e., they must be pharmaceutical equivalents), and they must have the same rate and extent of systemic drug absorption (i.e., the same bioavailability). The inactive ingredients or excipients may be different.

129. The answer is C (I and II). Theophylline is an agent that depends on the cytochrome P450 microsomal enzyme for its metabolism. Tobacco tars and phenobarbital are both considered to be enzyme inducers of the cytochrome P450 microsomal enzyme system; consequently, theophylline metabolism may be increased in patients taking these agents concurrently. The H_2-receptor antagonists cimetidine and ranitidine have both been shown to inhibit the P450 enzyme system and thus reduce theophylline metabolism.

130. The answer is B. Anemia is a common complication of chronic renal failure caused by a decrease in production of erythropoietin and endocrine product in the kidney. Erythropoietin, or epoetin α (Epogen, Procrit), stimulates red blood cell production in the bone marrow. This production is reflected by an increase in hematocrit and hemoglobin and a decrease in the need for blood transfusions. Recently, erythropoietin has been approved for the treatment of anemia in HIV-positive patients or for the prevention of anemia owing to zidovudine (AZT).

131. The answer is C. The most frequently reported adverse effects of raloxifene include hot flashes (up to 28% of women) and leg cramps (5.9%). Raloxifene has not been associated with irregular uterine bleeding or breast tenderness. GI complaints and allergic manifestations occur less frequently.

132. The answer is E (I, II, and III). Emulsifying agents, also known as wetting agents, surfactants, or surface-active agents (e.g., soaps, sodium lauryl sulfate, and dioctyl sodium sulfosuccinate), lower the surface and interfacial tension. These agents permit more intimate contact between an aqueous (water) phase and a lipid phase.

133. The answer is C. Amitiza (lubiprostone) is indicated for treatment of chronic idiopathic constipation in adults.

134. The answer is E (I, II, and III). Pyrimethamine, trimethoprim, and methotrexate act on the folic acid pathway to inhibit reduction of dihydrofolic acid to tetrahydrofolic acid by the enzyme dihydrofolate reductase.

135. The answer is D. Salicylic acid is commonly used externally as a keratolytic in corn and wart preparations (e.g., Wart-Off and Freezone) to remove the horny layers of the skin in a process known as desquamation.

136. The answer is D. Products containing benzoyl peroxide, sulfur, salicylic acid (3% to 6%), and resorcinol (1% to 2%) have been shown to be effective agents in the treatment of acne vulgaris. Benzoyl peroxide (Loroxide), salicylic acid (PROPA pH), sulfur (Liquimat), and resorcinol and sulfur (Rezamid Lotion) are available OTC anti-acne products. Carmol-HC, a urea-containing product that also contains hydrocortisone, is effective in treating dry skin.

137. The answer is B (III). Patients with type 1, or insulin-dependent, diabetes are normally younger; are not obese; have an absolute lack of insulin in the pancreas; and are predisposed to ketoacidosis if they do not receive insulin.

138. The answer is B. The choices are all steroids. Estrogenic steroids have an aromatic A ring. Progesterone and other progestins are derivatives of pregnane.

139. The answer is D. Any disturbance in the balance between dopaminergic receptors and cholinergic receptors seems to result in various movement disorders. Increases in acetylcholine and decreases in dopamine, norepinephrine, serotonin, or GABA have been linked to the development of various forms of Parkinson disease. These alterations may occur because of the aging process, infection, drug consumption, or trauma.

140. The answer is D. Paliperidone (Invega) labeling includes a warning regarding prolongation of the QT interval and associated risks of cardiac arrhythmias. Accordingly, paliperidone use should be avoided in patients taking other medications known to cause QT prolongation (e.g., procainamide, quinidine, amiodarone, sotalol, chlorpromazine, thioridazine, or moxifloxacin). Paliperidone is the major active metabolite of risperidone (Risperdal; not a prodrug). It appears to exhibit antipsychotic activity through a combination of central dopamine type 2 (D_2) and serotonin type 2 (5-HT_{2A}) antagonism. A change in GI transit time may alter the bioavailability of paliperidone (decreased bioavailability with decreased transit time as might occur with laxatives). The prolactin-elevating effect of paliperidone is similar to risperidone; galactorrhea, amenorrhea, gynecomastia, and impotence have been reported with their use.

141. The answer is D. Aminophylline, the parenteral form of theophylline, is commonly available as the dihydrate salt and contains approximately 80% theophylline. Enter this information into the calculation of the final serum concentration by first converting the aminophylline dose into the equivalent theophylline dose. The expected serum concentration then can be calculated by dividing the corrected theophylline dose by the volume of distribution and adding that to the initial level of 7.5 μg/mL in this patient. The calculations are as follows:

$$250 \text{ mg aminophylline bolus} = 200 \text{ mg theophylline}$$
$$250 \times 0.80 = 200$$
$$C = \text{Dose}/V_D = 200 \text{ mg}/0.5 \text{ L/kg} = 200 \text{ mg}/0.5 \text{ L/kg} \times$$
$$71.8 \text{ kg} = 200 \text{ mg}/36 \text{ L} = 5.55 \text{ } \mu\text{g/mL}$$
$$5.55 + 7.50 = 13.05 = 13.1 \text{ } \mu\text{g/mL}$$

142. The answer is E (I, II, and III). Drugs that follow two-compartment pharmacokinetics have a rapid distribution phase, followed by a slower elimination phase representing the elimination of the drug after equilibration with the body. The plasma drug concentration at any time is the sum of two first-order processes. The slope of the terminal elimination phase, b, is generally used in the calculation of a dosage regimen.

143. The answer is D. Competitive binding of cimetidine (and ranitidine) to the cytochrome P450 mixed-function oxidase metabolic pathway of the liver acts to interfere with the metabolism of other drugs dependent on this pathway.

Phenytoin, theophylline, phenobarbital, lidocaine, warfarin, imipramine, diazepam, and propranolol may be cleared more slowly and their effects may be accentuated if they are administered concomitantly with cimetidine or ranitidine.

144. The answer is B (III). First-order elimination kinetics is expressed as $C = C_0e^{-kt}$, where $C = 1.2$ mg/mL, $C_0 = 6.2$ mg/mL, and $t = 11$ hours. By substitution, $1.2 = 6.2e^{-k(11)}$; $k = 0.149$ hr^{-1}. The $t_{1/2}$ is estimated by the relationship, $t_{1/2} = 0.693/k$. Therefore, $t_{1/2} = 0.693/0.149 = 4.65$ hours. The dose and serum concentration must be known to determine the volume of distribution for this patient. The volume of distribution cannot be accurately calculated from C_{max}, as this is an IV infusion rather than an IV bolus. In order to calculate the Vd, we would need to know the infusion rate for the drug, R in order to use the equation; $Cp = (R/Vd \times k) \times (1-e^{-kt})$, where R = infusion rate, Cp, drug concentration after infusion for time t; k is obtained from $k = 0.693/t_{1/2}$.

145. The answer is D. The MIC for gentamicin returned back as 4, and based on the available serum levels and the need to exceed the MIC by four to five times; it would appear that gentamicin is not the appropriate agent in this patient. Tobramycin would be an appropriate alternative to the current gentamicin regimen with a returning MIC of 0.5 μg/mL.

146. The answer is B. True cross-reactivity between cephalosporin antibiotics and penicillin is considered rare. Commonly, the rate of cross-reactivity is approximately 10%, and the future use of a cephalosporin is dependent on the degree of reported previous reactions for a patient receiving a penicillin (local rash vs. anaphylaxis).

147. The answer is C. If the patient is receiving 16 mg theophylline per hour by IV infusion, then the patient should receive the oral dose of theophylline at the same approximate dosing rate:

$$\text{Theophylline dose} = 16 \text{ mg} \times 24 \text{ hours} = 384 \text{ mg}$$

Therefore, the patient should be given 400 mg of theophylline controlled-release product every 24 hours, initially with necessary follow-up.

148. The answer is E (I, II, and III). Conversion from IV to oral theophylline dosing should be accomplished using a sustained-release theophylline preparation designed to deliver a daily dose of theophylline comparable to the dose from the IV infusion. Due to potential variabilities among the absorption characteristics of orally administered products, there is a greater variability in drug concentrations for orally administered theophylline products as compared to IV infusions. A steady-state theophylline level is achievable if no doses are missed within the preceding 48-hour period. Reasonable sampling time should be within 3 to 7 hours of dosing.

149. The answer is C (I and II). To demonstrate bioequivalency of two products, both must be the same dosage form (e.g., both must be controlled-release tablets), both must contain the same amount of the same active ingredient, and both must be given in the same dose and via the same route of administration. This study is a relative bioavailability study to demonstrate the controlled-release characteristics of the extended-release tablet. Note: Bioequivalence implies that both drug products have the same rate and extent of systemic drug absorption. The pharmacist must consider whether the difference in pharmacokinetic profiles lead to differences in pharmacodynamic effects.

150. The answer is C. It is recommended that COPD patients receive influenza vaccine annually, usually in the fall. Frequent viral mutations require administration of the most current vaccine each year to ensure protection from the current virus strain(s) causing infections.

151. The answer is C (I and II). Dextromethorphan is a dextro-isomer of levorphanol, and many clinicians consider it equivalent to codeine as an antitussive. It depresses the cough center in the medulla. Diphenhydramine has both antitussive and antihistamine properties. Its antitussive effect results from direct medullary action. Dihydrocodeinone (hydrocodone) is a narcotic antitussive available only in prescription products.

152. The answer is E (I, II, and III). PTU and methimazole may help attain remission in hyperthyroid patients. Both agents inhibit iodide oxidation and iodotyrosyl coupling. PTU (but not methimazole) also diminishes peripheral deiodination of thyroxine (T_4) to triiodothyronine (T_3). These drugs can be used to induce remission by themselves or as adjunctive therapy with radioiodine. They can be used for preoperative preparation of hyperthyroid patients to establish and maintain a euthyroid state until definitive surgery can be performed. Dermatologic reactions (e.g., rash, urticaria, pruritus, hair loss, and skin pigmentation) are the most troublesome. Patients receiving either PTU or methimazole are at increased risk for developing agranulocytosis.

153. The answer is B (III). Atropine is a belladonna alkaloid that possesses anticholinergic properties. Vincristine and vinblastine are vinca alkaloids used in the treatment of various malignancies.

154. The answer is A. Spiriva (tiotropium bromide) is an anticholinergic agent used to treat bronchospasm associated with COPD that may aggravate narrow-angle glaucoma.

155. The answer is E (I, II, and III). Ampules, the oldest form of parenteral vehicle, are composed entirely of glass, which may break during transport. Because the ampule is cut open on use, glass particles may be mixed with the drug substance. Therefore, all drugs supplied in ampules must be filtered before use to remove any glass particles from the solution. Once broken open, the solution must be used to avoid contamination, and it is thus not a multiple-dose product.

156. The answer is B. Half-normal saline solution (0.45% sodium chloride) has an osmotic pressure less than that of blood and is referred to as a hypotonic solution. Isotonic and isosmotic solutions have osmotic pressures that are equal to blood. Normal saline solution, 0.9% sodium chloride, usually is given as an example of an isotonic solution. Hypertonic solutions have osmotic pressures greater than blood (e.g., high concentrations of dextrose used in total parenteral therapy).

157. The answer is A (I). Drug substances that have narrow therapeutic indexes (i.e., for which the difference between a therapeutic effect and a toxic effect is small, such as with heparin) may be given via the continuous infusion route. This method allows less fluctuation in blood levels of such drugs. Intermittent infusions, although used extensively in medicine, provide for greater differences between peak effects and trough effects compared to agents with narrow therapeutic indexes. Agents such as norepinephrine, nitroprusside, and dopamine, which have very short half-lives, are routinely given by continuous infusion to provide a continuous therapeutic effect, which would not be available from intermittent dosing.

158. The answer is B. Aluminum hydroxide (Amphojel) is used in patients with renal failure because it binds excess phosphate in the intestine, thereby reducing the serum phosphate concentration. The aluminum hydroxide can be in liquid or tablet form and is administered three or four times daily with meals.

159. The answer is A. Kayexalate, or sodium polystyrene sulfonate (SPS), is an ion-exchange resin that exchanges sodium ion for potassium in the intestines. SPS, with its potassium content, is excreted in the feces. The result is a decrease in potassium levels in the serum and other body fluids.

160. The answer is A. Chronic renal failure causes a normochromic, normocytic anemia, usually reflected in a decreased hemoglobin and decreased hematocrit. In most patients, the hematocrit is between 20% and 30%.

161. The answer is D (II and III). The major route of elimination for both digoxin and tobramycin (an aminoglycoside) is the kidney. Both medications require dosage adjustment in patients with acute or chronic renal failure. Haloperidol is mainly metabolized by the liver and, therefore, would not need dosage adjustment.

162. The answer is C. Calcitriol is 1,25-dihydroxycholecalciferol, the active form of vitamin D_2. Because of its increased efficacy, calcitriol is the preferred form of vitamin D therapy used in patients with renal failure. Vitamin D enhances calcium absorption from the gut and is used to treat the hypocalcemia that occurs in renal failure.

163. The answer is C (I and II). Aluminum hydroxide gel (Amphojel), which is used to treat the patient's hyperphosphatemia, and sodium polystyrene sulfonate (SPS; Kayexalate), which is used to treat his hyperkalemia, are both major causes of constipation.

164. The answer is A (I). Calcium chloride or gluconate is used to treat potassium-induced arrhythmias. Loop diuretics and sodium polystyrene sulfonate (SPS) do not have a significant effect on potassium in a short period to treat life-threatening arrhythmia. SPS and loop diuretics, along with dialysis, may be considered to remove potassium in the short term, preventing recurrence of arrhythmias.

165. The answer is B. The most common adverse reaction to haloperidol is extrapyramidal effects, which include dystonic reactions, akinesia, drug-induced parkinsonism, and tardive dyskinesia. Cardiovascular and anticholinergic side effects occur less frequently. Neuroleptic malignant syndrome is rare. A decreased seizure threshold is uncommon, except in patients with a history of seizures.

166. The answer is A (I). Antacids, when given at the same time as cimetidine, decrease the absorption of cimetidine from the stomach. No interaction occurs between cimetidine and Colace or ferrous sulfate.

167. The answer is E. Chemotherapeutic agents may cause dysfunction of many organ systems. Patients treated with daunorubicin, doxorubicin, and mitoxantrone are at greater risk for developing cardiotoxicity, ranging from electrocardiogram changes to cardiomyopathy. The risk is dose-related and cumulative. Total dose for daunorubicin should not exceed 550 mg/m^2.

168. The answer is B (III). Alopecia occurs 1 and 2 weeks after treatment with most chemotherapeutic agents. Neither cytarabine nor daunorubicin causes renal dysfunction or peripheral neuropathy.

169. The answer is B. When extravasation takes place, the needle is left in place and excess drug is drawn off with a syringe. A corticosteroid is injected to reduce local inflammation. Ice can also be applied. Sodium bicarbonate can be injected when the extravasation involves doxorubicin and other anthracyclines. Local anesthetics (e.g., potassium chloride) are not recommended and can cause local tissue damage.

170. The answer is C. Ortho-Novum 1/50 contains 50 mg estrogen. When it is continuously administered, the monthly menstrual period will be suppressed. After chemotherapy, thrombocytopenia and neutropenia can occur, and Ms. Peterson will be at risk for increased bleeding owing to thrombocytopenia.

171. The answer is C (I and II). The chemotherapeutic agents used to treat Ms. Peterson cause myelosuppression, with attendant infection and bleeding, usually 10 to 14 days after chemotherapy. White blood cell lines, leukocytes, granulocytes, and platelets are affected because of their shorter life span.

172. The answer is A. Chemotherapeutic agents may be toxic to the pharmacist if handled improperly; therefore, many organizations have developed special guidelines. A vertical (rather than horizontal) laminar flow hood should be used to prevent airborne particles from contaminating room air. Special techniques, equipment, and protective gowns and gloves are recommended.

173. The answer is A. Patients with hypertension should avoid the SNRIs venlafaxine and duloxetine because of the risk of increased blood pressure. Tricyclic antidepressants may interact with antihypertensive agents to either intensify or counteract their effects.

174. The answer is D. Ms. Peterson is allergic to penicillin. Cross-sensitivity between cephalosporins and penicillins is currently approximately 10%. The literature still recommends caution when cephalosporins are administered to patients with acute nonlymphocytic leukemia and an allergy to penicillin.

175. The answer is B (III). Gentamicin, an aminoglycoside, is excreted unchanged in the urine. The drug accumulates in the proximal tubule, causing renal damage in up to 25% of patients. The aminoglycosides do not cause hepatotoxicity or neurotoxicity.

176. The answer is D. The approved dosage of ranitidine for management of GERD is 150 mg four times a day. GERD treatment requires aggressive acid inhibition that will maintain the esophageal pH at 4 or greater around the clock. Higher doses of ranitidine have not been proven to improve outcomes in GERD patients; lower doses may provide some improvement in heartburn symptoms but are less effective in eliminating symptoms or healing erosive esophagitis.

177. The answer is B. Bleeding abnormalities result from vitamin K deficiency because of reduced formation of clotting factors II, VII, IX, and X.

178. The answer is B. BSA correlates with cardiac output, which determines renal and hepatic blood flow and thus affects drug elimination.

179. The answer is B. When weak acids are presented to the kidney for elimination, drugs that increase the ionization of these agents also increase their elimination. However, weak acids (e.g., methenamine) have their elimination delayed when agents such as aspirin decrease their ionization. This relative increase in un-ionized methenamine results in greater reabsorption of methenamine and, therefore, an increase in activity.

180. The answer is B. Boceprevir is contraindicated for use in conjunction with potent CYP3A4/5 inducers; such agents may reduce boceprevir plasma concentrations, resulting in reduced efficacy. These include carbamazepine, phenobarbital, phenytoin, rifampin, and St. John's wort. Boceprevir is also contraindicated in conjunction with CYP3A4/5 substrates for which elevated plasma concentrations are associated with serious and/or life-threatening events. These include alfuzosin, dihydroergotamine, ergonovine, ergotamine, methylergonovine, cisapride, lovastatin, simvastatin drospirenone, pimozide, triazolam, oral midazolam, and sildenafil and tadalafil when used in the treatment of pulmonary arterial hypertension.

181. The answer is D. Transdermal fentanyl is a controlled-release dosage form that is effective for a 72-hour period. All of the other drugs listed are effective for periods of 1 to 8 hours.

182. The answer is B. Burow's solution is an aluminum acetate solution commonly used as an astringent solution and as an astringent mouthwash and gargle. Aluminum acetate is found in products that treat diaper rash, athlete's foot, and poison ivy.

183. The answer is E (I, II, and III). Activase (recombinant tissue plasminogen activator) is a thrombolytic agent. Neupogen (granulocyte colony-stimulating factor [G-CSF]) is a cytokine that regulates the proliferation and differentiation

of white blood cells. Epogen (recombinant erythropoietin) stimulates the production of red blood cells.

184. The answer is A (I). Although anticholinergic agents have no proven value in ulcer healing, they have been used in conjunction with antacids for relief of refractory duodenal ulcer pain. An anticholinergic, propantheline can cause dry mouth, blurred vision, urinary retention, constipation, and pupillary dilation.

185. The answer is E (I, II, and III). The liver is the main organ for the synthesis of plasma proteins. During end-stage liver disease, a decrease in plasma albumin concentrations leads to less drug protein binding and more free Coumadin drug concentrations, causing a more intense pharmacodynamic effect and, therefore, an increase in prothrombin time.

186. The answer is C. To calculate the number of mEq KCl per tablet, divide the tablet strength (600 mg) by the molecular weight (74.5). Each tablet contains 8 mEq KCl. The woman needs to take four tablets to provide a dose of 32 mEq KCl.

187. The answer is B. The final suspension contains 8 g in 120 mL, which is 6.7% sucralfate (8/120 = 0.067 = 6.7%).

188. The answer is D. The amount of sucralfate in 10 mL of this product is 0.667 g (8 g sucralfate/120 mL = 10 mL = 0.667 g sucralfate).

189. The answer is E (I, II, and III). Passive diffusion follows Fick's principle of diffusion, in which the rate of diffusion depends on the concentration gradient, the partition coefficient (e.g., lipid solubility to water solubility ratio), and the surface area of the cell membrane. The extent of ionization relates the ratio of the nonionized or nonpolar species to the ionized or more water-soluble species.

190. The answer is B. Psyllium is one of the bulk-forming laxatives. These agents absorb intestinal water and swell, increasing the bulk and moisture content of the stool to promote peristalsis. They act in both the small and large intestines.

Case 1

The patient was a 22-year-old man who received the MMR (measles, mumps, rubella) vaccine as a requirement for starting college. His past medical history revealed that he was a hemophiliac and was HIV+. The MMR vaccine is a live attenuated vaccine, and his CD4 T-lymphocyte count should have been examined prior to administering the vaccine. Later laboratory tests revealed that his CD4 T-lymphocyte count was 150 cells/μL. Several months after his precollege immunization he developed a severe lung pneumonitis. He had no rash. Multiple laboratory tests to determine the cause of his infection were negative. Finally, a lung biopsy was performed and revealed "giant cells." Physicians were subsequently able to isolate measles virus of the type included in the vaccine from the clinical specimens.

1. This patient had measles pneumonitis as a result of the MMR vaccine. Why did he not develop the rash typical of measles infections?

    (A) The rash of measles is due to the immune response and he was immunodeficient because his CD4 T-lymphocyte count was low.
    (B) The rash of measles only occurs in infants.
    (C) The rash of measles is due to the clotting factors, and he lacked the clotting factors because of his hemophilia.
    (D) Measles virus was present in his body from the vaccine, but had not actually been growing, and therefore didn't result in a rash.
    (E) He had preexisting antibody directed to measles from his previous vaccinations, which prevented the development of the rash.

2. What were the giant cells observed from his lung tissue?

    (A) They were normal alveolar macrophages.
    (B) They were transformed (cancerous) cells due to the measles virus.
    (C) They were individual measles virions.
    (D) They were syncytia which were due to the fusion of neighboring measles-infected cells.
    (E) They were Negri bodies due to the replicating measles virus.

3. He acquired the infection because he was immunocompromised and should not have received the live attenuated vaccine. How are measles infections typically acquired?

    (A) From the MMR vaccine.
    (B) Via respiratory droplets from an infected individual.
    (C) Contact with the rash of an infected individual.
    (D) Through ingestion of virion particles from food handled by an individual with measles in the prodromal stage.
    (E) Through the bite of an infected mosquito.

4. This patient further developed a bacterial pneumonia and received antimicrobials to treat the bacterial infection. What features about the measles infection predisposed him to bacterial pneumonia?

    (A) The vaccine strain is more likely to result in a bacterial pneumonia.
    (B) The measles virus is able to replicate in gram-positive bacteria.
    (C) Measles infections are associated with immunosuppression and a high rate of complications including secondary infections.
    (D) His bacterial pneumonia is unrelated to his viral illness.
    (E) The sulfamethoxazole-trimethoprim he received to treat the measles led to the respiratory infection with highly resistant bacteria.

Answers to Case 1

1. The answer is A *[see 56.IV.E.2].*
Rashes (exanthems) are often due to the immune response directed to viral antigens, and thus to infected cells (e.g., measles, parvovirus B19). Without a functioning immune system the rash will not develop. Immunocompromised patients should not receive most live attenuated vaccines. However, it is important that patients who might otherwise have a weakened immune system develop immunity to infectious agents they might encounter. The current recommendation with regard to HIV+ individuals is that adults with CD4 T-lymphocyte counts < 200 cells/µL should not receive the MMR vaccine.

2. The answer is D *[see 56.IV.D.2].*
Viral infections, such as measles and respiratory syncytial virus, can lead to fusion of neighboring cells, forming giant multinucleated cells (syncytia). Other host cells infected by viruses might have unusual appearances, such as neural cells infected with rabies virus (Negri bodies). Measles virions would be too small in comparison to the eukaryotic cells, so the fused cells will not be measles virions. Macrophages are mononuclear cells.

3. The answer is B *[see Table 56-2].*
Measles is acquired through respiratory droplets from an infected individual.

4. The answer is C *[see 56.IV.E.3].*
Some viruses, such as measles, modulate the immune response, resulting in increased susceptibility to secondary infections. With measles, respiratory involvement is particularly common and respiratory complications can be due to primary viral invasion or secondary infection by bacteria, usually *Streptococcus pneumoniae*. Bacterial secondary infections are so commonplace that prophylactic antibiotic treatment is often practiced in endemic regions; however, that practice is not universally accepted. Measles is not treated with antibiotics that target bacteria. In areas of the world where individuals may be undernourished, vitamin A supplementation reduces the incidence of measles complications.

Case 2

JB was 5 years old when he was referred to the hospital with a severe sinus infection; he had a history of recurrent sinus infections since he was 8 months old. He was successfully treated for the sinus infection with intravenous antibiotics; however, his white cell count, particularly his polymorphonuclear leukocytes (PMNs), remained low. Laboratory analysis of his serum revealed low levels of immunoglobulin (Ig) G and IgA, and markedly high levels of IgM. A lymph node biopsy showed poorly organized structures with an absence of germinal centers.

1. JB was diagnosed with X-linked hyper-IgM syndrome (XHIM). What is the immunological defect that is the basis for his syndrome?

    (A) His B cells lack the Bruton's tyrosine kinase.
    (B) His antigen presenting cells lack class II major histocompatibility complex (MHC).
    (C) His lymph nodes lack germinal centers.
    (D) His T cells lack the CD40 ligand.
    (E) His T cells lacked T-cell receptor (TCR) antigen diversity.

2. JB was treated with intravenous gamma globulin (IVIG) and subsequently remained free of infection. What was the source of the IVIG?

    (A) pooled human sera
    (B) equine sera
    (C) monoclonal antibody
    (D) pooled human sera enriched for specific pathogen antibodies
    (E) sera collected from family members

3. Why did his frequent infections begin at 8 months rather than as soon as he was born?

    (A) He was just lucky.
    (B) He was protected from infections by passively acquired maternal IgG.
    (C) Expression of this particular gene does not occur until 8 months.
    (D) He was protected from infection by passively acquired maternal T cells.
    (E) Complement provided the necessary signals until 8 months.

4. Which of the following will be important to include in his continued medical care?

    (A) He will need regular IVIG injections, and prompt antimicrobial therapy when he has signs of an infection.
    (B) He will need prophylactic antibiotics.
    (C) It will be imperative that he receive all of the active immunizations recommended for his age, and prompt antimicrobial therapy when he has signs of an infection.
    (D) He will need to avoid all contact with other children, and receive prompt antimicrobial therapy when he has signs of an infection.
    (E) He won't need any further intervention for his disorder.

Answers to Case 2

1. The answer is D *[see 57.V.A.3.c].*
B cells from XHIM patients are functionally normal; however, their T cells lack a ligand necessary for the communication between the T cell and the B cell. T-cell communication is required for isotype switching and memory cell differentiation. Without this interaction, T-cell and B-cell interaction in the lymph node does not occur, and the germinal centers do not develop. The CD40 ligand is also important for activation of macrophages. Macrophages and the cytokines that they produce are also important for immune function.

2. The answer is A *[see 57.X.B.1.b].*
IVIG and IGIM are both produced from pooled human sera. Both formulations are mostly IgG.

3. The answer is B *[see 57.IV.F.2.c].*
In the last trimester of a pregnancy, maternal IgG is actively transported via FcRn receptors across the placenta into the developing fetus. At birth the infant will have the IgG antibody profile of the mother, and these passively acquired antibodies provide antibody protection for the infant, until the baby is able to make antibodies for himself.

4. The answer is A *[see 57.V.A.3.c; 57.X.B.1.b].*
Whereas active immunizations are a good idea for some primary immunodeficiencies, such as asplenia, this immunodeficiency (XHIM) will interfere with his ability to respond to the injected antigens. Without T-cell communication, as mediated by CD40:CD40 ligand interaction, he is unable to generate appropriate antibody isotypes and cannot generate a memory response. It might also seem that prophylactic antibiotics would be warranted; however, they should be avoided, because they increase the risk of infections with fungi or drug-resistant organisms. Injected IVIG will only provide formed antibodies, which will degrade over time. He will need regular injections (usually every 3 to 4 weeks). Bone marrow transplantation for XHIM patients can be performed, which would permanently reconstitute the immune system with functional T cells. Bone marrow transplantation is not without risks, so it is important to have an HLA-matched donor (preferably a sibling), and the patient should be in good condition prior to transplantation (young patient, without bronchiectasis or severe chronic infections).

Case 3

JD is a 25-year-old first-year pharmacy student who dreads seeing the end of the mild temperatures of fall. Every winter, he complains that his hands become extremely dry, leading to his skin cracking and itching. In addition, the past two winter seasons have caused JD to notice thin, gray-white flakes covering a large portion of his scalp. His mother gave him a bottle of Neutrogena T/Gel shampoo, but he's unsure if this is the best treatment option for him. The one thing JD won't miss about the upcoming holiday season is the need to walk the half-mile from his apartment to class every day. JD's new shoes have caused a painful area to develop on top of his left foot's small toe. JD is an otherwise healthy individual with no major medical concerns.

1. JD might consider using any of the following over-the-counter (OTC) products for his dry skin *except*

   (A) cytostatic agent.
   (B) colloidal oatmeal.
   (C) keratin-softening agent.
   (D) humectant.
   (E) topical hydrocortisone.

2. The most likely diagnosis of JD's scalp condition is

   (A) dandruff.
   (B) seborrheic dermatitis.
   (C) psoriasis.
   (D) xerosis.
   (E) pediculosis.

3. Is Neutrogena T/Gel shampoo an appropriate first-line treatment option for JD's condition?

   (A) yes
   (B) no

4. Which of the following statements regarding Neutrogena T/Gel shampoo is correct?

   (A) is odorless
   (B) contains selenium sulfide 1%
   (C) may stain hair and clothes
   (D) treatments should be separated by at least 5 days

5. The painful area on JD's left foot is most likely a

   (A) wart.
   (B) hard corn.
   (C) soft corn.
   (D) callus.

6. All of the following counseling points regarding the painful area on JD's foot are correct *except*

   (A) JD may find relief simply by discontinuing use of his new shoes.
   (B) Salicylic acid is the only FDA-approved OTC treatment option for JD's condition.
   (C) After soaking his foot in warm water for at least 5 minutes every day, JD may use a razor blade to remove excess skin from the area.
   (D) The area on JD's foot is most likely not viral in origin.

Answers to Case 3

1. The answer is A *[20.V.D.2].*
All of these agents would be considered appropriate treatment options for patients with dry skin except for cytostatic agents, which do not have a role in dry skin therapy.

2. The answer is A *[20.II.C.1].*
The most likely diagnosis of JD's condition is dandruff, which is primarily characterized by dry white/gray "flakes" scattered across the scalp. Dandruff is more severe in cooler months and less severe during summer months.

3. The answer is A *[20.II.C.2.b.(4).(a)].*
The active ingredient in Neutrogena T/Gel is coal tar, which is an appropriate first-line recommendation for the self-treatment of dandruff.

4. The answer is C *[20.II.C.2.b.(4).(a)].*
Important counseling points regarding the use of coal tar products include the following: may cause photosensitivity and folliculitis, and use on or near the groin, anus, and axillae should be avoided; can stain clothing and bedsheets, as well as skin and hair (particularly blonde, gray, and bleached hair); possesses a strong, unpleasant odor; and should be used at least twice weekly for the first 2 to 3 weeks of treatment.

5. The answer is B *[20.VIII.C.1.a].*
The painful area on JD's left foot is most likely a hard corn. Hard corns appear on areas over bony protrusions, such as the tops of toes or the bottom of the foot, and possess a glossy appearance with a cone-shaped center.

6. The answer is C *[20.VIII.D.1.a].*
Patients with corns and calluses may be instructed to soak the affected foot in warm water for at least 5 minutes every day, which helps to loosen dead skin. Although files and pumice stones may be used with great caution to remove the dead skin, any tool with a sharp blade (such as a razor) should be avoided altogether.

Case 4

A 60-year-old, 75-kg man, with serum creatinine of 2.0 mg/dL, is scheduled to start gentamicin intravenous (IV) therapy for a *Klebsiella* infection. Your colleague recommends a regimen of 2 mg/kg q12h. Assume the same pharmacokinetic parameters listed for tobramycin in Study Question 6.

1. Would you use therapeutic drug monitoring (TDM) as part of the procedure for following this patient?

   (A) yes
   (B) no

2. If your colleague decides to request serum concentration monitoring for the regimen, he tells you he wants his regimen to achieve target concentration goals of $C_{max,ss} = 8$ to 10 µg/mL and $C_{min,ss} = < 1.5$ µg/mL. Do you agree with him?

   (A) yes
   (B) no

3. Your colleague says he requests serum concentration measurements be obtained at 6 hours after the first dose of each day. Do you agree with him?

   (A) yes
   (B) no

4. Do you agree with your colleague's recommendation of 2 mg/kg q12h?

   (A) yes
   (B) no

Answers to Case 4

1. The answer is A *[see Table 26-1].*
TDM is frequently used for monitoring gentamicin regimens.

2. The answer is A *[see Table 26-1].*

3. The answer is B *[see 26.IV.D.3.b; 26.II.D].*
The $t_{1/2,ri}$ for this patient is estimated at ~ 7 hour. Therefore, steady state should be reached in 20 to 30 hours. So, your colleague's recommendation is likely incorrect for two reasons:

(1) It is more appropriate to obtain serum concentration measurements at $C_{max,ss}$ for gentamicin (Table 36-1) and that occurs very soon after a 30- to 60-minute injection. The colleague's recommendation of 6 hours postinjection will correspond more closely to $C_{avg,ss}$. (2) The first measurement that is expected to be after steady state is achieved will likely occur after the first dose on day 2.

4. The answer is B *[see 26.IV.D].*
The serum concentration estimates for your colleague's recommended regimen of 2 mg/kg q12h are $C_{max,ss} = 11.4$ µg/mL and $C_{min,ss} = 3.4$ µg/mL. The approach for calculating the concentrations is found in 26.IV.D and also the answer to Study Question 6.

$Cl_{cr} = (140 - 60 \text{ yr})(75 \text{ kg})/(2 \text{ mg/dL})(72) = 42 \text{ mL/min}$

$(2.5 \text{ hr})/(t_{1/2})_{ri} = 1 - 0.98 + 0.98(42/120) = \sim 7 \text{ hr}$

$\text{steady state}_{(90\%)} = 3 - 4 (t_{1/2}) = 3 - 4 (7 \text{ hr}) = \sim 20\text{--}30 \text{ hr}$

$\text{fraction lost}/\tau_{ri} = 1 - 10^{-0.3(12/7)} = \sim 0.7$

$D_L = (C_{max,ss})(V)(S)(f) = (8 \text{ µg/mL})(0.25 \text{ L/kg})(1)(1) = 2.3 \text{ mg/kg}$

$D_M/\tau_{ri} = (D_L)(\text{fraction lost}/\tau_{ri}) = (2.3 \text{ mg/kg})(0.7) = 1.6 \text{ mg/kg}$

Using your colleague's desired target concentration recommendations and the resulting predicted concentrations resulting from his regimen of 2 mg/kg q12h, $C_{max,ss} = 11.4$ µg/mL and $C_{min,ss} = 3.4$ µg/mL. These values are predicted to be too high for the maximum and much too high for the minimum. Using his recommended dose of 2 mg/kg but extending the interval to q24h yields more desirable concentration estimates of $C_{max,ss} = 8.8$ µg/mL and $C_{min,ss} = 0.8$ µg/mL.

Case 5

You are a pharmacist in a retail pharmacy when the father of EF, a 2-month-old infant, approaches the counter to ask for your advice. He tells you that she has had a fever to 101.3°F and his wife has called to tell him that their pediatrician has recommended that EF be given a dose of acetaminophen. Other than the fever and a clear nasal discharge that started earlier in the day, EF has been well. She was born at term and went home from the hospital on the second day of life. She is formula-fed and has been feeding without difficulty. EF's parents have never given her medication and her father needs guidance on selecting an acetaminophen product and administering it appropriately.

1. As you review the package label for acetaminophen oral suspension with EF's father, you call his attention to the dosing recommendations. Which of the following would *not* be included in pediatric acetaminophen labeling?

    (A) dosing according to patient's body surface area (BSA)
    (B) dosing according to patient's weight
    (C) the recommended length of treatment without a physician's approval
    (D) the recommended maximum number of doses per day
    (E) information on adverse effects

2. Peak serum concentrations of acetaminophen may be delayed in infants, particularly those born prematurely, due to which of the following factors affecting drug absorption?

    (A) elevated gastric pH
    (B) prolonged gastric emptying time
    (C) reduced pancreatic enzyme production
    (D) absence of gut microflora
    (E) reduced activity of intestinal metabolic enzymes

3. Acetaminophen metabolism changes with age. Which metabolic enzyme serves as the primary route of metabolism for a patient EF's age?

    (A) alcohol dehydrogenase
    (B) CYP1A2
    (C) CYP3A4
    (D) sulfotransferase
    (E) uridine 5′-diphosphate glucosyltransferase

4. When giving EF's father instructions for the preparation of a dose of acetaminophen, you recommend that the dose be administered by which of the following devices?

    (A) an oral dosing syringe
    (B) a dosing spoon
    (C) a dosing cup
    (D) a teaspoon
    (E) a tablespoon

5. If EF were unable to tolerate oral acetaminophen, which of the following would be the *most* appropriate alternative?

    (A) oral administration of aspirin
    (B) rectal administration of aspirin
    (C) topical administration of aspirin
    (D) rectal administration of acetaminophen
    (E) oral administration of ibuprofen

Answers for Case 5

1. The answer is A *[see 27.I.D].*
OTC products for infants and children should contain appropriate weight-based dosing recommendations. Acetaminophen dosing does not require calculation of BSA in order to provide a safe and effective dose. The labeling information should also include recommendations for the length of therapy, the maximum daily dose, and adverse effect information, including guidelines for when medical care should be sought immediately.

2. The answer is B *[see 27.I.B.2].*
The delay in acetaminophen absorption in early infancy is related to the delayed gastric emptying time seen in neonates, especially in those born prematurely. Acetaminophen absorption is not significantly affected by the higher gastric pH, reduced bile salt and pancreatic enzyme production, the absence of gut flora, or reduced intestinal metabolism.

3. The answer is D *[see 27.I.B.4].*
During infancy, acetaminophen is primarily metabolized through sulfation. Sulfotransferases develop in utero and remain the predominant means of conjugation during the first year of life. Glucuronidation via UGT1A6 and UGT1A9 becomes the primary means of acetaminophen metabolism during childhood.

4. The answer is A *[see 27.I.D.4].*
Oral syringes are the preferred means of measuring and administering medications to infants. The volume of most doses given during the first year of life are too small to be accurately measured with a dosing spoon or cup. In addition, the syringe allows placement of the medication between the cheek and gums, increasing the likelihood that the patient will swallow the dose. Household measuring devices, including those used for cooking, are often imprecise and can lead to over- or underdosing.

5. The answer is D *[see 27.I.B.2; 27.I.F].*
Rectal acetaminophen is a useful alternative when oral therapy is not tolerated. Neither aspirin nor the nonsteroidal anti-inflammatory agents are appropriate for a 2-month-old. Aspirin has been associated with the development of Reye syndrome in children and ibuprofen administration may predispose EF to renal impairment.

Case 6

Patient PO, an 88-year-old man with benign prostatic hyperplasia (BPH), was given finasteride (Proscar) 8 months ago and has demonstrated a positive response for that. However, recent complaints of wheezing from a bronchospastic attack resulted in the initiation of ipratropium inhalation for nebulizer treatment. Additionally, the patient was placed on a daily regimen of theophylline (Uniphyl) 400 mg. It was discovered during the initial H and P that the patient's grandson, a second-year medical student, brought over the OTC antihistamine chlorpheniramine (Chlor-Trimeton) to help his grandfather. Shortly after starting this regimen the patient could not urinate, had a distended bladder as shown by bladder catheterization (800 mL), blurred vision, and appeared a bit "out of touch."

Directions for questions 1–3: The questions and incomplete statements in this section can be correctly answered or completed by **one or more** of the suggested answers. Choose the answer, **A–E.**

(A) I only
(B) III only
(C) I and II
(D) II and III
(E) I, II, and III

1. What is the most likely cause of the patient's new onset symptoms?

   I. finasteride
   II. theophylline
   III. chlorpheniramine

2. What agent(s), due to its/their mechanism of action can interact with chlorpheniramine by causing an additive effect, which could be a significant problem in patient P.O.?

   I. finasteride
   II. theophylline
   III. ipratropium

3. Which of the following represent major reasons why the geriatric patient population is at risk for adverse drug reactions?

   I. age-related alterations in drug distribution
   II. reductions in renal blood flow and glomerular filtration rate (GFR)
   III. significant changes in phase II pathways within the liver

4. Which of the following statements regarding age-related changes is not correct?

   (A) Reductions in gastrointestinal (GI) motility and splanchnic blood flow in the elderly pose significant concerns for most orally administered drugs and must be considered for most agents administered.
   (B) Serum albumin levels may be reduced in elderly patients with chronic illness, which poses a potential problem for drugs such as phenytoin, which are highly protein bound.
   (C) Phase I reactions within the liver are reduced in the elderly, which poses a potential problem for long-acting agents like diazepam, which are dependent on phase I reactions for their metabolism.
   (D) Reductions in hepatic blood flow with advancing age poses a potential problem for drugs such as lidocaine (Xylocaine) and propranolol (Inderal), which have high extraction rates from the liver as part of their metabolism.
   (E) Reductions in renal blood flow and subsequent GFR in the elderly poses a potential problem for drugs such as digoxin, which are primarily eliminated by the kidney.

5. Which of the following groups of drugs would not pose a problem when administered to patient PO?

   (A) amitriptyline (Elavil), imipramine (Tofranil)
   (B) oxazepam (Serax), lorazepam (Ativan)
   (C) diazepam (Valium), flurazepam (Dalmane)
   (D) methyldopa (Aldomet), propranolol (Inderal)
   (E) hydroxyzine (Atarax), cyproheptadine (Periactin)

Answers to Case 6

1. The answer is D (II and III) *[see 28.I.C.2; Table 28.3].*
Patient PO is demonstrating several of the routine effects of anticholinergic drugs when administered to patients. Unfortunately for patient PO, the anticholinergic effects of chlorpheniramine may very well have contributed to the routine effects seen with the administration of agents possessing anticholinergic properties.

2. The answer is B (III) *[see 28.I.C.2; Table 28.3].*
Ipratropium, although used in the treatment of bronchospasm as an inhalational agent; its activity is due to its anticholinergic properties which can result in an additive effect in patient PO who is also receiving the antihistamine, chlorpheniramine, which possesses strong anticholinergic effects.

3. The answer is C (I and II) *[see 28.I.B.2–4].*
Reductions in lean body mass, total body water, and serum albumin concentrations results in changes in the manner in which drug disposition occurs in the elderly population. Additionally, documented reductions in renal blood flow with advancing age results in a decrease in GFR as such a reduction will necessitate changes in renally eliminated drugs. Phase II reaction pathways are not impacted with advancing age and, therefore, agents such as oxazepam and lorazepam do not have altered dosing requirements in the elderly population.

4. The answer is A *[see 28.I.B.1–4].*
Although it has been documented that advancing age does decrease GI mobility and splanchnic blood flow; the clinical impact which these changes occur do not result in significant adjustments necessary for patients receiving orally administered drugs.

5. The answer is C *[see 28.I.D.1–5; Table 28-2].*
Oxazepam and lorazepam are dependent on phase II reactions for their inactivation by the liver. However, such reactions are not altered with advancing and therefore do not create potential issues in elderly patients. Each of the other groups of drugs represent classes of drugs which either have demonstrable exaggerated effects in the elderly (propranolol and methyldopa), are associated with a high degree of anticholinergic effects (amitriptyline, imipramine, hydroxyzine, and cyproheptadine), or are dependent on a pharmacokinetic process, which is altered in the elderly population phase I reactions (diazepam, flurazepam).

Case 7

PH is a 63-year-old woman who complains of hot flashes throughout the day and night and feeling like she has to urinate all of the time. Sometimes she loses urine with little warning, other times she only loses urine when she laughs. She is most bothered by the sudden urge to go followed by the loss of urine. She's also heard about the latest osteoporosis medicines through the media. She has a family history of severe osteoporosis and would like to start therapy. She wants advice about her complaints and possibly medications to treat her primary symptoms.

1. What is the most effective therapy for her menopausal symptoms?

   (A) soy isoflavones
   (B) venlafaxine
   (C) estrogen
   (D) clonidine
   (E) black cohosh

2. Which of the following agents would *not* be helpful?

   (A) gabapentin
   (B) bupropion
   (C) methyldopa
   (D) paroxetine
   (E) phenytoin

3. What type of incontinence best describes her symptoms?

   (A) urge incontinence
   (B) overflow incontinence
   (C) stress incontinence
   (D) mixed incontinence
   (E) dual incontinence

4. She is most bothered by a sudden urge to urinate then losing urine. All of the following agents are useful to treat this type of incontinence *except*

   (A) tolterodine.
   (B) trospium.
   (C) solifenacin.
   (D) duloxetine.

5. Which of the following would be the best for her initial osteoporosis test?

   (A) a T score
   (B) a femur x-ray
   (C) a FRAX score
   (D) a heel ultrasound

6. She is especially concerned about hip fractures and wants to make sure her therapy will help prevent these. All of the following have been shown to decrease hip fractures *except*

   (A) teriparatide.
   (B) calcitonin.
   (C) denosumab.
   (D) alendronate.
   (E) estrogen therapy.

Answers to Case 7

1. The answer is C [see 29.VI.C.2].
Menopause symptoms can be relieved most effectively by replacing the deficient hormone, estrogen. Symptoms typically resolve within the first month of therapy. Phytoestrogens, such as soy isoflavones, have not been shown to be more effective than placebo in studies. Venlafaxine is effective and clonidine is also helpful in relieving hot flashes, but not other symptoms of menopause such as vaginal dryness. Black cohosh can be helpful, but therapy should be limited to less than 6 months.

2. The answer is B [see 29.VI.C.3].
Many agents have been studied for the treatment of vasomotor symptoms. The selective serotonin reuptake inhibitors (SSRIs) paroxetine and fluoxetine and the serotonin–norepinephrine reuptake inhibitor (SNRI) venlafaxine are all more effective than placebo as is gabapentin and methyldopa. The antidepressant bupropion has not been studied for this purpose.

3. The answer is D *[see 29.V.E–G].*
Her symptoms are best described as both stress incontinence and urge incontinence. Stress incontinence involves the loss of urine with increased intra-abdominal pressure. Urge incontinence can be described as a sudden sense of needing to void followed by the involuntary loss of urine. Treatment should focus on whichever component is more bothersome to the woman. Overflow incontinence is uncommon in women. This type of incontinence typically results in a continuous loss of small amounts of urine.

4. The answer is D *[see 29.V.F.1.b.(1)].*
Tolterodine, trospium, and solifenacin are all anticholinergic agents that will decrease bladder contractility, thus improving urge incontinence. Duloxetine exerts its effect on the urethra which will be more helpful in stress incontinence.

5. The answer is A *[see 29.VII.C].*
A T score is determined by a dual-energy x-ray absorptiometry (DXA) scan. The bone mineral density measurement from this scan is compared to that of a woman in her 30s. A T score less than -2.5 is indicative of osteoporosis. A traditional x-ray can detect low bone mass only after 20% to 30% loss. A FRAX score only predicts a woman's likelihood of having a fracture in the next 10 years. It does not diagnose osteoporosis. A heel ultrasound is a great screening tool and can have a T score assigned to the result, but this is not the gold standard nor is the measurement one of the two commonly used for the diagnosis of osteoporosis (hip and spine).

6. The answer is B *[see 29.VII.D; Table 29-4].*
Hip fractures have been shown to be reduced with estrogen, bisphosphonate, teriparatide, and denosumab therapies. Calcitonin has been shown to reduce vertebral fractures but not fractures elsewhere.

Case 8

Ralph is a 53-year-old man who presents to the hospital with shortness of breath and altered mental status. His past medical history is significant for end-stage renal disease secondary to lupus nephritis and hypertension. Of note, the patient has refused dialysis over the past year. He is currently nonadherent to his outpatient medication regimen. Current laboratory values are sodium 140 mEq/L, potassium 6.9 mEq/L, chloride 102 mEq/L, bicarbonate 22 mEq/L, blood urea nitrogen (BUN) 99 mg/dL, serum creatinine (SCr) 7.8 mg/dL, and glucose 106 mg/dL. In addition, an electrocardiogram (ECG) is obtained and shows peaked T waves and a prolonged PR interval.

1. What laboratory abnormality is Ralph presenting with that requires urgent attention?

   (A) elevated BUN
   (B) hyperkalemia
   (C) hyponatremia
   (D) hyperglycemia
   (E) elevated creatinine

2. What is the best treatment(s) to manage Ralph's condition?

   (A) sodium polystyrene sulfonate (SPS) 30 g by mouth (po) $\times$ 1
   (B) insulin 10 units intravenous (IV) + $D_{50}W \times 1$ plus SPS 30 g po $\times$ 1
   (C) calcium gluconate 1 g IV $\times$ 1 plus insulin 10 units IV $\times$ 1 + $D_{50}W$ plus SPS 30 g po $\times$ 1
   (D) albuterol 20 mg nebs plus furosemide 40 mg po $\times$ 1

3. Joe is a 75-year-old man who presents to the hospital with a productive cough and fever the past 2 days. His past medical history is significant for end-stage renal disease (receives hemodialysis MWF), hypertension, hyperlipidemia, and type 2 diabetes mellitus. His outpatient medications include amlodipine, furosemide, atorvastatin, and Lantus insulin. The following labs were obtained: sodium 136 mEq/L, potassium 4.8 mEq/L, chloride 98 mEq/L, bicarbonate 25 mEq/L, BUN 45 mg/dL, SCr 3.9 mg/dL, glucose 188 mg/dL, magnesium 2 mg/dL, phosphorus 6.3 g/dL, calcium 9.3 mg/dL, and albumin 3.2 g/dL. What laboratory abnormality is Joe presenting with that can be appropriately treated with drug therapy?

   (A) elevated creatinine
   (B) hyperphosphatemia
   (C) hypokalemia
   (D) hypocalcemia

4. Dan has been in the hospital for 2 days. His morning laboratory values on day 3 return and all are significantly different from his values the previous 2 days. Dan is clinically stable. All of the following are potential reasons for his abnormal lab values *except*

   (A) laboratory error.
   (B) the results reported are for a different patient.
   (C) Dan had a late dinner the evening prior.
   (D) the wrong collection tube(s) might have been used.

5. A patient with iron deficiency anemia would most likely have which of the following set of laboratory values?

   (A) low hemoglobin, hematocrit, and mean corpuscular volume (MCV)
   (B) high hemoglobin, hematocrit, and MCV
   (C) high hemoglobin, low hematocrit, and high MCV
   (D) high red blood cell (RBC) count, hematocrit, and low red cell distribution width (RDW)

Answers to Case 8

1. The answer is B *[see 30.IV.B.1–4].*
Although his BUN and SCr are significantly elevated above normal, they are consistent for a patient with end-stage renal disease who is not receiving hemodialysis. His sodium, chloride, and glucose values are normal. Potassium is significantly elevated putting him at risk for arrhythmias. His ECG changes are consistent with hyperkalemia requiring urgent intervention to "protect"/stabilize his heart to the effects of potassium and to lower serum potassium values.

2. The answer is C *[see 30.VII.B.2–6].*
The patient has severe hyperkalemia with ECG changes; therefore, he needs Ca gluconate to stabilize the heart and aggressive intervention to lower the serum potassium levels with a combination of a binding agent to remove potassium from the body (SPS) and an intervention to drive potassium into the cells quickly (insulin and glucose).

3. The answer is B *[see 30.VIII.B.1–2].*
His phosphate level is elevated mainly as a result of his renal failure. This is the only laboratory abnormality he has that can be managed with drug therapy. A non–calcium-based phosphate binding agent could be initiated such as sevelamer.

4. The answer is C *[see 30.I.A–D].*
Given the huge discrepancy in Dan's lab values from the previous 2 days without a change in his clinical status, the most likely reasons related to some type of error either laboratory, reporting, or collecting of samples. The effect of his late dinner would be very unlikely to impact all of his morning labs.

5. The answer is A *[see 30.II.A.1–5].*
Classic iron deficiency anemia is characterized by a low hemoglobin, hematocrit, MCV, and RBC. Other specific tests including ferritin, serum iron, and total iron-binding capacity (TIBC) are abnormal as well.

Case 9

A 55-year-old man arrives in the emergency room of the local hospital approximately 6 hours after developing chest pain with the signs and symptoms of an acute ST-segment elevated myocardial infarction (STEMI). This is the second such attack for this 50-kg white man within the last 4 months, and the patient has not altered his lifestyle to eliminate important risk factors. Previous therapy included a thrombolytic agent (name unknown), a blood thinner, daily aspirin, omeprazole to prevent GI bleeding, and metoprolol (Lopressor).

Directions for questions 1–3: The questions and incomplete statements in this section can be correctly answered or completed by **one or more** of the suggested answers. Choose the answer, **A–E.**

- **(A)** I only
- **(B)** III only
- **(C)** I and II
- **(D)** II and III
- **(E)** I, II, and III

1. Which of the following agents is recommended during the acute myocardial infarction to help prevent sudden death?

   I. atenolol (Tenormin)
   II. metoprolol (Lopressor)
   III. aspirin (Various)

2. The physician documents the administration of a fibrinolytic agent to the patient as a 30 mg IV × 1. Which of the following best represents the agent that the patient received?

   (A) tenecteplase (TNKase)
   (B) enoxaparin (Lovenox)
   (C) reteplase (Retavase)
   (D) fondaparinux (Arixtra)
   (E) alteplase (Activase)

3. Which agent has been shown to potentially predispose select cardiac patients to thrombosis despite being placed on clopidogrel?

   I. omeprazole (Various)
   II. eptifibatide (Integrilin)
   III. bivalirudin (Angiomax)

4. Which of the following would *not* represent initial therapy for our patient with a diagnosis of STEMI?

   (A) atenolol (Tenormin)
   (B) morphine
   (C) clopidogrel (Plavix)
   (D) eptifibatide (Integrilin)
   (E) reteplase (Retavase)

5. Which of the following would *not* represent recommended therapy for our patient, had he been documented with an NSTEMI?

   (A) atenolol (Tenormin)
   (B) ASA
   (C) clopidogrel (Plavix)
   (D) SL nitroglycerin (Various)
   (E) reteplase (Retavase)

Answers to Case 9

1. The answer is E (I, II, and III) *[see 31.III.H.4.a.(3)]*.
The most recently introduced guidelines for the treatment of STEMI patients include the use of β-adrenergic blocker therapy, such as atenolol or metoprolol initiated within the first 24 hours, assuming that there are no contraindications for their use (heart failure, heart block, asthma, etc.). Additionally, aspirin continues to be a very important part of the initial therapy for STEMI patients. The most recent guidelines provide a Class I recommendation for the administration of aspirin as early as possible, pending no contraindications in a dose of 162 to 325 mg.

2. The answer is A *[see 31.III.H..4.a.(2).(a-c.)]*.
Tenecteplase is a fibrinolytic indicated in the treatment of STEMI patients, and its major benefit is the ease of administration. For our patient, weight less than 60 kg, a single IV dose of 30 mg is used for treatment. Of the remaining choices, only alteplase and reteplase are considered fibrinolytic agents, with alteplase being given IV over 90 minutes as a bolus followed by a 60-minute infusion; and reteplase given as two 10-unit IV doses 30 minutes apart from each other.

3. The answer is A (I only) *[see 31.II.H.5.c.(1)]*.
During recent years, concern has resulted in conflicting concerns regarding the potential interaction between select proton pump inhibitors (PPIs) such as omeprazole and the antiplatelet agent clopidogrel. Reports have shown the potential for a drug interaction, which could reduce the efficacy of clopidogrel in cardiac patients and predispose them to thrombosis. The most recent national guidelines addressing the issue presented the following recommendations that no evidence has established clinically meaningful differences in outcomes; however, clinically significant interaction cannot be excluded in subgroups who are poor metabolizers of clopidogrel.

4. The answer is D *[see 31.III.G.2.d]*.
The most recent national guidelines for the treatment of STEMI include the use of fibrinolytics within 30 minutes of hospital presentation, or primary percutaneous coronary intervention (PCI) within 90 minutes of first medical as part of the management of patients with STEMI. Additionally, adjunctive therapies suggested for patients treated for STEMI include the analgesic morphine, the antiplatelet clopidogrel, and a β-adrenergic blocker such as atenolol an initial therapy in patients with STEMI. Eptifibatide, as a glycoprotein IIB/IIIA receptor blocker, is indicated for patients undergoing PCI. However, it is not considered as an initial therapy in STEMI patients.

5. The answer is E *[see 31.III.G.2.d]*.
The treatment of acute coronary syndrome provides specific guidelines for unstable angina (UA), STEMI, and non-ST elevated myocardial infarction (NSTEMI). A major difference between the treatment of STEMI and NSTEMI is the indication for fibrinolytics such as reteplase in the acute treatment of STEMI but, to date, not yet shown benefit in patients with NSTEMI.

Case 10

Patient AM is an 83-year-old white man with a 6-week history of worsening dyspnea. Annual cardiac exams have been normal since a previous diagnosis of atrial fibrillation for which he was started on sotalol AF (Betapace AF) 80 mg po every 12 hours without problems. He has since been without cardiac issues till his most recent cardiac evaluation, which appeared to demonstrate signs and symptoms of heart failure with an ejection fractions of 30%. Ramipril 5 mg every A.M. had been added to his list of prescriptions as a result of his most recent cardiac evaluation.

1. Which of the following recommendations would you agree with as patient AM now presents to the clinic where you are practicing?

   I. Increase sotalol dose to 120 mg.
  II. Decrease the sotalol dose and increase the ramipril dose.
 III. Discontinue the sotalol and utilize an alternative for atrial fibrillation.

  (A) I only
  (B) III only
  (C) I and II
  (D) II and III
  (E) I, II, and III

2. Which of the following drugs might be a satisfactory alternative for patient AM in the treatment of atrial fibrillation with preexisting heart failure?

  (A) propafenone (Rythmol)
  (B) disopyramide (Norpace)
  (C) dronedarone (Multaq)
  (D) dofetilide (Tikosyn)
  (E) verapamil (Calan)

3. The decision is made to discontinue the sotalol prescription and initiate amiodarone (Cordarone). How would you recommend starting amiodarone therapy?

   I. 10 mg/kg/day for 10 to 14 days po; followed by 300 mg/day for 4 weeks and then 200 mg daily po thereafter
  II. 400 mg po three times daily × 5 to 7 days; then 400 mg daily × 1 month; then 200 mg daily thereafter
 III. IV or IO push of 300 mg followed by 150 mg; then 1 mg/min for 6 hours followed by 0.5 mg/min for up to 18 hours to thoroughly load patient adequately

  (A) I only
  (B) III only
  (C) I and II
  (D) II and III
  (E) I, II, and III

4. Which of the following choices accurately represents the drugs included within the respective Vaughan Williams classification classes?

   I. amiodarone (Cordarone), ibutilide (Corvert), sotalol (Betapace)
  II. mexiletine (Various), lidocaine (Xylocaine) flecainide (Tambocor)
 III. propranolol (Inderal), verapamil (Calan), diltiazem (Cardizem)

  (A) I only
  (B) III only
  (C) I and II
  (D) II and III
  (E) I, II, and III

5. This has been defined as a polymorphic ventricular tachycardia with a twisting QRS complex morphology, which sometimes occurs with drugs that prolong ventricular repolarization and has since seen an expansion of drugs—both antiarrhythmics and nonantiarrhythmics, which are capable of causing it.

  (A) torsades de Gateau
  (B) torsades de pointes
  (C) pointe de l'Eglise
  (D) pointe des Galets
  (E) torsades de necklace

Answers to Case 10

1. The answer is B (III) *[see 32.II.C.4.b; 32.II.C.5.b].*
Although sotalol is included in the Class III antiarrhythmics, due to its effect to prolong the action potential, it still possesses the attributes of other β-adrenergic receptor blockers. In patient AM this is revealing itself through its negative inotropic effects, which is responsible for his dyspnea and need for ramipril. A decision to discontinue the sotalol and employ another agent for atrial fibrillation might result in the ability to remove the ramipril as well, depending on cardiac status. The first step would be to stop the sotalol and evaluate cardiac response while initiating another agent for atrial fibrillation.

2. The answer is D *[see 32.II.A.4.g; 32.II.C.1.d; 32.II.E.5.b].*
Each of the agents has received a recommendation in the treatment of atrial fibrillation. However, only dofetilide (Tikosyn) would be a suitable alternative to sotalol in this patient who also suffers from heart failure, and does not possess the concerns demonstrated with the other agents for patients with heart failure. The recent focused guidelines algorithm includes dofetilide for those patients with atrial fibrillation accompanied by heart failure. The negative inotropic effects associated with each of the other agents listed make them not useful in such patients.

3. The answer is C (I and II) *[see 32.II.C.3.a].*
Amiodarone has been indicated for treatment of various arrhythmias, including the ventricular arrhythmias as well as atrial and supraventricular arrhythmias. With various indications, various regimens for maximizing the administration of amiodarone to patients have appeared. However, many different regimens have been recommended, based on such indications. For atrial fibrillation, which is an unlabeled indication for amiodarone, several recommendations have been made that provide the drug in a less than "emergency" manner through the slow administration titration of the drug over a period of weeks to months—as compared to the treatment of serious ventricular tachycardias, where the goal is to administer larger amounts of drug over a shorter time period in order to correct an emergency critical situation.

4. The answer is A (I) *[see Table 32-1].*
The Vaughan Williams classification has been used to provide a structure for placing antiarrhythmics into categories based on the effect which each drug has on the cardiac action potential. Currently, four classes of drugs are used (Class I, II, III, IV); with Class I agents broken down into three respective groups (Group Ia, Ib, Ic), based on specific actions on the fast-channel sodium conduction. Choice I accurately represents the Class III agents; choice II represents Class Ib (mexiletine and lidocaine) and Class Ic (flecainide) agents, and choice III represents Class II β-adrenergic receptor blockers (propranolol) and Class IV calcium-channel blockers (diltiazem) agents.

5. The answer is B *[see 32.I.C.3.a–d].*
Torsades de pointes, from the French for "twisting of the points," continues to receive increased attention as a major proarrhythmic event, which has been reported with antiarrhythmic drug therapy as well as nonantiarrhythmic therapy. The attention has resulted in an ongoing list of a registry site where health care providers can add additional drugs, which have demonstrated such effects, as a way to try and minimize the use of such agents, in combination. Currently, the registry contains four categories of drugs based on the risk for their association with causing torsades.

Case 11

Patient HY Tension is a 62-year-old healthy white man who, upon his recent visit to his licensed medical practitioner, was diagnosed with "prehypertension" with a blood pressure of 130/85 mm Hg, and started on an initial regimen to treat this entity. All other aspects of the patient's health and well-being are normal, but he is extremely concerned over the need to begin treatment for "prehypertension."

1. Which of the following choices best represents the recommended initial regimen, which HY Tension should receive?

   (A) Thiazide diuretic, such as chlorothiazide, as this patient has no other compelling issues to address.
   (B) Angiotensin-converting enzyme (ACE) inhibitor, such as captopril (Capoten), in order to prevent the long-term effects of hypertension on the kidneys and heart.
   (C) Treatment should center around "lifestyle modifications" which will reduce his future need for hypertensive therapy.
   (D) Treatment should center around a combination of drugs, which could include a thiazide diuretic plus an ACE inhibitor to prevent the development of hypertension.
   (E) The patient does not require any treatment regimen as he does not have hypertension.

2. When the JNC-7 guidelines refer to "compelling issues," which of the following does *not* accurately reflect one of them?

   (A) diabetes mellitus
   (B) obesity
   (C) post-MI
   (D) recurrent stroke prevention
   (E) high-risk cardiovascular history

3. After a lengthy follow-up phone call with Mr. HY Tension, it is discovered that his father had an MI at age 54 and his mother has been treated for angina pectoris since the age of 60; a decision is made to initiate drug therapy. Which of the following would *not* be appropriate additions to Mr. HY Tension treatment regimen?

   (A) chlorothiazide
   (B) ramipril (Altace)
   (C) carvedilol (Coreg)
   (D) felodipine (Plendil)
   (E) prazosin (Minipress)

4. Aliskiren (Tekturna) is a relatively new addition to the antihypertension drug arsenal, and represents a new class of drugs with a distinct mechanism of action to aid in the reduction of blood pressure. What best describes the mechanism of action?

   (A) direct acting inhibitor of angiotensin II resulting in reduced vasoconstriction
   (B) direct acting angiotensin I inhibitor resulting in reduced levels of angiotensin II
   (C) direct acting renin inhibitor resulting in reduced production of angiotensin II
   (D) direct acting aldosterone antagonist resulting in reduced sodium levels and increased potassium
   (E) direct acting inhibitor of catechol-O-methyltransferase resulting in decreased norepinephrine levels

For the following question, please answer in the following manner:

   (A) I only
   (B) III only
   (C) I and II
   (D) II and III
   (E) I, II, and III

5. The patient arrives in the pharmacy to fill the prescription, which was telephoned in by his physician. After being greeted by the pharmacist, the patient asks for information on this new "super pill," which he has heard about at work, wondering if it might be for him. As the pharmacist, what super pill might you discuss with the patient as it relates to the treatment of hypertension?

   I. Exforge HCT
   II. Tribenzor
   III. Amturnide

Answers to Case 11

1. The answer is C *[see Table 33-1].*
"Prehypertension" was a newly introduced category into the most recent JNC-7 treatment guidelines, and represents an intent to deal with predisposing lifestyle factors, which play a part in the future development of hypertension in such patients. The guideline assumes that by treating those factors which can be altered in patients who are predisposed to hypertension that hypertension can be avoided. Currently, the recommendation does not include drug therapy; unless the patient has a compelling reason for doing so.

2. The answer is B *[see Table 33-1; Table 33-2].*
The JNC-7 report provides a listing of six clinical entities, which are recognized as significant enough in the lives of hypertensive patients, that their therapy needs to be highly prioritized in patients presenting with one of them. Clinical entities such as heart failure, post-myocardial infarction (MI), high coronary artery risk history, chronic kidney failure, diabetes mellitus, and recurrent stroke prevention have been included in the list of designated compelling issues. Each issue has a group or groups of selected drugs for treatment, which are then added to the specific regimen for such patients. Obesity is a modifiable risk factor for hypertension, but by itself is not considered a compelling issue needing select treatment in a hypertensive patient.

3. The answer is E *[see Table 33-1].*
The added information regarding the patient's strong family history of cardiovascular events would suggest a compelling reason to initiate therapy for "prehypertension." In this case with the use of diuretics, ACE inhibitors, β-adrenergic blockers, and calcium-channel blockers (CCBs) such as chlorothiazide, ramipril, carvedilol, and felodipine would be consistent with the guidelines based on a "high-risk cardiovascular lifestyle"; however, prazosin, a peripheral α_1 adrenergic blocker, is not considered an initial therapy for hypertension and would not be used in this patient at this time.

4. The answer is C *[see 33.III.B.8.b].*
Recognizing the successes which have been described with the use of ACE inhibitors and angiotensin II receptor blockers (ARBs) in the treatment of hypertension, the ability to directly inhibit the enzyme responsible for producing the end product angiotensin II would appear to be a good step in the effective treatment of hypertension. Because angiotensin II acts as a potent vasoconstrictor as well as stimulator for the subsequent release of aldosterone from the adrenal cortex, it would appear that the inhibition of the enzyme responsible for that would add value in the treatment of hypertension. Currently, there is one single entity product on the market with aliskiren; however, to date, additional combination products have already been marketed with other therapeutic categories used in the treatment of hypertension.

5. The answer is E (I, II, and III) *[see Table 33-5].*
Substantial attention has focused on the development of combination products during the last few years. Referred to as super pills, the products contain different types of drugs, which are indicated for differing types of diseases as well as combinations of drugs used to treat a single disease state, such as hypertension. Each of the responses represents a combination of three separate drugs with different antihypertensive treatment classes in one tablet, with the goal being to improve patient compliance. The three drugs included in each product contain the following:

(A) Amlodipine/valsartan/hydrochlorothiazide (Exforge HCT): CCB, ARB, thiazide diuretic
(B) Amlodipine/olmesartan/hydrochlorothiazide (Tribenzor): CCB, ARB, thiazide diuretic
(C) Aliskiren/amlodipine/hydrochlorothiazide (Amturnide): renin inhibitor, CCB, thiazide diuretic

Case 12

Patient EL is a 71-year-old white woman with no known allergies, who visits her physician with a 30-year history of hypertension for which she has been taking diltiazem (Cardizem) 30 mg by mouth three times daily, and bisoprolol (Zebeta), 10 mg by mouth daily. All laboratory work is within normal limits. Relevant vital signs include blood pressure of 150/85 mm Hg and heart rate 50 beats per minute (bpm). On physical examination, patient appears a bit anxious, is short of breath, and easily fatigue upon questioning. Patient also states that of late, she has had a bit of difficulty staying asleep because she wakes up in the middle of the night with difficulty in breathing, which improves when she places several pillows under her head.

Directions for questions 1–3: The questions and incomplete statements in this section can be correctly answered or completed by **one or more** of the suggested answers. Choose the answer, A–E.

(A) I only
(B) III only
(C) I and II
(D) II and III
(E) I, II, and III

1. Which of the following might be responsible for the current clinical state which patient EL is in at this time?

   I. diltiazem (Cardizem)
   II. bisoprolol (Zebeta)
   III. long-standing hypertension

2. Which of the following might be reasonable recommendations based on the initial findings?

   I. DC diltiazem and slowly titrate the patient off of the bisoprolol
   II. initiate therapy with a thiazide diuretic
   III. initiate therapy with an ACE inhibitor

3. Based on patient EL's presenting symptoms suggestive for heart failure, which choice would best represent the findings on EL?

   I. left-sided heart failure
   II. right-sided heart failure
   III. high-output heart failure

4. A recently approved drug for treating heart failure has been given a Class I, Level A recommendation by several cardiology associations, for its use in patients with Stage C heart failure. Which of the following represents the recommendations made by the cardiology groups?

   (A) risk exceeds the benefit, while studied in large multiple populations
   (B) benefit far exceeds the risk, while studied in multiple populations of patients
   (C) benefit far exceeds the risk, while studied in very limited populations of patients
   (D) risk exceeds the benefit, while studied in very limited populations of patients
   (E) benefit greater than the risk, while studied in limited populations of patients

5. Based on the most recent national guidelines, what role does digoxin (Lanoxin) *not* have?

   (A) no current role based on national guidelines
   (B) continues to play a role in the treatment of heart failure
   (C) strong role with a Class IIa, Level B recommendation for patients with current heart failure symptoms
   (D) small role due to a Class IIb, Level C recommendation for patients with heart failure and normal ejection fractions
   (E) strong role as it received a Class IIa, Level A recommendation to control ventricular rate in heart failure patients with atrial fibrillation

Answers to Case 12

1. The answer is E (I, II, and III) *[see 34.IV.F.5–6; 34.IV.J; 34.I.F.3.e].*

Patient EL has been treated for hypertension with a combination of CCB (diltiazem) and β-adrenergic receptor blocker (bisoprolol). Although these agents in combination might be helpful in the treatment of hypertension, they are not routinely suggested as initial therapy in the JNC-7 guidelines. CCBs and β-adrenergic receptor blockers are not considered initial therapy for hypertension unless the patient has a compelling issue, which might warrant the use of such agents. This, owing to the negative inotropic effects of the combination, has a resultant ability to cause drug-induced heart failure. Additionally, long-standing hypertension is a major cause for heart failure in many patients.

2. The answer is C (I and II) *[see Table 34-4].*

As it appears, the combination of diltiazem and bisoprolol have put the patient in a heart failure state, without adequate reduction in blood pressure it would appear necessary to alternate the therapy, based on national guidelines. This would result in a discontinuation in both the bisoprolol and diltiazem. However, remember to slowly titrate the patient off of the β-blocker. Additionally, as per the JNC-7 guidelines, a thiazide diuretic would be considered the initial treatment for this patient. As there appear to be no compelling issues for using other therapies instead of a β-blocker, the thiazide diuretic should be the only agent added to this patient's regimen. As the patient might be experiencing drug-induced heart failure, this might become a compelling reason to initiate therapy with an ACE inhibitor or ARB, if no adequate response from the diuretic.

3. The answer is A (I only) *[see 34.I.F.1–2; Fig. 34-1].*

Patients do not routinely present with either left-sided or right-sided heart failure but the terms are useful in helping to identify which side of the heart is responsible for the respective signs and symptoms which patients present with. In the current patient, EL, signs suggestive of left-sided heart failure include the pulmonary signs of shortness of breath, fatigue, and orthopnea—based on the number of pillows necessary when in the reclining position. This is in comparison to right-sided findings which would reflect peripheral edema, resulting in pedal edema, jugular venous distension, a positive hepatojugular reflux, etc. It is also clear that this patient does not have high-output failure, where one would expect the patient to have normal or high ejection fractions, as well as tachycardia (findings that are consistent with anemias, hyperthyroidism, etc.).

4. The answer is B *[see 34.I.G.4.c].*

A Class I, Level A recommendation is the best recommendation one can receive for any given treatment/intervention, based on the grading criteria used by the respective American Cardiology Associations. Such a recommendation would favorably recommend its use based on the benefit far exceeding the risk for use, and the level of evidence available demonstrating such benefit.

5. The answer is B *[see 34.IV. I.1–3].*

Digoxin continues to find routine usefulness in the heart failure patient population, despite the level of evidence, which appears to be shifting away from its routine usage. It has been used for its inotropic effects, despite the potential for significant side effects upon its use. Therapeutic monitoring for changes in renal function, altered fluid, and electrolytes will maximize the therapeutic effects while minimizing the side effects associated with its use.

Case 13

A patient is referred to a cardiologist and is diagnosed with atrial fibrillation. The patient starts oral warfarin therapy, but is concerned about the potential risk of bleeding complications and the need for frequent anticoagulation monitoring and asks her cardiologist if there is an available alternative to warfarin therapy.

1. An alternative to warfarin that is currently available and FDA approved to reduce the risk of stroke and systemic embolism in patients with nonvvalvular atrial fibrillation is

    I. oral direct Factor IIa (thrombin) inhibitor, dabigatran.
    II. oral direct Factor Xa inhibitor, rivaroxaban.
    III. oral direct Factor Xa inhibitor, fondaparinux.

    (A) I only
    (B) III only
    (C) I and II
    (D) II and III
    (E) I, II, and III

2. When queried by patient or physician regarding a necessity to perform routine monitoring of the international normalized ratio (INR) or activated partial thromboplastin time (aPTT), how would you respond?

    I. Routine monitoring of the INR is necessary for this drug class.
    II. Routine monitoring of the aPTT is necessary for this drug class.
    III. Routine monitoring of the INR and aPTT are not necessary for drug class.

    (A) I only
    (B) III only
    (C) I and II
    (D) II and III
    (E) I, II, and III

Answers to Case 13

1. **The answer is C (I and II)** *[see 35.V.F.1.a]*.
At present time, there are two FDA approved alternatives to warfarin to reduce the risk of stroke and systemic embolism in patients with nonvvalvular atrial fibrillation. The oral direct Factor IIa (thrombin) inhibitor [dabigatran] and the oral direct Factor Xa inhibitor [rivaroxaban]. With respect to safety, dabigatran has been demonstrated to statistically significantly reduce the likelihood of intracranial hemorrhage, life-threatening bleeding, and any bleeding when compared to warfarin. There was a statistically significant increase for the potential of major gastrointestinal bleeding—favoring warfarin. Major bleeding event rates were comparable between the two drugs (dabigatran and warfarin). For rivaroxaban—there was demonstrated non-inferiority to warfarin for prevention of stroke in the setting of nonvvalvular atrial fibrillation with comparable rates of major bleeding when comparing rivaroxaban to warfarin. Less critical organ bleeding (primarily intracranial hemorrhage) and less fatal bleeding were observed with rivaroxaban than with warfarin. There is no INR monitoring of either of these two drugs.

2. **The answer is B (III)** *[see 35.V.E.5.b; 35.V.F.5.b]*.
The routine monitoring of the INR or aPTT is not necessary for either the oral direct Factor Xa inhibitor or the oral direct Factor IIa (thrombin) inhibitor, which is considered a convenience relative to the requisite monitoring of the oral vitamin K antagonist (warfarin).

Case 14

JR is an 87-year-old man with a chief complaint of shortness of breath, productive cough, and fever. This is his second admission to the hospital in the last month for a similar complaint. His past medical history includes BPH, congestive heart failure (CHF), and hypertension. His home medications are fluconazole, citalopram, furosemide, metoprolol, aspirin, and lisinopril. JR is admitted with nasal cannula oxygen. His diagnosis is pneumonia. Labs are pertinent for creatinine clearance of 41 mL/min and sputum culture positive for *Pseudomonas aeruginosa*. Bacterial sensitivities are not back yet.

1. The optimal choice of antibiotic(s) for the treatment of JR's pneumonia is (are)

   (A) cefuroxime.
   (B) sulfamethoxazole.
   (C) ceftaroline.
   (D) doxycycline.
   (E) doripenem.

2. JR is not responding to your choice of antibiotics and the physician adds tobramycin to the regimen. Using the ODA method, his tobramycin peak at steady state is 17.2 μg/mL and trough of 1.4 μg/mL. Based on these levels, the best recommendation would be to

   (A) hold tobramycin and restart at a lower dose/ frequency.
   (B) increase tobramycin frequency but keep dose the same.
   (C) continue tobramycin at the same dose and frequency.
   (D) discontinue tobramycin and start amikacin.
   (E) discontinue tobramycin and start ciprofloxacin.

3. Five days later, JR complains of flank pain and pain on urination. His urine culture is positive for *Enterococcus faecium*. The best choice to treat his urinary tract infection is

   (A) cefepime.
   (B) azithromycin.
   (C) piperacillin/tazobactam.
   (D) telavancin.
   (E) linezolid.

4. After 2 days on his new antibiotic, JR has developed a major drug interaction. Which of the following is the major sign/symptom of this drug interaction?

   (A) thrombocytopenia
   (B) serotonin syndrome
   (C) torsades de pointe
   (D) hypertensive crisis
   (E) jaundice

5. JR is ready for discharge from the hospital when he develops multiple episodes of diarrhea. Stool culture is positive for *Clostridium difficile*. The optimal initial treatment of choice is

   (A) vancomycin.
   (B) clofazimine.
   (C) clindamycin.
   (D) metronidazole.
   (E) moxifloxacin.

Answers to Case 14

1. The answer is E *[see 36.II.C.2]*.
Only doripenem has broad-spectrum activity including the treatment of *P. aeruginosa*. All other agents have a limited spectrum of activity against gram-negative bacteria.

2. The answer is C *[see 36.II.B.4.e]*.
The optimal therapeutic range for ODA using tobramycin is a peak of 16 to 20 μg/mL and trough of < 2 μg/mL.

3. The answer is E *[see 36.III.C.2.b.(3)]*.
Telavancin has activity against *Enterococcus* but only *faecalis*. Of all the other agents, only linezolid has good activity against *E. faecium*.

4. The answer is B *[see 36.II.K.8.e]*.
The use of citalopram in combination with linezolid results in a serious drug interaction producing the serotonin syndrome. Risk rating X—avoid this combination.

5. The answer is D *[see 36.V.C.2.b]*.
This agent is the recommended initial treatment of choice for mild-to-moderate *C. difficile*.

Case 15

AA is a 34-year-old white woman with no known allergies who presents to your pharmacy with the following new prescriptions:

> tenofovir 300 mg, take one tab po daily with breakfast, dispense #30
> emtricitabine 200 mg, take one capsule po daily with breakfast, dispense #30
> efavirenz 600 mg, take one tablet po daily with breakfast, dispense #30

AA tells you that she was diagnosed with HIV 2 weeks ago following a visit to a free clinic offering rapid HIV screening tests. She has never had any symptoms or opportunistic infections (OIs). She then visited Dr. Smith, a physician specializing in HIV care, who examined her, performed lab work and counseling, and initiated the above treatment regimen. She notes that she is sexually active and does not use contraception.

1. Which of AA's prescriptions requires clarification from Dr. Smith to determine the proper time for dosing?

   (A) tenofovir
   (B) emtricitabine
   (C) efavirenz
   (D) none of the prescriptions requires clarification with Dr. Smith

2. Which of the following combination products contain the three antiretroviral therapies (ARTs) that AA has been prescribed?

   (A) Trizivir
   (B) Atripla
   (C) Epzicom
   (D) Truvada
   (E) Combivir

3. AA returns to the pharmacy 2 weeks later, complaining of vivid nightmares that are intolerable. Which of AA's medications is the *most* likely cause of this adverse effect?

   (A) tenofovir
   (B) emtricitabine
   (C) efavirenz
   (D) none of AA's medications cause nightmares

4. Four weeks later, Dr. Smith notifies you that he needs to discontinue AA's efavirenz due to elevated AST and ALT values. After reviewing AA's case, which of the following medications do you recommend that Dr. Smith add to AA's regimen in place of the efavirenz?

   (A) nevirapine 200 mg po daily for 14 days, followed by 200 mg po bid
   (B) delavirdine 400 mg po daily
   (C) etravirine 200 mg po bid
   (D) raltegravir 400 mg po bid
   (E) lamivudine 150 mg po bid

5. Four months later, Dr. Smith informs you that AA needs a change in her ART regimen because she wishes to become pregnant. Which of the following regimens is most appropriate for use in AA if she becomes pregnant?

   (A) lopinavir/ritonavir + zidovudine + lamivudine
   (B) raltegravir + tenofovir + emtricitabine
   (C) tipranavir/ritonavir + tenofovir + emtricitabine
   (D) darunavir/ritonavir + tenofovir + emtricitabine
   (E) efavirenz + zidovudine + lamivudine

Answers to Case 15

1. The answer is C *[see 36.VII.C.4.b.(3).(a)].*
Tenofovir and emtricitabine may be dosed at any time of day, without regard to meals. Efavirenz should be dosed on an empty stomach at bedtime to permit optimal absorption and minimization of adverse effects.

2. The answer is B *[see 36.VII.C.4.b.(2)].*
Atripla is the only combination product containing two nucleoside reverse transcriptase inhibitors (NRTIs) and one nucleotide NRTI (NNRTI). The other combination products listed are NRTI-only combinations.

3. The answer is C *[see 36.VII.C.4.b.(3).(a)].*
Efavirenz causes central nervous system (CNS) adverse effects in approximately 52% of patients who take it. Typically, patients experience dizziness, drowsiness, and vivid nightmares. Tenofovir and emtricitabine do not cause CNS adverse effects.

4. The answer is D *[see 36.VII.C.4; Table 36-6].*
NNRTIs are metabolized through the liver and require cautious use in hepatic dysfunction. In this case, the NNRTIs (nevirapine, etravirine, delavirdine) should be avoided due to the patient's elevated liver function tests (LFTs). The patient should receive a protease inhibitor (PI) or an integrase inhibitor in place of the efavirenz. Addition of lamivudine is not an option, as it is an NRTI. Raltegravir is the appropriate agent to use in this situation.

5. The answer is A *[see Table 36-6].*
The preferred regimen for pregnant patients is lopinavir/ritonavir plus zidovudine and lamivudine, as each of these agents have the most clinical data for use in pregnancy. Efavirenz should be avoided in pregnancy due to its teratogenic potential.

Case 16

WX is admitted to your hospital due to acute psychosis. He is currently experiencing visual hallucinations and is acutely agitated. He is being loud and physically aggressive. The team gave him an intramuscular (IM) injection of olanzapine 10 mg approximately 1 hour ago with some benefit.

1. When can the team give the next IM injection?

   (A) 1 hour
   (B) 2 hours
   (C) 3 hours
   (D) 4 hours

2. What is the maximum 24-hour amount of IM olanzapine?

   (A) 15 mg
   (B) 20 mg
   (C) 30 mg
   (D) 40 mg

3. After receiving the IM injections, the patient calmed down. The team would now like to switch him to an oral medication but they think he may spit it out. Which of the following medications is a sublingual tablet?

   (A) Asenapine
   (B) Haloperidol
   (C) Ziprasidone
   (D) Lurasidone

4. The patient has been hospitalized for 2 weeks and is no longer acutely psychotic. The team would like to try a long-acting injectable antipsychotic. They want to know which of the choices below can be given in a loading dose strategy. You pick which choice?

   (A) Fluphenazine
   (B) Risperidone consta
   (C) Aripiprazole
   (D) Paliperidone palmitate

5. The team agrees with your decision. The attending states that paliperidone palmitate requires the patient to be monitored for 3 hours following injection. What is your response?

   (A) yes, paliperidone palmitate requires a patient to be monitored for a 3-hour period
   (B) no, risperidone consta requires a patient to be monitored for a 3-hour period
   (C) no, olanzapine pamoate requires a patient to be monitored for a 3-hour period
   (D) no, no long-acting antipsychotics require a patient to be monitored for a 3-hour period

Answers to Case 16

1. The answer is B *[see 39.IV.C.7.b]*.
IM olanzapine can be given every 2 hours for a maximum of 30 mg in 24-hour period.

2. The answer is C *[see 39.IV.C.7.b]*.
IM olanzapine can be given every 2 hours for a maximum of 30 mg in 24-hour period.

3. The answer is A *[see 39.IV.C.7.a]*.
Asenapine is given sublingually. Its bioavailability significantly decreases if the tablet is swallowed.

4. The answer is D *[see 39.IV.D.4]*.
Paliperidone palmitate is initiated with a loading dose of 234 mg followed by a second injection of 156 mg 1 week later. Subsequent doses are given every 4 weeks and range from 39 to 234 mg.

5. The answer is C *[see 39.IV.D.5]*.
Olanzapine pamoate can only be administered at a registered health care facility and patients must be monitored for at least 3 hours following injection. This monitoring is required due to delirium/sedation syndrome.

Case 17

WY is a 20-year-old man admitted to your hospital for acute mania. In addition to being manic, he is agitated and has not slept for the past 3 days. He has no other medical or psychiatric illnesses other than bipolar disorder. The team would like your help in managing this patient. Please select the correct answer for each of the questions below.

1. The team would like to use valproic acid (VPA) to treat his acute manic episode. You recommend which dosing strategy?

   (A) 5 mg/kg/day
   (B) 10 mg/kg/day
   (C) 60 mg/kg/day
   (D) 20 mg/kg/day

2. When should the team first measure the VPA level?

   (A) 3 days
   (B) 6 days
   (C) 9 days
   (D) 12 days

3. After 1 day of receiving VPA, the patient is still agitated and not sleeping. The team wants to start an adjunctive medication. You recommend which of the following?

   (A) lithium (Lithobid)
   (B) lorazepam (Ativan)
   (C) carbamazepine (Tegretol)
   (D) lamotrigine (Lamictal)

4. The team wants to know if there are any side effects from VPA they should be watching for in this patient. You mention which of the following to the team?

   (A) polydipsia
   (B) hypothyroidism
   (C) hyponatremia
   (D) sedation

5. The team wants to know if they should be monitoring any laboratory values in this patient prescribed VPA. You mention which of the following?

   (A) liver function panel
   (B) renal function panel
   (C) thyroid panel
   (D) VPA does not require any laboratory values to be monitored

Answers to Case 17

1. The answer is D *[see 40.II.D.b.3].*
The appropriate loading dose for an acutely manic patient started on VPA is 20 to 30 mg/kg/day. The maximum weight-based dose is 60 mg/kg/day. The recommended dose in a nonmanic patient is 5 to 10 mg/kg/day.

2. The answer is A *[see 40.II.D.b.3.a].*
A VPA level can be drawn 3 to 5 days after starting VPA. Using a loading dose strategy allows for VPA to reach steady state quicker than in a nonloaded patient. Therefore, you can draw a VPA level at day 3.

3. The answer is B *[see 40.II.D.h].*
Benzodiazepines, which lorazepam is, are useful in the short term because they help in treating agitation and insomnia. Because benzodiazepines are not effective in the treatment of bipolar disorder, they should be stopped once the patient is no longer acutely manic or experiencing symptoms of agitation or insomnia.

4. The answer is D *[see 40.II.D.b.4].*
Sedation is an early side effect of VPA therapy especially when it is prescribed at higher dose (i.e., loading dose strategy used in this patient). The other side effects listed are caused by lithium and carbamazepine.

5. The answer is A *[see 40.II.D.b.4.b].*
VPA can cause hepatotoxicity early on in treatment, therefore baseline and follow-up monitoring of liver function panel is recommended. A renal and thyroid function panels are recommended for lithium therapy.

Case 18

AB is a 65-year-old woman with chronic obstructive pulmonary disease (COPD), coronary artery disease (CAD), insulin-dependent diabetes mellitus (IDDM), and a current smoker. She has required antibiotics and prednisone twice in the last 12 months for COPD exacerbations. Her home medications are tiotropium one inhalation q24h; Duoneb (ipratropium, albuterol) via nebulization qid prn; formoterol DPI 1 inhalation twice daily; Lantus 16 units q P.M.; Lispro 3 units with meals; isosorbide dinitrate 30 mg daily; and ASA 81 mg q24h. She has very severe COPD based on spirometry and clinical history.

1. Which of the following is the best choice to modify her bronchodilator regimen?

   (A) DC the tiotropium and continue other meds
   (B) DC the ipratropium and continue albuterol qid via nebs
   (C) DC the formoterol and continue other meds
   (D) continue all current meds

2. Which of the below choices is the best option to decrease further COPD exacerbations?

   (A) no changes will further decrease exacerbations
   (B) change formoterol to a formoterol/ICS combination (Symbicort or Dulera)
   (C) discontinue formoterol and replace with an ICS such as fluticasone MDI (Flovent)
   (D) add sustained-release theophylline

3. Which of the following is true regarding β-blockers in COPD?

   (A) β-blockers are contraindicated in COPD
   (B) selective or nonselective β-blockers can be used in COPD
   (C) selective β-blockers have been shown to improve cardiovascular outcomes in COPD
   (D) none of the above are true

4. Prednisone has which of the following effects on the patient's blood sugars?

   (A) no effect on blood glucose
   (B) increases blood glucose shortly after administration, especially with higher doses
   (C) increases blood glucose only after numerous days of oral prednisone
   (D) decreases blood glucose

5. Which of the following would be the best intervention to increase the likelihood of the patient quitting smoking?

   (A) state strongly that she should quit smoking
   (B) recommend that she talk to her doctor
   (C) recommend an intensive smoking cessation counseling program for the patient
   (D) recommend an intensive smoking cessation counseling program and a smoking cessation drug therapy such as nicotine replacement therapy

Answers to Case 18

1. The answer is B *[see 41.II.G.1.d.(3).(d).(ii)]*.
Ipratropium and tiotropium should not be administered concomitantly due to increased anticholinergic ADRs and little additive bronchodilation when combined. As tiotropium is a more potent bronchodilator in COPD, preferable to stop ipratropium.

2. The answer is B *[see 41.II.G.1.h.(2).(f)]*.
ICS are well documented to decrease COPD exacerbations in combination with long-acting β-agonists. ICS should not be used without long-acting β2-agonists in COPD (in contrast to asthma, where ICS can be used as monotherapy). Theophylline is unsafe due to CAD.

3. The answer is C *[see 32.II.B.4.a.(1); 41.I.I.1.f.(8).(b)]*.
β-Adrenergic blockers, especially selective agents, have been shown to improve cardiovascular mortality in COPD. Selective β-blockers can be used in asthma, but should be administered cautiously, such as in a controlled environment (e.g., hospital) and in patients where mortality benefits outweigh the risk of worsened bronchospasm.

4. The answer is B *[see 41.I.I.2.d.(1).(a)]*.
Systemic steroids routinely increase blood glucose within 24 hours in patients with diabetes mellitus.

5. The answer is D *[see 41.II.G.2.e]*.
Brief interventions such as (**A**) or (**B**) are less effective than more intensive counseling. Addition of drug therapy and intensive counseling has highest probability of cessation.

Case 19

Betty is 65 years old, obese, and has type 2 diabetes, renal insufficiency, hypertension, and a history of deep vein thrombosis. She works as a seamstress. She was active as a younger woman, played several sports, and skied. She injured her right knee in a skiing accident. Her chief complaint is bilateral hand pain and stiffness and right knee pain which is worse in the morning (< 30 minutes) and after sitting for prolonged periods. Some crepitus is heard on joint manipulation of her right knee. Her medications include glipizide, lisinopril, hydrochlorothiazide, warfarin, and acetaminophen 1 g qid × 1 month.

1. All of the following nonpharmacological treatments should be recommended to improve Betty's osteoarthritis (OA) symptoms *except*

    (A) retire as a seamstress.
    (B) weight loss.
    (C) rest.
    (D) aerobic exercise.
    (E) assistive devices (e.g., cane).

2. For additional OA pain relief, which of the following agents is relatively contraindicated?

    (A) oral tramadol
    (B) oral glucosamine
    (C) oral oxycodone
    (D) oral naproxen sodium
    (E) intra-articular triamcinolone

3. Glucosamine

    (A) treats the acute pain associated with osteoarthritis.
    (B) is most effective when combined with chondroitin.
    (C) promotes the synthesis of glycosaminoglycans.
    (D) inhibits stores of substance P.
    (E) must be given intramuscularly to achieve maximum benefit.

4. Characteristics of osteoarthritis include all of the following *except*

    (A) short-term stiffness (< 30 minutes).
    (B) articular crepitus.
    (C) joint space narrowing.
    (D) diminished range of motion.
    (E) diffuse joint inflammation.

Answers to Case 19

1. The answer is A *[see 42.III.E.2]*.
Although repetitive stress can be a risk factor for OA, retiring from the job, unless pain is severe and disability exists, is not recommended.

2. The answer is D *[see 42.III.E.3.b.(4)]*.
With her history of renal insufficiency and hypertension combined with the drugs lisinopril, hydrochlorothiazide, and warfarin, the NSAID would not be the "best" choice and relatively contraindicated.

3. The answer is C *[see 42.III.E.3.c.(5).(a)]*.
Glucosamine acts as a substrate for and promotes the synthesis of glycosaminoglycans, which is essential for the extracellular matrix in cartilage.

4. The answer is E *[see 42.III.A]*.
Osteoarthritis is not considered a disease of inflammation. Although there are times of minor inflammation (e.g., OA flare), it is localized to the affected joint(s).

Case 20

A 48-year-old man (LN) is seen in the clinic with the diagnosis of an acute attack of gouty arthritis. He has severe pain in his left big toe. His serum uric acid is elevated (9.5 mg/dL with the normal range being 3 to 7 mg/dL). This is his first attack and he apparently has no other medical problems, although he was told once that he had "borderline high blood pressure." He is overweight, and could use shedding a few pounds.

1. Of the following possible treatment approaches, which would be the *best treatment plan* for this patient?

   (A) give one of several NSAIDs at the maximal dose for 3 weeks
   (B) give colchicine 1.2 mg stat, followed by 0.6 mg in 1 hour
   (C) give recommended doses of naproxen and taper the dose over 7 days along with febuxostat 40 mg/day
   (D) administer po indomethacin 50 mg three times a day for 2 days, then increase the dose over the next few days as the patient responds
   (E) administer no drugs yet until the 24-hour urinary uric acid level is obtained

2. All of the following statements concerning LN's gout are correct *except*:

   (A) keeping the affected joint immobilized would be very important to his comfort.
   (B) his age and sex do not match the usual gouty arthritis profile.
   (C) he is like most patients as his first attack involved a single joint.
   (D) his attack most likely occurred in the middle of the night.
   (E) if LN is like most patients, he is an "underexcreter" of uric acid.

3. LN developed a second attack 6 months after the first one. It is now 12 months after the first attack and he has developed yet another attack in his right big toe this time. His serum uric acid level is now 10 mg/dL. All of the following statements concerning the treatment of hyperuricemia and gout in this patient are correct *except*:

   (A) giving him large initial doses of acetaminophen and then tapering the dose would be a good treatment approach here.
   (B) he has met the criteria for starting urate lowering drug therapy with the onset of this third attack.
   (C) as with most patients, the eventual goal for the serum uric acid level for LN is at or below 6 mg/dL.
   (D) once the attack is controlled, LN would be a candidate for low-dose prophylactic colchicine or an NSAID.
   (E) an intra-articular injection of corticosteroid in the big toe could be given this time.

4. LN is begun on low-dose colchicine and then a month later he is begun on allopurinol 100 mg/day to start. Four months later, he has yet another attack of acute gouty arthritis. He is on colchicine 0.6 mg once a day and allopurinol 300 mg/day. He has been on this dose for 3 months and claims that he takes his medication regularly. His serum uric acid is 7.5 mg/dL. Which of the following statements below *best describes* a current important point about the use of allopurinol in the treatment of hyperuricemia?

(A) LN's "standard 300 mg/day dose" is inadequate and should be increased.
(B) It needs to be dosed three times daily in this patient.
(C) It can only be used in patients who are overproducers of uric acid.
(D) It is the only available uricosuric agent in the United States.
(E) It should be taken with plenty of fluid to prevent uric acid precipitation in the kidney.

5. LN follows his physician's next therapeutic regimen which includes some counseling about his diet. All of the following will likely produce a decrease in the serum uric acid level which may prevent another attack for LN *except*:

(A) cutting back some on red meat and fish.
(B) getting LN to lose some weight.
(C) drinking a couple of beers daily.
(D) taking a 500 mg vitamin C tablet daily.
(E) drinking low-fat milk as a source of protein.

Answers to Case 20

1. The answer is B *[see 43.III.E.2.b].*
NSAIDs are generally the first-line agents, but will only be needed for a few days, not 3 weeks. For (**B**), this is the new effective dosage regimen for colchicine. Do not give anything (febuxostat) that would alter the serum uric acid as this will likely prolong the attack. Take care of the patient's acute attack—we don't care about the uric acid level initially. Can give oral indomethacin 50 mg tid, but then *decrease* the dose, don't increase it. The uric acid has been elevated probably for several months, but don't worry about it, take care of the patient's pain—failing to start pain management as soon as possible will likely decrease the effectiveness of the pain management therapy.

2. The answer is B *[see 43.I.B].*
(**A**), (**C**), (**D**), and (**E**) are correct statements related to acute gouty arthritis. Gouty arthritis occurs most often in men (seven to nine times more often than women) and he is almost right at the usual age of onset.

3. The answer is A *[see 43.III.E.2].*
Acetaminophen has no anti-inflammatory properties and, therefore, would not be useful in treating this patient's acute gouty arthritis attack. This agent is not included amongst the specific agents to treat acute gouty arthritis. (**B**) through (**E**) are all correct statements.

4. The answer is A *[see 43.IV.C.3.b.(1)].*
This most common dose of 300 mg/day is often inadequate. The drug can be given in daily doses up to 800 mg/day. The drug can be dosed once daily (long acting oxypurinol metabolite), it can be used for both overproducers or under-excretors, it is a xanthine oxidase inhibitor (not a uricosuric), and plenty of fluids are only warranted for the uricosuric, probenecid.

5. The answer is C *[see 43.IV.C.1].*
Beer can increase the serum uric acid level. Meat and fish have high levels of purines which can elevate the serum uric acid, so *decreasing* these in the diet will likely decrease the serum uric acid. Weight loss decreases the serum uric. Taking agents that have uricosuric activity (vitamin C) will decrease the serum uric acid level and using low-fat milk as a source of dietary protein is a good approach and will have a positive effect on lowering his serum uric acid level.

Case 21

ER is a 61-year-old man admitted to the emergency department with a chief complaint of hematuria for 2 days. History of present illness (HPI): ER awoke at night 2 days ago with abdominal pain, bloating, and two episodes of emesis which progressed to hematemesis. His past medical history is significant for hypertension, acute MI, gastroesophageal reflux disease (GERD), type 2 diabetes, and obesity. Home medications included omeprazole, lisinopril, glyburide, aspirin, naproxen, simvastatin, and metoprolol. ER is currently not allowed anything by mouth (NPO) with IV fluids running and no subsequent episodes of hematemesis.

1. ER is diagnosed and admitted to the hospital with erosive esophagitis. Which of the following agents would be the best treatment of choice?

   (A) omeprazole 20 mg oral bid
   (B) esomeprazole 30 mg IV daily
   (C) lansoprazole 40 mg suspension bid
   (D) pantoprazole 40 mg IV daily
   (E) dexlansoprazole 30 mg oral daily

2. ER's 5-year-old daughter, JR, comes to visit with his wife. She tells her husband that their daughter was just diagnosed with GERD. What is the best agent to treat JR with?

   (A) rabeprazole
   (B) dexlansoprazole
   (C) pantoprazole
   (D) transoprazole
   (E) lansoprazole

3. The most common adverse effects of the PPIs that JR's parents should be educated about include all of the following *except*

   (A) nausea and vomiting.
   (B) elevated liver enzymes.
   (C) headache.
   (D) abdominal pain.
   (E) diarrhea.

4. Prior to admission, ER frequently encountered episodes of nocturnal GERD even on his daily PPI. JR asks his physician what the optimal regimen to use for this when he is discharged. The best choice is

   (A) pantoprazole 40 mg oral daily plus ranitidine 150 mg at bedtime.
   (B) rabeprazole 30 mg oral bid.
   (C) omeprazole 20 mg oral bid.
   (D) esomeprazole 30 mg oral bid.
   (E) lansoprazole 20 mg oral daily plus famotidine 20 mg at bedtime.

5. ER is discharged home with a prescription for a PPI and misoprostol. All of the following are true statements *except*

   (A) misoprostol is indicated for the prevention of NSAID-induced duodenal ulcer.
   (B) misoprostol has both mucosal and antisecretory properties.
   (C) the most frequent adverse effect of the drug is diarrhea.
   (D) this drug should not be prescribed in women of childbearing potential.
   (E) no significant drug–drug interactions have been reported with this drug.

Answers to Case 21

1. The answer is D *[see 44.II.A.6.b.(11)]*.
Although all of these agents are effective in the treatment of erosive esophagitis, intravenous pantoprazole at this dose and frequency is the best treatment choice in an NPO patient.

2. The answer is E *[see 44.II.A.6.a.(6)]*.
Only omeprazole, esomeprazole, and lansoprazole are approved for use in infants and children with GERD.

3. The answer is B *[see 44.II.A.6.c]*.
All are commonly associated adverse drug effects except elevation of liver enzymes.

4. The answer is C *[see 44.II.A.6.b.(13)]*.
In patients with frequent episodes of nocturnal GERD already on a daily PPI, the addition of an evening dose has been shown to be effective.

5. The answer is A *[see 44.II.A.5.b]*.
Misoprostol is indicated for the prevention of NSAID-induced gastric, not duodenal ulcers, in patients 60 years or older.

Case 22

Varda Torkey is a 33-year-old woman seen in clinic today for worsening ulcerative colitis (UC). She was first diagnosed with UC 8 years ago. In the time since, she has successfully managed her symptoms with loperamide for occasional diarrhea and acetaminophen for occasional pain. Her chief complaints include increased bowel movements (now 6 per day, some of which appear bloody) and abdominal cramping. She also mentions new "aches" in her knees and shoulders which she feels are job-related.

Ms. Torkey's labs indicate mild anemia and mild dehydration. Stool cultures are negative. Her vital signs are within normal limits although she has lost 7 lb in the last 2 months without intent. The remainder of her physical exam is unremarkable.

Just prior to this visit, Ms. Torkey underwent a colonoscopy. That exam revealed mucosal changes characteristic of moderate UC. The extent of involvement included rectum and descending colon just below the splenic flexure. There was no evidence of cancer or precancerous lesions.

Ms. Torkey has no known medication allergies. Her current medications include loperamide up to 8 mg/day, acetaminophen up to 4 g/day, daily multivitamin with iron, amitriptyline 30 mg daily, and recently ibuprofen 200 mg up to six times daily as needed for joint pain, and diphenhydramine nightly for sleep. Ms. Torkey is a single parent. She has a new (1 month) part-time job as a janitress.

1. It is possible that Ms. Torkey's UC was worsened due to use of which of the following medications?

   (A) amitriptyline 30 mg/day
   (B) acetaminophen max of 4 g/day
   (C) ibuprofen max of 1200 mg/day
   (D) diphenhydramine at bedtime
   (E) loperamide

2. A decision is made to initiate therapy to control the current flair of UC. Which of the following would be the best choice for Ms. Torkey (patient indicates no preference)?

   (A) oral azathioprine plus mesalamine suppository
   (B) oral mesalamine plus mesalamine enemas
   (C) oral mesalamine plus corticosteroid enemas
   (D) oral corticosteroid plus corticosteroid enemas
   (E) oral corticosteroid plus mesalamine enemas

3. After 6 weeks of treatment, the UC flare-up has subsided. A decision is made to initiate continued therapy to lessen the chance of future flare-ups. Which of the following would be the best choice for Ms. Torkey?

   (A) low-dose oral corticosteroid
   (B) corticosteroid enema on M, W, F
   (C) sulfasalazine 1 g/day
   (D) mesalamine 2.4 g/day
   (E) prednisone 5 mg/day

4. In 1 year's time on the maintenance regimen above, Ms. Torkey had three flare-ups of her UC. An alternative therapy is needed for maintenance of her UC going forward. Which of the following would be the best choice for her?

   (A) higher dose corticosteroid
   (B) metronidazole three times daily
   (C) azathioprine daily
   (D) ciprofloxacin daily
   (E) rifaximin

5. Ms. Torkey heard something about the use of probiotics for UC from an internet support group. She would like to know more. Which of the following statements would best summarize the use of probiotics?

   (A) The efficacy of probiotics has been clearly defined in clinical trials, you should feel reassured using them.
   (B) Probiotics have only been shown effective in patients with Crohn disease; as you have UC, they would be of no benefit to you.
   (C) There is some evidence of benefit when probiotics are combined with prescription therapies; you should talk with your doctor before using them.
   (D) Probiotics have been shown in clinical studies to be more effective at treating flare-ups than preventing them; consider using them for you next flare-up.
   (E) Probiotics clearly have no value in irritable bowel disease (IBD).

Answers to Case 22

1. The answer is C *[see 45.I.F.1.i]*.
Ibuprofen and other NSAIDs are the most commonly implicated class of drugs inducing IBD-like symptoms. Other drugs implicated include gold compounds, oral contraceptives, enteric potassium supplements, pancreatic enzymes, and phosphosoda bowel preps.

2. The answer is B *[see 45.II.B.2]*.
Patients with mild-to-moderate acute distal UC respond well to oral or topical 5-ASA (i.e., mesalamine). Topical 5-ASA plus oral 5-ASA is superior to either alone and may induce remission more quickly than either route alone.

3. The answer is D *[see 45.II.B.3.b]*.
Corticosteroids, topical or oral, are not effective in maintaining remission of UC and should not be used. Data suggest total daily doses of 5-ASA less than 2 g are less effective than doses greater than 2 g. Mesalamine 2.4 g/day is the proper choice.

4. The answer is C *[see 45.II.A.2; 45.II.A.3; 45.II.A.7]*.
No specific infectious agent has been identified as a single causative factor for UC. Use of broad-spectrum antibiotics in UC is limited to fulminant disease or in patients with toxic megacolon, where short-term use of antibiotics can be justified due to the increased risk of perforation or bacteremia. Use of select antibiotics with a goal of remission of acute IBD is controversial. Systemic corticosteroids as a rule are not accepted as long-term therapy due to risks of adverse events and questionable therapeutic effect. Azathioprine has been useful as a long-term option.

5. The answer is C *[see 45.II.A.8]*.
Controlled trials of probiotic therapy in IBD have yet to clearly define clinical utility. There is little evidence to support their use in acute IBD. However, recent meta-analyses suggest potential benefit of probiotics, when combined with conventional therapies, for maintenance of UC but not Crohn disease.

Case 23

A 38-year-old Hispanic male presents with complaints of frequent urination, "cotton mouth," and blurry vision. He does not have a fever and denies gastrointestinal symptoms. His vitals and laboratory tests are as follows:

Objective Data
Blood Pressure: 132/88   Pulse: 86   Height: 63 inches   Weight: 179 lbs   BMI: 31.7 kg/m^2

Laboratory Tests (random)

Glucose = 326	A1c = 7.5%	Na = 133	K = 4.6	Cl = 97
CO2 = 23	BUN = 15	SCr = 1.3	eGFR = 54 ml/min/1.73m^2	
eCrCl = 62 ml/min (Salazar-Corcoran)		Alb = 2.7	AST = 22	ALT = 14
Total Cholesterol = 222		LDL = 162	HDL = 36	Triglycerides = 149
Islet cell antibodies = negative		Albumin:Creatinine ratio: <30		

1. Which is the most likely diagnosis for this individual?

   (A) Type 1 Diabetes (T1DM)
   (B) Latent Autoimmune Diabetes of the Adult (LADA)
   (C) Type 2 Diabetes (T2DM)
   (D) Hyperosmolar Hyperglycemic State (HHS)

2. Which would be the most appropriate agent to initiate for home management of the blood glucose?

   (A) Biguanide
   (B) Thiazolidinedione
   (C) Long-acting insulin
   (D) Pre-mixed 70/30 insulin

3. Which non-glycemic target should be addressed first?

   (A) Albumin to creatinine ratio
   (B) Triglyceride level
   (C) LDL level
   (D) HDL level

4. If the blood pressure measurement was a continued trend, which would be the most appropriate initial agent?

   (A) Lisinopril
   (B) Amlodipine
   (C) Hydrochlorothiazide
   (D) Aliskiren

5. How much rapid-acting insulin should be injected in-office today to bring the blood glucose level to a target of 120 mg/dL?

   (A) 2 units
   (B) 5 units
   (C) 10 units
   (D) 12 units

Answers to Case 23

1. The answer is C *[see 46.I.B]*.
The individual is at risk for T2DM because of his ethnic origin and his weight. Additionally, his islet cell antibodies (ICA) are negative, which further confirms the suspicion of T2DM. Individuals with either LADA or T1DM typically present with positive antibodies to insulin, glutamic acid decarboxylase, and/or pancreatic islet β cells. HHS is a form of hyperglycemic crisis that usually presents with blood glucose levels greater than 600 mg/dL.

2. The answer is A *[see 46.VI.A.1.a]*.
Metformin, a biguanide, is the recommended initial agent for the management of T2DM, unless contraindications (e.g., significant renal or hepatic impairment, alcoholism, unstable heart failure) exist. A thiazolidinedione could be initiated, but is not the preferred initial agent. At this time, insulin is not indicated for long-term management of the blood glucose.

3. The answer is C *[see 46.X.A.1; X.C.1.a.(1)]*.
Neither the albumin to creatinine ratio, nor the triglyceride level is above goal. The HDL is too low and the LDL is too high, but the LDL should be the primary focus at this time.

4. The answer is A *[see 46.X.A.2]*.
ACE inhibitors or ARBs should be first line treatment for hypertension in the individual with diabetes, unless contraindications exist. Thiazide diuretics may be added for additional blood glucose lowering. Aliskiren is for adjunctive therapy rather than monotherapy.

5. The answer is B *[see 46.V.A.7.a]*.
It would take either 5-6 units to bring the blood glucose to target based on the following calculations:

$$TDD = (0.6 \times \text{weight in kg}) = (0.6 \times 81) = 48.6 \approx 49$$

Rule of 1800 to determine correction factor (CF):
$$CF = 1800/TDD = 1800/49 \approx 37$$

Point-of-care calculation to determine # of units to inject to bring BG to target = (Current blood glucose − target blood glucose)/CF = $(326 − 120)/37 \approx 5.6$ units

Case 24

A 55-year-old woman has a history of uncontrolled hypertension for years and sporadically uses captopril and hydrochlorothiazide. The patient has noticeable edema in her legs and some difficulty breathing. Her blood pressure is 165/110 mm Hg, pulse is 90 bpm, and her temperature is 97°F. Her labs show a BUN of 44 mg/dL, SCr of 3.8 mg/dL, serum potassium of 6.2 mg/mL, and a hematocrit of 22. Specific gravity of the urine is 1.010. The patient believes she is experiencing fatigue due to a respiratory infection.

1. What could be the explanation for the patient's current condition?

   (A) chronic renal failure due to uncontrolled hypertension
   (B) pneumonia
   (C) acute renal failure due to captopril
   (D) chronic renal failure due to acetaminophen use
   (E) dehydration

2. What may be contributing to the patient's difficulty breathing?

   (A) pneumonia
   (B) allergies
   (C) use of hydrochlorothiazide
   (D) pulmonary edema
   (E) hypertension

3. Does captopril appear to be *ineffective* in this patient?

   (A) yes, the blood pressure is still 165/110 mm Hg
   (B) yes, the blood pressure has not been controlled for years
   (C) no, the patient is not compliant with the medication
   (D) no, the patient has a blood pressure reading within range
   (E) difficult to say at this point due to lack of information

4. All of the following items could be used as an initial treatment of the patient's edema *except*

   (A) fluid restriction.
   (B) hemodialysis.
   (C) furosemide.
   (D) metolazone.
   (E) torsemide.

5. Treatment of anemia may involve all of the following *except*

   (A) calcitriol.
   (B) epoetin alfa.
   (C) darbepoetin.
   (D) transfusion with packed red blood cells.
   (E) IV iron.

Answers to Case 24

1. The answer is A *[see 48.II.D.1]*.
In addition to the uncontrolled hypertension over many years, the fluid and electrolyte status of the patient, the specific gravity of the urine, and fatigue suggest chronic renal failure. Acetaminophen does not lead to chronic renal failure, but may lead to chronic hepatic failure.

2. The answer is D *[see 48.II.D.1.e]*.
Respiratory problems including dyspnea when CHF is present and pulmonary edema may be present in patients with chronic renal failure due to accumulation of fluid in the lungs.

3. The answer is C *[see 48:II.F.1.a]*.
ACE inhibitors are effective in lowering blood pressure in patients with chronic kidney disease (CKD). However, patients must be compliant for their effects to be realized. In this patient, she has stated that she has not been compliant with her medications for years.

4. The answer is B *[see 48.II.F.1,2]*.
Hemodialysis should be reserved until conservative treatments do not work.

5. The answer is A *[see 48.II.F.5.a]*.
Calcitriol is a vitamin D supplement that is used in the treatment of hypocalcemia in CKD. All of the other agents can aid in treating anemia in CKD.

Case 25

A 25-year-old woman presents to the emergency department after ingesting an unknown number of acetaminophen tablets. The time of ingestion is unknown. She states that she wants to end her life. Her heart rate is 100 bpm, blood pressure is 100/75 mm Hg, and temperature is 98°F. Her plasma acetaminophen level is 160 μg/mL. She has a history of depression and is currently taking Lexapro and Wellbutrin.

1. What substance is contained in the liver that helps the patient detoxify the toxic metabolite of *N*-acetyl-p-aminophenol (APAP)?

   (A) glutathione
   (B) *N*-acetyl-p-benzoquinone imine (NAPQI)
   (C) ALT
   (D) AST
   (E) bilirubin

2. Ideally, activated charcoal is given within what period of time?

   (A) prior to ingestion of APAP
   (B) within 1 hour of ingestion of APAP
   (C) it is never given
   (D) within 12 hours of ingestion of APAP
   (E) within 6 hours of ingestion of APAP

3. The physicians decide to administer *N*-acetylcysteine. How does it work to protect the liver in an APAP overdose?

   (A) binding to APAP
   (B) inactivating the P-450 system
   (C) increasing urinary elimination
   (D) reversing damage to injured hepatocytes
   (E) increasing stores of glutathione

4. What oral dose of *N*-acetylcysteine should be administered to this patient?

   (A) 140 mg/kg followed by 70 mg/kg every 4 hours for 17 doses
   (B) 140 mg/kg for one dose
   (C) 50 mg/kg every 6 hours
   (D) 150 mg/kg followed by 110 mg/kg every 8 hours for 10 doses
   (E) inappropriate to use

Answers to Case 25

1. The answer is A *[see 49.II.A.3]*.
Glutathione in the liver normally detoxifies NAPQI. An acute overdose of APAP depletes glutathione stores which results in an accumulation of NAPQI that causes hepatocellular necrosis.

2. The answer is B *[see 49.II.C.1.a]*.
Activated charcoal can bind unabsorbed APAP. Ideally, it is administered within 1 hour of ingestion, but may be of benefit as long as 3 to 4 hours after ingestion.

3. The answer is E *[see 49.II.C.2.a]*.
N-acetylcysteine is a precursor for glutathione and decreases APAP toxicity by increasing glutathione hepatic stores. It does not reverse damage to liver cells that have already been injured. Ideally begin treatment within 8 hours of ingestion. It may be of value 48 hours or more after ingestion.

4. The answer is A *[see 49.II.C.2.c]*.
The adult oral dose of *N*-acetylcysteine is 140 mg/kg, followed by 70 mg/kg every 4 hours times 17 doses.

Case 26

TJ is an 18-year-old young woman who was recently diagnosed with osteosarcoma. After her case was evaluated, it was decided that she would undergo neoadjuvant chemotherapy, followed by surgical resection of the primary tumor, and then receive adjuvant chemotherapy. Her chemotherapy will include three different cycles given in a rotation fashion. The chemotherapy she will receive includes cycles of high-dose methotrexate, cycles of high-dose cisplatin plus doxorubicin, and cycles of ifosfamide plus etoposide. You are about to counsel the patient regarding the potential toxicities of each of the agents. Answer the following questions based on the potential toxicity.

1. Chronic cardiac toxicity is most likely associated with which of the following agents?

   (A) methotrexate
   (B) cisplatin
   (C) doxorubicin
   (D) ifosfamide
   (E) etoposide

2. Severe acute and delayed nausea and vomiting, especially if appropriate antiemetics are not administered, is most likely associated with which of the following agents?

   (A) methotrexate
   (B) cisplatin
   (C) doxorubicin
   (D) ifosfamide
   (E) etoposide

3. The metabolite acrolein and the development of hemorrhagic cystitis is associated with which of the following agents?

   (A) methotrexate
   (B) cisplatin
   (C) doxorubicin
   (D) ifosfamide
   (E) etoposide

4. Hypersensitivity reactions and infusion-related hypotension have been associated with which of the following agents?

   (A) methotrexate
   (B) cisplatin
   (C) doxorubicin
   (D) ifosfamide
   (E) etoposide

5. The use of leucovorin should be used to rescue normal, healthy cells from the cytotoxic effects of which agent?

   (A) methotrexate
   (B) cisplatin
   (C) doxorubicin
   (D) ifosfamide
   (E) etoposide

Answers to Case 26

1. The answer is C *[see 50.V.H]*.
Chronic cardiac toxicity which presents as irreversible left-sided heart failure is commonly associated with the anthracyclines, such as doxorubicin.

2. The answer is B *[see 50.V.C; Table 50-3]*.
High-dose cisplatin (doses ≥ 50 mg/m^2) has been associated with significant nausea and vomiting in both the acute and delayed setting.

3. The answer is D *[see 50.V.K]*.
Acrolein is a toxic metabolite of ifosfamide (and cyclophosphamide). It is known to cause irritation of the bladder wall and hemorrhagic cystitis. Measures that can be used to minimize the risk of this toxicity include the co-administration of hydration and mesna.

4. The answer is E *[see 50.V.I; Table 50-1]*.
Etoposide has been associated with hypersensitivity reactions and infusion-related hypotension, likely due to the polysorbate 80 (Tween 80) contained in the injectable product.

5. The answer is A *[see 50.IV.D]*.
Leucovorin rescue should always be administered following high-dose methotrexate to minimize cytotoxic damage to normal, healthy cells. Omission of leucovorin in this setting can have fatal consequences.

Case 27

A 39-year-old man with documented alcoholic cirrhosis was admitted to the hospital's intensive care unit (ICU). He lost 25 lb over the last 5 months and has become weak and unable to take in adequate amounts of oral feedings. He also presents with increased pedal edema and significant electrolyte abnormalities.

1. The physician prescribes enteral tube feedings to meet his caloric and protein requirements. The primary reason for selecting this mode of nutrient delivery is to

   (A) prevent intestinal atrophy.
   (B) enhance his immune function.
   (C) provide the optimal route of nutrient delivery for ICU patients with chronic liver disease.
   (D) reverse his alcoholic cirrhosis.
   (E) C and D

2. After 3 days of enteral tube feedings, the patient is now presenting with persistent vomiting with episodes of hematemesis and diarrhea but is not encephalopathic. The ICU physician places him on central glucose system parenteral nutrition (PN). Which one of the following statement(s) is true in regard to his PN program?

   (A) Protein intake should be restricted to 0.8 to 1.2 g/kg/day.
   (B) Protein requirements should not be restricted to reduce the risk of developing hepatic encephalopathy.
   (C) A PN formulation enriched in essential amino acids should be the modality of choice.
   (D) A standard PN formulation that would meet his caloric and protein requirements would be appropriate in this patient.
   (E) B and D

3. The patient develops hepatic encephalopathy 4 days after initiation of his PN program. Which of the following is the most appropriate initial step to manage this adverse event?

   (A) Administer a PN formulation enriched in branched-chain amino acids and low in aromatic amino acids.
   (B) Supplement the current PN formulation with glutamine.
   (C) Provide a PN formulation that is enriched in essential amino acids.
   (D) Treat with luminal acting antibiotics and lactulose.
   (E) Discontinue PN for 3 to 4 days.

4. The patient responded to treatment for hepatic encephalopathy but he further deteriorates clinically with the development of renal failure. He now presents with decreased urinary output, elevated serum creatinine, and abdominal distention and tenderness. Which of the following would be the most appropriate strategy for the nutritional support of this ICU patient?

   (A) provide a low nitrogen, high caloric density PN formula
   (B) administer a PN formula enriched in aromatic amino acids and low in branched-chain amino acids
   (C) discontinue the PN until the renal failure resolves
   (D) provision of hemodialysis or continuous renal replacement therapy on a regular basis in order to provide adequate protein to achieve positive nitrogen balance
   (E) administer a PN formulation where the lipid component would comprise 40% to 50% of the nonprotein calories

5. The most appropriate base solution PN formula for this ICU patient would be

   (A) 4% HepatAmine/25% dextrose
   (B) 2% standard amino acids/47% dextrose
   (C) 4.25% essential amino acids/25% dextrose
   (D) 4.25% high–branched-chain amino acids/25% dextrose
   (E) 4.25% standard amino acids/25% dextrose

Answers to Case 27

1. The answer is C *[see 52.V.C.2]*.
Enteral nutrition (EN) is recommended whenever feasible as the optimal route of nutrient delivery for ICU patients with acute and/or chronic liver disease. EN has been shown to improve nutritional status, reduce complications, and prolong survival in liver disease patients.

2. The answer is E *[see 52.V.C.3]*.
Protein requirements in ICU patients should not be restricted as a clinical management strategy to reduce the risk of developing hepatic encephalopathy. The protein dose should be determined in the same manner as the general ICU patient. Standard formulas have not demonstrated definitive clinical differences in morbidity and mortality than the more expensive specialty formulations enriched in branched-chain amino acids and low in aromatic amino acids.

3. The answer is D *[see 52.V.C.1]*.
Enriched branched-chain amino acid formulations should be reserved for the rare encephalopathic patient who is refractory to standard treatment with luminal acting antibiotics and lactulose.

4. The answer is D *[see 52.V.B.3]*.
Dialysis therapy should not be avoided or delayed to provide ICU patients in renal failure adequate protein doses of 1.5 to 2.5 g/kg/day to achieve positive nitrogen balance.

5. The answer is E *[see 52.V.B.3]*.
Standard glucose system formulations (4.25% amino acid/25% dextrose) can generally be used in renal failure patients receiving hemodialysis or continuous replacement therapy (CRRT) on a regular basis. This formulation is particularly useful in critically ill ICU patients because it can provide adequate protein to attain positive nitrogen balance, which is not possible with renal failure PN.

Case 28

A recent trial compared the use of bivalirudin (Angiomax) to that of eptifibatide (Integrilin) and heparin in patients undergoing a percutaneous coronary intervention (PCI). A total of 6,114 patients were entered into the study, with 2,100 receiving bivalirudin, 2,005 receiving heparin, and 2,009 receiving eptifibatide. The success rates for each study population was 70% for bivalirudin; 65% for heparin; and 80% for eptifibatide. Associated costs for each group were as follows: bivalirudin, $10,000 for successes, $14,000 for failures; heparin, $13,500 for successes, $15,500 for failures; and eptifibatide, $12,000 for successes, $16,000 for failures.

1. Which of the following would be a useful approach to evaluating the above trial?

   (A) cost-utility analysis
   (B) cost of illness
   (C) decision analysis

2. Which of the following statements best represent the clinical and/or financial outcomes associated with the three treatment groups in the study?

   (A) Bivalirudin had the lowest average costs per patient and eptifibatide had the highest average costs per patient.
   (B) Heparin had lower average costs per patient compared to bivalirudin.
   (C) Eptifibatide had the lowest average costs per patient compared to heparin.
   (D) Eptifibatide represents the most cost-effective of the three treatment arms.
   (E) Bivalirudin provided the best quality-adjusted life years.

3. Which of the following choices represents the average costs with each arm of the trial?

   (A) bivalirudin costs were $11,200; heparin costs were $14,720; eptifibatide costs were $14,200
   (B) bivalirudin costs were $14,720; heparin costs were $11,200; eptifibatide costs were $14,200
   (C) bivalirudin costs were $11,200; heparin costs were $14,720; eptifibatide costs were $14,200
   (D) bivalirudin costs were $11,200; heparin costs were $14,200; eptifibatide costs were $14,720
   (E) bivalirudin costs were $14,200; heparin costs were $14,720; eptifibatide costs were $14,200

4. The process utilized to calculate the above answer is referred to as

   (A) decision analysis.
   (B) decision tree modeling.
   (C) averaging out and folding back.
   (D) monte carlo simulation.
   (E) multiattribute utility theory.

5. Based on the results of the above clinical trial, when evaluating all patients included in the trial, what was the average cost associated with the 6,114 patients treated in the trial?

   (A) $12,921
   (B) $13,240
   (C) $13,352
   (D) $13,373
   (E) $13,600

6. A pharmacoeconomic technique is frequently used in assessing utilities, in which several attributes can be used, in order to assess clinical, financial, and quality-of-life effects. Each attribute can be weighted from the perspective of each respective decision maker, in order to identify the most preferable therapy, service, etc. The technique is referred to as

   (A) cost-utility analysis.
   (B) cost-benefit analysis.
   (C) cost-effectiveness analysis.
   (D) multiattribute utility theory.
   (E) cost-minimization analysis.

Answers to Case 28

1. The answer is C *[see 54.V].*
Decision analysis is a systemic approach to decision making, which enables decision makers to compare therapies and assess the outcomes associated with each option, in order to choose the option with the best payoff.

2. The answer is A *[see 54.V.E].*
Bivalirudin costs = ($10,000 × .7% Success) + ($14,000 × .3% Failure) = $11,200 per patient

Heparin costs = ($13,500 × .65% Success) + ($15,500 × .35% Failure) = $14,200 per patient

Eptifibatide costs = ($12,000 × .80% Success) + ($16,000 × .20% Failure) = $14,720 per patient

3. The answer is D *[see 54.V.E].*
See above calculations.

4. The answer is C *[see 54.V.E].*
Averaging out and folding back is the process which is used after completing a decision tree, in order to calculate the respective outcomes for each decision made within the evaluation and the associated consequences of such decisions. The decision maker is able to compare the respective therapies, interventions, in order to formalize the clinical and financial outcomes associated with them.

5. The answer is C *[see 54.V.E].*
Average costs per PCI patient = ($ bivalirudin × % total population) + ($ heparin × % total population) + ($ eptifibatide × % total population)

Average costs per PCI patient = ($11,200 × .34%) + ($14,200 × .33%) + ($14,720 × .33%)

Average costs per PCI patient = ($3,808) + ($4,686) + ($4,858)

Average costs per PCI patient = $13,352

6. The answer is D *[see 54.IV.A–G].*
Multiattribute utility therapy is one technique utilized, which allows the decision maker to include more than two attributes into a single decision-making model, and provides the decision maker with the flexibility of assigning weights for the decision based on how important each of the attributes is in the final decision-making process. A key aspect of this is the identification of the "perspective" being taken; as the weight-based response will be impacted by the respective priorities for each attribute given by each potential decision maker.

Case 29

The patient is a 61-year-old obese woman with limited activity due to hip pain scheduled to undergo surgery for an elective hip replacement. Past medical history is significant for hypertension for 9 years, which is adequately controlled with pharmacologic therapy. She has documented chronic renal impairment with a stated creatinine clearance (Clcr) of 40 mL/min. Body mass index (BMI) is 33. She is a nonsmoker, no history of other cardiovascular disease, and no history of personal or familial DVT.

1. Which of the **new** oral agents would be appropriate for thromboprophylaxis against DVT/PE after the planned elective hip replacement surgery?

   (A) Dabigatran 150 mg by mouth administered twice daily for 10 days.
   (B) Rivaroxaban 10 mg by mouth administered once daily for 10 days.
   (C) Dabigatran 150 mg by mouth administered twice daily for 35 days.
   (D) Rivaroxaban 10 mg by mouth administered once daily for 35 days.

Directions for questions 2–3: The questions and incomplete statements in this section can be correctly answered or completed by **one or more** of the suggested answers. Choose the answer, **A–E**.

   (A) I only
   (B) III only
   (C) I and II
   (D) II and III
   (E) I, II, and III

2. Which of the **new** oral agents appropriate for prophylaxis against DVT/PE would *not* require dose adjustment for the stated Clcr of 40 mL/min?

   I. Rivaroxaban 10 mg by mouth administered once daily.
   II. Dabigatran 75 mg by mouth administered twice daily.
   III. Dabigatran 150 mg by mouth administered twice daily.

3. Which of the following conditions are there contraindication(s) or lack of clinical trials outcome data to support the use of the **new** oral agents?

   I. hypersensitivity
   II. active pathologic bleeding
   III. pregnancy and lactation

Answers to Case 29

1. The answer is D [*see 35.V.E.1.a; 35.V.E.5.a*].
At present time, only the oral direct factor Xa inhibitor (rivaroxaban) is approved for thromboprophylaxis against DVT/PE after the planned elective hip replacement surgery. Rivaroxaban is administered 10 mg by mouth once daily for 35 days based on the manufacturer's FDA-approved package insert. Dabigatran is approved by FDA to reduce the risk of stroke and systemic embolism in patients with nonvalvular atrial fibrillation.

2. The answer is A (I) [*see 35.V.E.6.b.(1)*].
Rivaroxaban is currently the only FDA approved new oral agent for prophylaxis against VTE after total joint replacement. For this patient with Clcr 40 mL/min, no dosage adjustment would be necessary.

3. The answer is E (I, II, and III) [*see 35.V.E.6.a.(1); 35.V.F.6.a.(1)*].
Both rivaroxaban and dabigatran are contraindicated in patients with known hypersensitivity reactions and in the presence of active pathologic bleeding. Rivaroxaban is contraindicated in the setting of pregnancy and lactation. Dabigatran lacks adequate well-controlled studies to support its use in the setting of pregnancy and lactation.

Case 30

TY is a 30-year-old Caucasian male recently diagnosed with obsessive compulsive disorder (OCD). His doctor would like you to help him treat TY's symptoms. The doctor has the following questions for you regarding OCD treatment.

1. TY's doctor would like your help selecting an initial medication to treat his symptoms. You recommend which of the following?

   (A) lorazepam (Ativan)
   (B) fluvoxamine (Luvox)
   (C) venlafaxine XR (Effexor XR)
   (D) olanzapine (Zyprexa)

2. An adequate medication trial for a patient diagnosed with OCD should be how long?

   (A) 2 to 4 weeks
   (B) 4 to 6 weeks
   (C) 6 to 8 weeks
   (D) 8 to 12 weeks

3. TY's doctor wants to know when clomipramine is recommended for OCD treatment. You tell her which of the following?

   (A) Clomipramine is a first-line treatment option.
   (B) Clomipramine should be used after failure of two to three trials of an SSRI.
   (C) Clomipramine should be used after failure of one trial with an SSRI.
   (D) Clomipramine is not recommended for OCD treatment.

4. What is the starting dose of clomipramine?

   (A) 25 mg
   (B) 50 mg
   (C) 100 mg
   (D) 150 mg

5. TY's doctor wants to know how long medication therapy should be continued for a patient following symptom remission of his or her initial episode. You tell her which of the following?

   (A) 3 to 6 months
   (B) 6 to 12 months
   (C) 12 to 24 months
   (D) Indefinitely

6. Which of the following statements about ADHD treatment is correct?

   (A) First-line treatment for moderate-to-severe symptoms is cognitive behavioral therapy (CBT).
   (B) First-line treatment for moderate-to-severe symptoms is stimulants.
   (C) First-line treatment for moderate-to-severe symptoms is nonstimulants.
   (D) First-line treatment for moderate-to-severe symptoms is pemoline (Cylert).

7. Which of the following statements about ADHD treatment is correct following the failure of a single trial with a stimulant medication? The medication trial was mixed amphetamine salt (Adderall).

   (A) The next treatment is to switch to cognitive behavioral therapy (CBT).
   (B) The next treatment is to switch to atomoxetine (Strattera).
   (C) The next treatment is to switch to bupropion (Wellbutrin SR).
   (D) The next treatment is to switch to a methylphenidate containing stimulant.

8. Which of the following nonstimulant medications is FDA approved for the treatment of adult ADHD?

   (A) bupropion (Wellbutrin SR)
   (B) extended-release guanfacine (Intuniv)
   (C) pemoline (Cylert)
   (D) atomoxetine (Strattera)

9. Which of the following is a contraindication to atomoxetine (Strattera) use in ADHD?

   (A) Combination with a stimulant medication
   (B) Clinical/laboratory evidence of liver injury
   (C) Stable cardiovascular disease
   (D) Depression

Answers to Case 30

1. The answer is B *[see 40.IV.D.3.a.1].*
Of the answers listed, fluvoxamine is a first-line treatment option for OCD.

2. The answer is D *[see 40.IV.D.4.a].*
The use of antidepressants treatment in OCD is longer, 8 to 12 weeks, compared to length of treatment with antidepressants used in order psychiatric illnesses, usually 4 to 8 weeks.

3. The answer is B *[see 40.IV.D.3.a.2].*
Clomipramine is recommended only after a patient fails two to three trials of SSRIs. Clomipramine has been shown to be as effective as the SSRIs; however, because of its adverse effect profile, it is recommended only after failure of SSRIs.

4. The answer is A *[see 40.IV.D.3.a.3].*
The starting dose of clomipramine is 25 mg. The maximum dose is 250 mg.

5. The answer is C *[see 40.IV.D.4.c].*
Following symptom remission medication should be continued for a period of 12 to 24 months. Patients who have multiple relapses of OCD symptoms throughout their life may require lifelong treatment.

6. The answer is B *[see 40.VI.D].*
Stimulant medications are recommended as first-line treatment because approximately 70% to 90% of patients will have a symptom response. Stimulants have a larger effect size and a lower number needed to treat compared to nonstimulants. Although pemoline is a stimulant medication, its use has fallen out of favor due to concerns over hepatotoxicity.

7. The answer is D *[see 40.VI.D.2.c].*
A trial of two stimulants (one methylphenidate and one amphetamine) is recommended as a first-line treatment before switching to a nonstimulant medication.

8. The answer is D *[see 40.VI.D.3.a].*
All of the choices are nonstimulant medications, but only atomoxetine is FDA approved for adult ADHD.

9. The answer is B *[see Table 40-10].*
Patients with evidence of clinical/laboratory evidence of liver injury is only contraindication listed to the use of atomoxetine.

Case 31

RT is a 6-year-old child who is currently experiencing signs and symptoms indicating a possible diagnosis of ADHD. He is currently in good health with no other medical or psychiatric comorbidities. His primary care physician would like to treat him for ADHD and asks your help.

1. RT's physician wants your recommendation for an initial treatment for RT. You recommend which of the following?

   (A) immediate release methylphenidate (Ritalin).
   (B) methylphenidate patch (Daytrana).
   (C) atomoxetine (Strattera).
   (D) long-acting methylphenidate (Ritalin LA).

2. RT's physician wants to know what is the usual dose range of your choice on previous number. You tell her which of the following?

   (A) 5 mg to 10 mg
   (B) 10 mg to 15 mg
   (C) 10 mg to 20 mg
   (D) 20 mg to 30 mg

3. On a 1-year follow-up visit, RT's mother states that he has not being doing well at school. She is worried the medication is no longer working. RT's physician would like to treat with another medication. Which of the following treatments is the next best option for a patient who failed only a single trial with a stimulant previously?

   (A) The next treatment is to switch to intermediate-acting methylphenidate (Methylin ER).
   (B) The next treatment is to switch to atomoxetine (Strattera).
   (C) The next treatment is to switch to bupropion (Wellbutrin SR).
   (D) The next treatment is to switch to a mixed amphetamine salt (Adderall).

4. RT's mom states that he is also very aggressive at time. His physician wants to know if any of the FDA-approved treatments help with aggression. You recommend which of the following?

   (A) bupropion (Wellbutrin SR).
   (B) atomoxetine (Strattera).
   (C) extended-release guanfacine (Intuniv).
   (D) mixed amphetamine salt (Adderall).

5. His doctor wants to begin a mixed amphetamine salt. She wants to know the difference in duration of effect between an immediate-release amphetamine salt (Adderall) versus a long-acting amphetamine salt (Adderall XR). You tell her which of the following?

   (A) 2 to 4 hrs with immediate-release amphetamine salt (Adderall) versus 6 to 8 with a long-acting amphetamine salt (Adderall XR)
   (B) 4 to 6 hrs with immediate-release amphetamine salt (Adderall) versus 6 to 8 with a long-acting amphetamine salt (Adderall XR)
   (C) 6 to 8 hrs with immediate-release amphetamine salt (Adderall) versus 8 to 10 with a long-acting amphetamine salt (Adderall XR)
   (D) 4 to 6 hrs with immediate-release amphetamine salt (Adderall) versus 8 to 12 with a long-acting amphetamine salt (Adderall XR)

6. Which of the following statements about insomnia treatment is correct?

   (A) First-line treatment for moderate-to-severe symptoms is zolpidem (Ambien).
   (B) First-line treatment for moderate-to-severe symptoms is mirtazapine (Remeron).
   (C) First-line treatment for moderate-to-severe symptoms is valerian root.
   (D) First-line treatment for moderate-to-severe symptoms is diphenhydramine.

7. Which of the following medications is melatonin-receptor agonist of melatonin receptors MT1 and MT2?

   (A) estazolam (ProSom)
   (B) trazodone (Desyrel)
   (C) ramelteon (Rozerem)
   (D) doxepin (Silenor)

8. Comparing benzodiazepines to benzodiazepine-receptor agonists, which of the following is correct?

   (A) Benzodiazepine-receptor agonists may have less rebound insomnia.
   (B) Benzodiazepine-receptor agonists may have greater potential for abuse.
   (C) Benzodiazepine-receptor agonists may have greater potential for rebound insomnia.
   (D) Benzodiazepine-receptor agonists offer no additional benefits compared to benzodiazepines.

9. Which pregnancy category do the 5 FDA-approved benzodiazepines belong?

   (A) Pregnancy category A
   (B) Pregnancy category B
   (C) Pregnancy category D
   (D) Pregnancy category X

Answers to Case 31

1. The answer is A *[see 40.VI.D.2.b]*.
Treatment with stimulants is started at the lowest possible dose and titrated slowly up to the maximal tolerated dose. Initiation of therapy usually starts with an immediate-release stimulant and then changes to an extended-release agent to minimize the number of doses per day.

2. The answer is C *[see Table 40-9]*.
The usual dosage range is 10 to 20 mg.

3. The answer is D *[see 40.VI.D.2.c]*.
A trial of two stimulants (one methylphenidate and one amphetamine) is recommended as a first-line treatment before switching to a nonstimulant medication.

4. The answer is C *[see 40.VI.D.3.c]*.
Extended-release guanfacine works by inhibiting central release of norepinephrine and by increasing blood flow to the prefrontal cortex. Benefit in disruptive behavior, aggression, and sleep may also be experienced with this medication.

5. The answer is D *[see Table 40-9]*.
Four to 6 hrs with immediate-release amphetamine salt (Adderall) versus 8 to 12 with a long-acting amphetamine salt (Adderall XR).

6. The answer is A *[see 40.VII.C.3.a]*.
Prescription medication for insomnia centers on the benzodiazepines and benzodiazepine-receptor agonists. Zolpidem is the only one listed that belongs to either of these two medication classes.

7. The answer is C *[see 40.VII.C.3.c]*.
Ramelteon is a melatonin-receptor agonist selectively targeting the melatonin receptors MT1 and MT2 located in the hypothalamus. Stimulating these receptors is thought to affect the sleep–wake cycle and promote sleep. This is the first and only agent in this medication class.

8. The answer is A *[see 40.VII.C.3.b.4]*.
Benzodiazepine-receptor agonists may have less rebound insomnia, potential for abuse and dependence, hangover effect, and rebound insomnia upon drug discontinuation compared to nonselective benzodiazepines.

9. The answer is D *[see 40.VII.E.1]*.
Benzodiazepines FDA approved for insomnia are all pregnancy category X.

Case 32

TR is a 46-year-old male who is currently experiencing difficulty falling and maintaining sleep indicating a possible diagnosis of insomnia. He is currently in good health with no other medical or psychiatric comorbidities. His primary care physician would like to treat him for insomnia and asks your help.

1. TR's physician wants to start eszopiclone (Lunesta). He wants to know the recommended usual dosage range and the half-life of this medication. You tell him which of the following?

   (A) Usual dosage range of 1 to 3 mg; half-life of 7 hrs
   (B) Usual dosage range of 3 to 5 mg; half-life of 5 hrs
   (C) Usual dosage range of 5 to 10 mg; half-life of 3 hrs
   (D) Usual dosage range of 3 to 5 mg; half-life of 14 hrs

2. TR's physician starts eszopiclone (Lunesta) and wants to know which of the following side effects to counsel the patient about. You tell him which of the following?

   (A) Rebound insomnia
   (B) Unpleasant taste
   (C) Anticholinergic side effects
   (D) Increased prolactin

3. After receiving benefit for 2 months with eszopiclone (Lunesta), TR would like to switch to a nonbenzodiazepine medication. TR's physician wants to start ramelteon (Rozerem) but wants to know what contraindications exist for this medication. You tell him which of the following?

   (A) Comorbid substance use disorder
   (B) Renal failure
   (C) Glaucoma
   (D) Hepatic failure

4. What is the usual dosage of ramelteon (Rozerem)?

   (A) 2
   (B) 4
   (C) 6
   (D) 8

5. What counseling points would you tell the patient about ramelteon (Rozerem)?

   (A) Take with a high-fat meal; take 1 hr prior to bed.
   (B) Do not take with a high-fat meal; avoid concomitant medications that induce CYP1A2 hepatic enzymes.
   (C) Take 30 mins prior to bed; ramelteon has no drug–drug interactions.
   (D) Ramelteon can cause anticholinergic side effects such as constipation and blurry vision.

Answers to Case 32

1. The answer is A *[see Table 40-11]*.
The usual dosage range of eszopiclone is 1 to 3 mg with a half-life of 7 hrs.

2. The answer is B *[see Table 40-11]*.
Eszopiclone is the only agent of this medication class to have an unpleasant taste listed as a side effect.

3. The answer is D *[see Table 40-11]*.
Ramelteon is contraindicated in patients with hepatic failure.

4. The answer is D *[see Table 40-11]*.
Ramelteon dose is 8 mg at bedtime.

5. The answer is B *[see 40.VII.C.3.c.5]*.
Ramelteon is a noncontrolled medication. It is metabolized by CYP1A2 hepatic enzymes. Do not take with a high-fat meal or use in a patient with severe hepatic impairment.

OTC and Related Questions

1. When a patient monitors his or her blood pressure at home, on average how many millimeters of mercury (mm Hg) is it different from in the office?

   (A) 5 mm Hg higher
   (B) 10 mm Hg higher
   (C) 3 mm Hg lower
   (D) 5 mm Hg lower
   (E) 10 mm Hg lower

2. Which of the following can be used to detect if a woman is ovulating?

   (A) vaginal pH kits
   (B) saliva test for estrogen
   (C) saliva test for progesterone
   (D) urinary test for human chorionic gonadotropin (hCG)
   (E) urinary test for ketones

3. When selecting a blood pressure monitoring device for a patient who lives alone and has dexterity issues, which of the following is most important to consider?

   (A) blood pressure cuff size
   (B) capability to store readings
   (C) cost of the monitoring device
   (D) size of the display monitor
   (E) use of the device with one hand

4. What is the difference between an oral temperature versus a rectal temperature?

   (A) Oral is 1°F higher than rectal.
   (B) Oral is 1°F lower than rectal.
   (C) Oral is 3°F higher than rectal.
   (D) Oral is 3°F lower than rectal.
   (E) There is no difference.

5. Which of the following products would be most appropriate for an individual who needs a crutch and has little or no hand strength (difficulty gripping a handle)?

   (A) axillary crutch
   (B) Canadian crutch
   (C) forearm crutch
   (D) quad crutch
   (E) platform crutch

6. Which of the following compounds may cause tooth discoloration with continuous use?

   (A) stannous fluoride
   (B) sodium fluoride
   (C) dibasic sodium citrate
   (D) sodium monofluorophosphate
   (E) sodium lauryl sulfate

7. Which of the following is a solution that is used to clean and moisten the surface of the contact lens while the lens is still in the eye?

   (A) cleaning solution
   (B) soaking solution
   (C) rewetting solution
   (D) conditioning solution

8. Which of the following is a true statement about the treatment of otic conditions?

   (A) The recommendation of a nonprescription otic product for self-care of vertigo is appropriate.
   (B) Ear candles are appropriate for the removal of cerumen if the wax is heated prior to insertion in the ear.
   (C) Swimmer's ear may be prevented by using a carbamide peroxide product prior to each water activity.
   (D) Isopropyl alcohol 95% in anhydrous glycerin is appropriate for self-care in a person with water-clogged ears.

9. A 60-year-old man presents to the pharmacy counter looking for a product to treat "floaters" in his eye. He denies other ocular symptoms, just the continuous presence of floaters when he looks in different directions. Which of the following would be the best recommendation for this person?

   (A) The lens has likely become detached from the eye and emergency medical treatment should be sought.
   (B) An ophthalmic demulcent should be recommended to assist in the dry eye that is causing the floater.
   (C) The floaters are likely due to the depletion of the vitreous humor and no treatment is necessary.
   (D) The symptoms are typical of macular degeneration and currently there are no over-the-counter (OTC) treatments.

10. An individual complains of itchy eyes associated with seasonal allergies. Which of the following would be the most appropriate recommendation for the ophthalmic symptoms?

    (A) ophthalmic demulcent
    (B) ophthalmic emollient
    (C) ophthalmic vasoconstrictor
    (D) ophthalmic antihistamine

11. Which of the following medications should alert you that a patient is not a candidate for self-care with nicotine replacement therapy (NRT)?

    (A) lisinopril (hypertension)
    (B) metoprolol (hypertension)
    (C) isosorbide dinitrate (severe angina)
    (D) levothyroxine (hypothyroidism)
    (E) metformin ER (diabetes mellitus)

12. JP is a 62-year-old man requesting self-care for smoking cessation. He currently smokes slightly over 1 pack/day; his first cigarette is about 10 minutes after he wakes. He has no diagnosed medical conditions and has dentures. Which of the following is the most appropriate recommendation for JP?

    (A) nicotine gum 2 mg
    (B) nicotine patch 7 mg
    (C) nicotine lozenge 2 mg
    (D) nicotine patch 21 mg
    (E) nicotine gum 4 mg

13. Which of the following patients would be appropriate to self-treat insomnia with doxylamine?

    (A) An 8-year-old girl whose parents just passed away.
    (B) A 90-year-old woman who naps consistently during the day.
    (C) A 56-year-old man with hypertension and diabetes.
    (D) A 64-year-old man with benign prostatic hypertrophy.

14. Which of the following patients would be an appropriate candidate for self-care with orlistat?

    (A) An individual who is 12 years old.
    (B) A patient diagnosed with bulimia.
    (C) A patient with a body mass index (BMI) of 20 kg/m^2.
    (D) A patient who is 40 lb overweight.

15. Which of the following would be the best self-care smoking cessation plan for an individual who currently smokes 2 to 3 packs/day with the first cigarette immediately upon awakening?

    (A) initiate two 14-mg nicotine patches
    (B) initiate a 21-mg nicotine patch
    (C) initiate 2-mg nicotine lozenges
    (D) initiate 14-mg patch and 2-mg gum
    (E) initiate no NRT agent for self-care

16. An individual with type 1 diabetes, BPH, and significantly uncontrolled hypertension requests a product for nasal congestion. Which of the following would be the best recommendation?

    (A) chlorpheniramine
    (B) topical phenylephrine
    (C) levmetamfetamine
    (D) oral phenylephrine
    (E) pseudoephedrine

17. A 28-year-old woman complains of nasal itching, rhinorrhea, and excessive sneezing, which she encounters every year. She typically does not treat the symptoms, but she needs to stay focused for her upcoming exams. She currently takes no other medications. Which of the following would be the best treatment to recommend?

    (A) diphenhydramine
    (B) cetirizine
    (C) pseudoephedrine
    (D) oxymetazoline
    (E) saline nasal spray

18. A mom requests a product to help with a productive cough and nasal congestion for her 12-month-old son. Which of the following represents the best recommendation?

    (A) pseudoephedrine
    (B) oxymetazoline
    (C) topical phenylephrine
    (D) saline nasal spray
    (E) guaifenesin

19. A 42-year-old man complains of nasal congestion and a sore throat. He regularly sees a chiropractor for neck pain. He has no other disease states and only takes Vicodin for his pain. Which of the following is the *best* recommendation for his congestion and sore throat?

    (A) chlorpheniramine
    (B) acetaminophen
    (C) pseudoephedrine
    (D) phenol spray
    (E) oral phenylephrine

20. Which of the following medications should be avoided in a patient who frequently takes Maalox (aluminum, magnesium, simethicone)?

    (A) fexofenadine
    (B) chlorpheniramine
    (C) loratadine
    (D) diphenhydramine
    (E) cetirizine

21. Which of the following self-care treatments would be appropriate to recommend for a child < 6 years old for constipation?

    (A) glycerin suppositories
    (B) polyethylene glycol
    (C) bisacodyl
    (D) mineral oil

22. All of the following are true regarding senna/sennoside laxatives *except*

    (A) sennosides may cause the urine to turn pink or red in color.
    (B) senna has demonstrated cathartic colon with extended use.
    (C) senna is appropriate for self-care in individuals over the age of 2 years.
    (D) sennosides are derived from the senna leaves.

23. All of the following agents would be an appropriate self-care recommendation for a person with heart failure *except*

    (A) sodium phosphate.
    (B) senna/sennosides.
    (C) docusate sodium.
    (D) glycerin.

24. Which of the following would be the most appropriate recommendation for an 8 year old who complains of diarrhea for several hours with no other symptoms, recent travel history, or dietary excursions?

    (A) loperamide
    (B) bismuth subsalicylate (BSS)
    (C) *Lactobacillus acidophilus*
    (D) lactase

25. Which of the following statements is true regarding the self-treatment of diarrhea?

    (A) Self-care is only appropriate for 7 days.
    (B) BSS may cause darkening of the tongue.
    (C) Loperamide is appropriate for individuals ≥ 2 years.
    (D) Prebiotics may be recommended as an antidiarrheal.

26. All of the following hemorrhoidal agents are acceptable to recommend for an individual with cardiovascular disease *except*

    (A) witch hazel.
    (B) mineral oil.
    (C) phenylephrine.
    (D) hydrocortisone.

27. Which of the following individuals would be an appropriate candidate for the recommendation of self-care with nonprescription levonorgestrel?

    (A) A 15-year-old girl who was sexually assaulted 3 hours ago.
    (B) A 32-year-old woman who intends on having intercourse tonight.
    (C) A 19-year-old woman who had unprotected intercourse 2 days ago.
    (D) A 22-year-old woman who had unprotected intercourse 6 days ago.
    (E) A 21-year-old woman who thinks she may be pregnant.

28. A woman complains of abdominal cramping and pain on the first day of menstruation. Which of the following would be the most appropriate recommendation?

    (A) acetaminophen
    (B) naproxen sodium
    (C) pamabrom
    (D) pyrilamine

29. A woman completed the 1-day treatment for vulvo-vaginal candidiasis 2 days ago but is still complaining of symptoms. Which of the following is the most appropriate recommendation?

    (A) Repeat treatment with the 1-day treatment.
    (B) Seek medical care to rule out bacterial infection.
    (C) Retreat with a 7-day treatment course.
    (D) No additional action is necessary at this time.

30. A perimenopausal female complains of constant vaginal dryness. She is single and has not had intercourse for the past 15 years. Which of the following would be the most appropriate recommendation for her vaginal dryness?

    (A) Petroleum jelly
    (B) Replens
    (C) Astroglide
    (D) K-Y INTRIGUE

31. Which of the following is an appropriate counseling point for a woman purchasing a basal thermometer?

    (A) Temperature should be taken each evening prior to bed.
    (B) The thermometer should obtain an accurate otic reading.
    (C) A temperature rise notes the start of the most fertile period.
    (D) Tension and stress may affect the temperature reading.

32. Which of the following male condoms is most likely to allow the transmission of HIV?

    (A) lambskin
    (B) latex
    (C) polyurethane
    (D) polyisoprene

Answers to OTC and Related Questions

1. The answer is D *[see 18.III]*.
A patient's blood pressure measured at home is typically 5 mm Hg lower than when measured in the office.

2. The answer is B *[see 18.V.4]*.
Fertility microscopes allow women to determine their most fertile time of the month by the appearance of a ferning pattern of their dried saliva. When estrogen levels rise with peak ovulation, there is an increase in the patient's salt levels in the saliva, resulting in a fernlike pattern in dried saliva.

3. The answer is E *[see 18.III]*.
The type of monitor to be selected or recommended should be determined by the patient's ability to use the product. In this patient who lives alone and has dexterity issue, the most important factor to consider is the ability for the patient to use the device with one hand. Selecting a monitoring device where the blood pressure cuff has a D-ring would enable this patient to use the device independently.

4. The answer is B *[see 18.XI.B.2]*.
The rectal temperature is 1°F higher and an axillary temperature is 1°F lower than an oral temperature. It is important when assessing a patient's temperature to know the location it was taken (oral vs. rectal vs. axillary).

5. The answer is E *[see 18.I.B.2]*.
An axillary, Canadian or forearm, and quad crutch all require the user to use their hands to grip the handle. A platform crutch is attached to the forearm with belts and does not require the user to grip them with their hands.

6. The answer is A *[see 19.II.B.2.d(1)]*.
The possibility of tooth discoloration may occur with the continuous use (2 to 3 months) of stannous fluoride. The staining is not permanent and may be removed by having a professional cleaning. The product is not recommended for patients less than 12 years old.

7. The answer is C *[see 19.III.F.2]*.
A rewetting solution is used to clean and moisten the surface of the contact lens while the lens is still in the eye.

8. The answer is D *[see 19.I.B]*.
Vertigo should be treated under the care of a medical provider. Ear candles are never an appropriate recommendation and carbamide peroxide is used for ear wax removal, not prevention of swimmer's ear. Isopropyl alcohol 95% in anhydrous glycerin 5% is appropriate for the treatment of water-clogged ears.

9. The answer is C *[see 19.III.A.7]*.
As one ages, the vitreous humor is lost and shadows are cast by various cells, giving the illusion of "floaters." There are no OTC treatments for this condition.

10. The answer is D *[see 19.III.C]*.
Ophthalmic demulcents and emollients are used to symptoms of dry eye, whereas ophthalmic vasoconstrictors reduce eye redness. Ophthalmic antihistamines are appropriate for ophthalmic conditions associated with allergic rhinitis.

11. The answer is C *[see 21.III.F.2.a]*.
Patients with acute cardiovascular disease (e.g., stroke, acute myocardial infarction, or severe angina) are not candidates for self-treatment with NRT products and should be referred to a health care provider.

12. The answer is D *[see 21.III.F.3]*.
Nicotine gum is inappropriate for this patient because he has dentures. The strength of the lozenge must be 4 mg because the patient smokes within 30 minutes of waking in the morning. The 7-mg patch is not an appropriate starting dose for a patient smoking over 1 pack/day.

13. The answer is C *[see 21.II.B.5.b.(1–2)]*.
Appropriate use of self-care for insomnia is for patients older than 12 years of age. Antihistamines such as doxylamine should be avoided in patients who are elderly, at high risk for falls, have benign prostatic hyperplasia (BPH), or narrow-angle glaucoma. However, there are no contraindications to the use of this agent in patients with hypertension or diabetes.

14. The answer is D *[see 21.I.B.2]*.
Appropriate use of self-care with orlistat is a patient who is greater than 18 years of age who is mildly to moderately overweight (BMI of 25 to 28). It is not appropriate for self-care in patients with diagnosed eating disorders.

15. The answer is E *[see 21.III.F.1; III.F.3]*.
On the basis that a cigarette contains approximately 1 mg of nicotine, self-care with NRT is appropriate for individuals who smoke less than 1.5 packs/day. Based on current practice recommendations, dual NRT therapy is not recommended for self-care, nor is doubling of nicotine patches. The doses of the 21-mg patch and the 2-mg lozenge are insufficient for this patient who smokes 2 to 3 packs/day with the first cigarette immediately in the morning. This patient should be referred for a prescription product or be instructed to cut back to at least 1.5 packs/day for improved success with NRT.

16. The answer is C [*see 22.II.F.1.b*].
All topical and oral decongestants should be used with extreme caution in patients with disease states that are sensitive to adrenergic stimulation (e.g., type 1 diabetes, hypertension, difficulty in urination owing to an enlarged prostate gland). Levmetamfetamine lacks vasopressor effects and can therefore be used in such patients.

17. The answer is B [*see 22.III.E.2*].
Pseudoephedrine and oxymetazoline are inappropriate recommendations because they treat nasal congestion. Saline nasal spray will only moisten the nasal passages for easier removal of congestion. Diphenhydramine is a first-generation antihistamine and will likely cause significant sedation. Cetirizine is a second-generation antihistamine and will likely treat the symptoms without significant sedation.

18. The answer is D [*see 22.II.F.1; II.F.5; II.F.7*].
The only answer choice that is appropriate to recommend for self-care for individuals less than the age of 2 is saline nasal spray.

19. The answer is C [*see 22.II.F.1; Table 22-1*].
Likely, the sore throat the patient is experiencing is attributable to nasal drainage. Treating the sore throat alone with phenol spray will do little to alleviate the nasal congestion. Acetaminophen should not be recommended due to therapeutic duplication with his Vicodin. Pseudoephedrine has better bioavailability than oral phenylephrine, thus serves as a better recommendation for treatment of the nasal congestion. This patient does not appear to have any contraindications to the use of pseudoephedrine.

20. The answer is A [*see 22.III.E.2.b.(2)*].
Concomitant administration of aluminum and magnesium-containing acids (e.g., Maalox) may decrease the absorption and peak plasma concentrations of fexofenadine.

21. The answer is A [*see 23.I.B.2*].
Glycerin suppositories can be used in ages 2 and older, but polyethylene glycol (e.g., MiraLAX) is not appropriate for self-care in those < 17 years old and bisacodyl is not appropriate in those < 6 years old. Mineral oil should not be recommended in the pediatric population as self-care for constipation.

22. The answer is B [*see 23.I.B.2.c*].
Senna is appropriate for individuals over the age of 2 and may cause discoloration of the urine. Sennosides are derived from the senna leaves. Although senna has been associated with cathartic colon when used for extended periods of time, no evidence exists that this does occur.

23. The answer is A [*see 23.I.B.2*].
Sodium phosphate is a saline laxative which should be avoided in individuals with sodium restricted diets, such as individuals with heart failure. Although docusate sodium contains sodium, it is an insignificant amount and does not require caution with use in a person with heart failure. Senna and glycerin are both appropriate to use in persons with heart failure.

24. The answer is A [*see 23.II.C.2*].
Loperamide is approved for those over the age of 6, whereas BSS is only approved for ages 12+ years for self-care. Lactase is only appropriate for individuals with a lactase deficiency, which is not demonstrated in this case. *L. acidophilus* is a probiotic, which may be recommended for maintenance of normal gastrointestinal function, but is not a prudent recommendation for treatment of acute, nonspecific diarrhea.

25. The answer is B [*see 23.II.C.2*].
Self-care for diarrhea should be limited to 2 days with BSS or loperamide. Loperamide is approved for those ≥ 6 years of age and prebiotics have no role in the management of diarrhea. BSS may cause a harmless darkening of the tongue and stools.

26. The answer is C [*see 23.III.F.2*].
At recommended doses, the risk of individuals receiving enough systemic absorption from hemorrhoidal vasoconstrictors (phenylephrine) to develop cardiovascular or central nervous system effects is minimal; however, in those with cardiovascular disease, anxiety disorders, or thyroid disease, an agent that does not contain a vasoconstrictor is a prudent recommendation.

27. The answer is C [*see 24.III.B.7*].
Levonorgestrel as emergency contraception is appropriate for nonprescription purchase only for individuals ages 17 and older. It is not appropriate to be used prior to intercourse, as it is not a method of birth control. It should be used within 72 hours of intercourse and is not effective once implantation has occurred.

28. The answer is B [*see 24.I.B.1.d.(2)*].
Nonsteroidal anti-inflammatory drugs (NSAIDs) are the drug of choice for dysmenorrhea. Acetaminophen lacks an effect on prostaglandins and thus would not be appropriate. Pamabrom is a diuretic and pyrilamine is an antihistamine.

29. The answer is D *[see 24.II.A.4.d.(3)]*.
It typically takes 5 to 7 days for the symptoms of vulvovaginal candidiasis (VVC) to resolve, despite treatment with a 1-, 3-, or 7-day course of therapy. The 1- and 3-day treatments are for convenience only and should not be misinterpreted as the time to symptom resolution. If symptoms have not cleared up within 7 days, the woman should consult the care of a medical professional.

30. The answer is B *[see 24.II.B.2–3]*.
Vaginal lubricants (e.g., K-Y INTRIGUE and Astroglide) are for immediate relief of vaginal dryness and are mostly used prior to intercourse. The vaginal dryness presented in this patient is chronic vaginal dryness. Thus, a vaginal moisturizer such as Replens would be more appropriate. Petroleum jelly is an oil-based lubricant that can harbor bacteria in the vagina and lead to infections.

31. The answer is D *[see 24.III.B.1.b]*.
The basal body temperature (BBT) should be taken in the morning prior to arising from bed. Temperature can be taken orally, vaginally, or rectally, depending on the thermometer purchased. A rise in temperature notes ovulation, thus the fertile time period has passed. Changes in the BBT may be due to infection, tension, a restless night, or any type of excessive movement.

32. The answer is A *[see 24.III.B.3]*.
Lambskin condoms have pores which may allow the transmission of HIV or hepatitis B.

1. How much zinc oxide powder should you add to 2 oz (AV) of 5% zinc oxide (ZnO) ointment to make a 10% ZnO ointment?

   (A) 1.6 g
   (B) 3.15 g
   (C) 3.46 g
   (D) 2.84 g
   (E) 95 g

2. How many milliliters of gentamicin injection (40 mg/mL) would you need to give a 7 mg/kg of body weight dose via an intravenous infusion to a 200-lb adult patient?

   (A) 1.6 mL
   (B) 8.0 mL
   (C) 15.9 mL
   (D) 32.0 mL
   (E) 35.0 mL

3. What is the ratio strength of a 0.04% mass/volume (w/v) solution of gentian violet?

   (A) 4:1
   (B) 4:100
   (C) 1:4,000
   (D) 1:2,500
   (E) 1:10,000

4. How many milliliters of a 20% potassium chloride (KCl) solution are to be given to an 80-kg patient who has been ordered a single 30 mEq dose? (KCl molecular weight [mw] = 74.5.)

   (A) 11.2 mL
   (B) 15.0 mL
   (C) 20.0 mL
   (D) 22.0 mL
   (E) 40.0 mL

5. The formula below is for an oral mixture used to treat pain and infections in the mouth. How many units of nystatin would be in a usual two teaspoonful dose given to a patient?

   Rx
   Nystatin 100,000 units/mL   60 mL
   Solu-Cortef   240 mg
   Benadryl Elixir   qs 480 mL

   (A) 37,500 units
   (B) 62,500 units
   (C) 100,000 units
   (D) 125,000 units
   (E) 1,000,000 units

6. How much does 3 lb of glycerine cost if you paid $4.75 per pint (specific gravity [SG] of glycerine is 1.25)?

   (A) $4.75
   (B) $5.97
   (C) $10.95
   (D) $17.10
   (E) $21.88

7. Calculating doses is frequently based on the patient's weight, but the actual, ideal body weight (IBW), or adjusted body weight (ABW) may be used. Formulas are shown below:

   IBW (Men) = 50 kg + 2.3 kg (# of inches greater than 60 in height)

   IBW (Women) = 45 kg + 2.3 kg (# of inches greater than 60 in height)

   ABW = IBW + 0.4 (actual weight − IBW)

   What is the adjusted body weight for a 6 ft 2 in. man who weighs 112 kg?

   (A) 94 kg
   (B) 112 kg
   (C) 11.9 kg
   (D) 82 kg

8. How many grams of hydrocortisone (HC) and how many grams of Eucerin ointment (EU) are needed to make 120 g of 3% HC in Eucerin ointment?

   (A) HC = 3.6 g, EU = 120.0 g
   (B) HC = 3.0 g, EU = 97.0 g
   (C) HC = 3.7 g, EU = 120.0 g
   (D) HC = 3.6 g, EU = 116.4 g

9. The patient in 3 East has been receiving aminophylline at 45 mg/hr and achieved a steady-state theophylline level of 16 mg/L. Which of the following schedules for Theo-Dur will come the closest to producing the 16 mg/L blood levels? Note: Theo-Dur in scored 100-mg, 200-mg, or 300-mg tablets provide approximately constant rate delivery for about 12 hours and has a usual bioavailability of 100%. Aminophylline is 80% theophylline.

   (A) Theo-Dur 900 mg po at 9 A.M. daily.
   (B) Theo-Dur 450 mg (1.5 of the 300-mg tabs) po q12h
   (C) Theo-Dur 400 mg po q8h
   (D) Theo-Dur 350 mg (1 × 300 mg, ½ of 100 mg) q8h

10. What is the # of mL/hr infusion rate to provide 10 μg/min of nitroglycerine if the bottle has 50 mg of NTG per 500 mL?

    (A) 6 mL/hr
    (B) 10 mL/hr
    (C) 12 mL/hr
    (D) 20 mL/hr

11. What is the creatinine clearance for Bill, using the full C-G equation below, if his ideal body weight is 62 kg, he is 72 years old, with a serum creatinine of 2.8 mg/dL?

    CrCl = [(140 − age in years)(IBW)] / [(SrCr)(72)]

    (A) 24 mL/min
    (B) 120 mL/min
    (C) 21 mL/min
    (D) 72 mL/min

12. Most practice areas have a standard protocol for heparin infusions and adjustments based on results. What mL/hr infusion rate is to be used for your protocol, which starts with 18 units/kg per hour, for a 62-kg patient? The heparin infusion contains 25,000 units per 500 mL.

    (A) 22.3 mL/hr
    (B) 1,120.0 mL/hr
    (C) 10.1 mL/hr
    (D) 62.0 mL/hr

13. With all of the national back orders in pharmacy today, you are not surprised to hear that your wholesaler will not be able to fill your order for methylprednisolone (Medrol) tablets for at least 8 weeks. What dose of prednisone, from the following equivalency table, would you recommend for a patient on 8 mg of Medrol po bid?

GLUCOCORTICOID INTERMEDIATE-ACTING COMPARISON

Drug	Equivalent Dose in mg	Anti-inflammatory Potency	Mineralo-corticoid Potency
Methylprednisolone	4	5	0
Prednisone	5	4	1
Prednisolone	5	4	1
Triamcinolone	4	5	0

   (A) 5 mg po bid meals
   (B) 20 mg po bid meals
   (C) 10 mg po bid meals
   (D) 6 mg po bid meals

14. Augmentin (amoxicillin/K clavulanate) is available in an ES form containing 600 mg/5 mL (amoxicillin component) and is generally dosed at 90 mg/kg per day, divided q12h. What is the dose in milliliters that will be given every 12 hours to a 40-lb patient?

    (A) 3.0 mL
    (B) 13.5 mL
    (C) 3.0 mL
    (D) 6.8 mL

15. The MD orders "Lovenox per protocol for treatment of DVT." You determine that an appropriate dose could be 1 mg/kg SQ bid for this patient, who has good renal function. What is the approximate dose to be injected twice daily for a 248-lb patient?

    (A) 80 mg
    (B) 110 mg
    (C) 248 mg
    (D) 220 mg

16. You own a compounding-able pharmacy and are presented with a prescription for fortified gentamicin eye drops 5 mg/mL. You have in stock gentamicin injection at 40 mg/mL and a 5 mL gentamicin eye drop labeled to contain 3 mg/mL of gentamicin. How many milliliters of the injection should be added to the 5 mL of the commercial eye drop to give it a 5 mg/mL "fortified" concentration?

    (A) 0.29 mL
    (B) 0.25 mL
    (C) 1.00 mL
    (D) 0.50 mL

17. A refrigerator in your pharmacy is set at 4°C. What is this temperature in degrees Fahrenheit?

    (A) 7.2°F
    (B) 34.4°F
    (C) 39.2°F
    (D) 64.8°F

18. A prescription calls for 1/8 gr of drug in each fluid dram of a liquid product. How many milligrams are in each 100 mL of the product?

    (A) 2.20
    (B) 3.39
    (C) 27.60
    (D) 220.00

19. If the specific gravity of glycerine is 1.25, what is the cost of 1 pt of glycerine bought at $8.23 per pound?

    (A) $6.86
    (B) $8.57
    (C) $10.72
    (D) $13.04

20. A prescription calls for 4 mg of atropine on a balance where 180 mg is the least weighable quantity with the precision desired. Which of the following choices will provide the 4 mg correctly, using lactose as the diluent?

    (A) weigh 180 mg drug, dilute with 8100 mg of lactose, and weigh 180 mg of mixture
    (B) weigh 100 mg drug, dilute with 2400 mg of lactose, and weigh 100 mg of mixture
    (C) weigh 180 mg drug, dilute with 8820 mg of lactose, and weigh 200 mg of mixture
    (D) weigh 180 mg drug, dilute with 4320 mg of lactose, and weigh 100 mg of mixture

21. A hospital pharmacist is asked to prepare an intravenous infusion of dopamine. Based on the patient's weight, the pharmacist calculates a dose of 500 μg/min for continuous infusion. The concentration of a premixed dopamine infusion is 400 mg/250 mL. How many milligrams of dopamine is the patient to receive in the first hour of treatment?

    (A) 0.5 mg
    (B) 18.75 mg
    (C) 30 mg
    (D) 30,000 mg

22. A proper dose of methylprednisolone for pediatric patients is 2 mg/kg/day divided into 4 doses given every 6 hours. How many milliliters of a 5 mg/mL stock solution should be used for each dose for a 38-lb patient?

    (A) 1.7 mL
    (B) 3.8 mL
    (C) 6.9 mL
    (D) 8.6 mL

23. How many milliliters of sulfuric acid labeled 96% w/w, s.g. 1.80 will be needed to make 12 fl oz of 5% w/v sulfuric acid?

    (A) 10.3
    (B) 18.5
    (C) 24.2
    (D) 33.3

24. Rx benzalkonium chloride 17% w/v   qs

    Water qs   120 mL

    M. ft. solution such that 2 tbsp added to a pint of water will yield a 1:750 solution.

    How many milliliters of the 17% w/v stock solution will be needed to prepare the 120 mL?

    (A) 2.68
    (B) 7.90
    (C) 15.80
    (D) 20.40

25. A treatment for a patient diagnosed with cancer includes the use of methotrexate at a starting dose of 360 mg/m^2 except in patients with decreased renal function, in which case this dose is reduced by 30%. How many milligrams of methotrexate should a patient with decreased renal function and a body surface area of 0.93 m^2 receive?

    (A) 252
    (B) 234
    (C) 108
    (D) 300

26. A multidose vial of penicillin contains 5,000,000 units per 10 mL after reconstitution. How many milliliters of this solution would be needed to give the patient a 25,000 unit test dose of penicillin?

    (A) 0.005
    (B) 0.05
    (C) 2
    (D) 20

27. How many milliliters of 50% dextrose solution should be added to 250 mL of 10% dextrose solution to yield a 12.5% dextrose solution (assume volumes are additive)?

    (A) 16.7
    (B) 62.5
    (C) 25.0
    (D) 12.5

28. A Terazol vaginal cream contains 0.8% (w/w) of terconazole. If 40 mg of drug is administered in each applicatorful of cream, calculate the weight, in grams, of each applicatorful.

    (A) 0.04 g
    (B) 5 g
    (C) 500 g
    (D) 5000 g

29. How many milliliters of a 1:50 w/v boric acid solution can be prepared from 500 mL of a 12% w/v boric acid solution?

    (A) 30
    (B) 1200
    (C) 2500
    (D) 3000

30. Determine if the following commercial product is hypertonic, approximately isotonic, or hypotonic, using sodium chloride equivalent values.

    Mannitol 5% w/v intravenous solution
    (E value for mannitol is 0.18)

    (A) hypotonic
    (B) approximately isotonic
    (C) hypertonic
    (D) cannot be determined from this data

31. Rx lithium carbonate 300 mg

    Dispense #60
    Sig: 1 cap po qid

    How many milliequivalents of lithium are provided daily to the patient by the prescription above? (Lithium carbonate, Li_2CO_3, MW = 74) (Li, MW = 7).

    (A) 4.06
    (B) 16.2
    (C) 155
    (D) 32.4

Answers to Practice Calculations

1. The answer is B, 3.15 g. The key point in this problem is that the weight of the added ZnO powder must be included in the total weight of the final product.

2. The answer is C, 15.9 mL. This is solved primarily by unit analysis and ratio and proportion.

3. The answer is D, 1:2,500.

4. The answer is A, 11.2 mL. This is solved by % w/v and electrolyte calculation. Students and pharmacists are generally expected to remember most basic chemicals and valences.

5. The answer is D, 125,000 units. This is characteristically an increase or decrease formula size question, simply handled by ratio and proportion.

6. The answer is C, $10.95. To solve this problem, you must refer to definitions of SG and convert volume to weight, then use ratio and proportion for determining cost. Although a "calculation," this is an important process to determine if the pharmacy is being reimbursed appropriately for a particular compounded product.

7. The correct answer is A, 94 kg.

> IBW = 50 kg + (14) 2.3 kg, equals 82.2 kg male, 14 in over 5 ft tall
> ABW = 82.2 kg + 0.4 (112 kg − 82.2 kg), equals 94 kg

8. The correct answer is D, HC = 3.6 g, EU = 116.4 g. For HC, 3% = 3 g/100 g, or 3.6 g/120 g, qs to 120 g with EU.

9. The correct answer is B, Theo-Dur 450 mg (1.5 of the 300 mg tabs) po q12h. Calculate theophylline equivalent from aminophylline per 24 hours. Give q12h or more frequently with this product.

> 45 mg/hr Aminophylline is 1080 mg aminophylline per day
> Theophylline = 80% of 1080 mg or 864 mg/day
> Closest answer is 450 mg po bid

10. The correct answer is A, 6 mL/hr. Be careful with mg to microgram conversion.

> 10 µg/min = 600 µg/hr
> 50 mg per 500 mL = 50,000 mcg/500 mL, or 100 µg/mL
> (600 µg/hr)(1 mL/100 µg) = 6 mL/hr

11. The correct answer is C, 21 mL/min. Remember these are "empirical equations" so units do not divide out as anticipated.

$$\text{CrCl} = [(140 - 72)(62)]/[(2.8)(72)] = 21 \text{ mL/min}$$

12. The correct answer is A, 22.3 mL/hr.

> (18 units/kg per hour)(62 kg) = 1,116 units/hr
> 25,000 units/500 mL = 50 units/mL
> (1,116 units/hr)(1.0 mL/50 units) = 22.3 mL/hr

13. The correct answer is C, 10 mg po bid meals. Simple ratio/proportion, look up the data in national publications.

14. The correct answer is D, 6.8 mL. Convert to kilogram, and either use 45 mg/kg per dose or 90 mg/kg per day and then divided by 2. Example calculation:

> (40.0 lb) (1 kg/2.2 lb) = 18.2 kg
> (45 mg/kg per dose)(18.2 kg) = 818 mg per dose

$$\frac{600\ mg}{818\ mg} = \frac{5\ mL}{X\ mL}$$

$$X = 6.8 \text{ mL}$$

15. The correct answer is B, 110 mg. Convert patient's weight to 110 kg.

16. The correct answer is A, 0.29 mL. Please note you are not to qs to 5 mL but adding to the 5 mL. Use alligation which adjusts for the added volume. You may use either mg/mL concentration or % (example for % shown below). Note: The 0.3% is the original eye drop, the 4.0% is the 40 mg/mL injection, and the 0.5% is the 5 mg/mL desired final concentration.

0.3%	3.5 parts	
	0.5%	
4.0%	0.2 parts,	total = 3.7 parts

Then you solve the ratio proportion that:

$$\frac{3.5\ parts}{0.2\ parts} = \frac{5\ mL}{X\ mL}$$

$$X = 0.29 \text{ mL}$$

17. The correct answer is C, 39.2°F.

> Use standard equation, F = (9/5) C + 32

18. The correct answer is D, 220 mg. A fluid dram is 3.69 mL.

$$\frac{\left[(1/8 \ gr)\left(\dfrac{65 \ mg}{grain}\right)\right]}{X \ mg} = \frac{3.69 \ mL}{100 \ mL}$$

19. The correct answer is C, $10.72.

1 pt = 473 mL = 473 g if water, but 1.25 × 473 g = 591 g if glycerine

$$\frac{591 \ g}{454 \ g} = \frac{\$Y}{\$8.23}$$

20. The correct answer is C, weigh 180 mg drug, dilute with 8820 mg of lactose, and weigh 200 mg of mixture.

$$\frac{4 \ mg \ of \ drug \ desired}{180 \ mg \ of \ drug \ weighed} =$$

$$\frac{200 \ mg \ of \ mixture \ weighed}{(180 \ mg \ of \ drug + 8820 \ mg \ of \ diluent) \ made}$$

21. The correct answer is C, 30 mg. Note: The bag concentration is not needed.

$$\left(\frac{500 \ \mu g}{1 \ min}\right)[60 \ min]\left[\frac{1 \ mg}{1000 \ \mu g}\right] = Z$$

22. The correct answer is A, 1.7 mL. Use string identities, multiplied together.

$$(38 \ lb)\left(\frac{1 \ kg}{2.2 \ lb}\right)\left(\frac{2 \ mg}{kg}\right)\left(\frac{1 \ day}{4 \ doses}\right)\left[\frac{1 \ mL}{5 \ mg}\right] = Z \ mL/dose$$

23. The correct answer is A, 10.3 mL. Use s.g. to convert % w/v to % w/w.

12 fl oz = 354.8 mL
100 mL = 100 g if water, 180 g if the s.g. = 1.8
180.00 g × 0.96 = 172.80 g of sulfuric acid in 100 mL
or 172.8% w/v
(172.8%)(Y) = (354.8 mL)(5%)
Y = 10.3 mL

24. The correct answer is C, 15.8 mL. This is a multistep problem. First is to find how much drug is in diluted solution. Note: The 2 tbsp were added to a pint.

$$\frac{1 \ g}{Y} = \frac{750 \ mL}{(473 \ mL + 30 \ mL)}, Y = 0.671 \ g$$

This is also the amount of drug in 2 tbsp of 120 mL preparation.

Therefore, amount in 120 mL is 4 × 0.671 g or 2.683 g.
Finally, you have a 17% stock solution from which to get the 2.683 g,

$$\frac{2.683 \ g}{17 \ g} = \frac{X \ mL}{(100 \ mL)}, X = 15.8 \ mL$$

25. The correct answer is B, 234 mg. The 0.7 is from the adjustment for renal function.

$$\left(\frac{360 \ mg}{m^2}\right)(0.93 \ m^2)(0.7) = 234 \ mg$$

26. The correct answer is B, 0.05 mL. Use ratio/proportion.

$$\frac{5,000,000 \ units}{25,000 \ units} = \frac{10 \ mL}{Q \ mL}, Q = 0.05 \ mL$$

27. The correct answer is A, 16.7 mL. Use an alligation or complex algebra solution. Must consider you are adding to the 250 mL.

50.0%   2.5 parts
          12.5%
10.0%   37.5 parts,   total = 40.0 parts

$$\frac{250 \ mL}{x \ mL} = \frac{37.5 \ parts}{2.5 \ parts}$$

28. The correct answer is B, 5 g. Use ratio/proportion.

0.8% = 0.8 g/100 g so 0.04 g (which is 40 mg) is in X g, or X = 5 g

29. The correct answer is D, 3000 mL. Convert ratio strength to % w/v, then (C1)(V1) = (C2)(V2)

1:50 is 1 g in 50 mL, or 2 g in 100 mL, or 2%
therefore (500 mL) 12% = 2% (x mL), or 3000 mL

30. The correct answer is B. approximately isotonic.

5% mannitol = 5 g/100 mL, 5 g × (E value of 0.18) = 0.9 g
of NaCl that the 5 g of mannitol is equivalent to 0.9 g NaCl
per 100 mL = 0.9% = isotonic

31. The correct answer is D, 32.4 mEq.

Milliequivalent weight is MW divided by valence. Qid dosing of 300 mg = 1200 mg dose daily
1 mEq of lithium carbonate is 74 mg / valence of 2 for the compound; 1200 mg/37 mg per mEq is 32.4 mEq.

Additional review problems from *Pharmaceutical Calculations*, 14e, by Howard Ansel.

A. FUNDAMENTAL SYSTEMS AND METHODS OF PHARMACEUTICAL CALCULATIONS

Weighing Accuracy

1. What is the least amount that should be weighed on Class A prescription balances with the following sensitivity requirements (SRs) and maximum errors?

   (A) SR 5 mg; error NMT 5%
   (B) SR 6 mg; error NMT 5%
   (C) SR 7 mg; error NMT 4%

2. Calculate the percentage error in the following weighings:

   (A) 6 mg in 120 mg weighing
   (B) 10 mg in 115 mg weighing

3. Rx   Drug A   0.5 mg
       Lactose   300
       M. ft. such caps # 12

   Using a torsion prescription balance with a sensitivity requirement of 6 mg, explain how to obtain the correct amount of drug A with an error not greater than 5%.

International System of Units and Intersystem Conversions

4. Perform the following equivalencies:

   (A) 5 mg/dL = _____ μg/mL
   (B) 40 mg/kg = _____ mg/lb
   (C) 0.04 μg/μL = _____ mg/mL
   (D) 500 g = _____ kg
   (E) 12 ℨ = _____ mL
   (F) 1½ pt = _____ mL
   (G) 40°F = _____ °C

5. How many grams of levothyroxine sodium (Synthroid; Abbott Laboratories, Abbott, IL) would a manufacturing pharmacist need to manufacture a batch of 250,000 tablets, each containing 25 μg of the drug?

6. A certain injectable solution contains 30 mg of a drug substance in 30 mL. How many milliliters of the solution would provide 100 μg of the drug substance?

7. How many grams of codeine phosphate are left in an original 5-g bottle after the amount required to prepare 100 capsules, each containing 15 mg of codeine phosphate, is used?

8. Ibandronate sodium (Boniva; Genentech, South San Francisco, CA) tablets are available in 2.5-mg and 150.0-mg strengths. The 2.5-mg tablets are taken daily, whereas the 150.0-mg tablets are taken once per month. Calculate the difference in the quantity of drug taken during a 30-day month.

   (A) 37.5 mg
   (B) 0.075 g
   (C) 137.5 mg
   (D) 0.150 g

9. Premature octuplets born in 1998 ranged in weight from the smallest, 10.3 oz, to the largest, 1 lb 9.7 oz. Convert these weights to grams.

10. A 240-mL serving of cough syrup contains 0.6 g of diphenhydramine hydrochloride. Which of the following strengths is correct?

    (A) 0.025 g/100 mL
    (B) 2500 μg/mL
    (C) 0.74 g/fl oz
    (D) 1.25 mg/tsp

11. If 30 mL of an injection containing metoclopramide (Reglan; Wyeth Pharmaceuticals, Madison, NJ), 5 mg/mL, are used to prepare 50 mL of an intravenous infusion, calculate the concentration of metoclopramide, on a mg/mL basis, in the infusion.

12. The fatal dose of cocaine has been approximated at 1.2 g for a 150-lb person. Express this effect on a mg/kg basis.

13. If a patient is determined to have 100 mg blood glucose/100 mL of blood, what is the equivalent concentration in terms of mg/dL?

14. Calculate the difference, in μg/mL, between two injections, each containing filgrastim (Neupogen; Amgen, Thousand Oaks, CA), one at 0.3 mg/0.5 mL and the other 480 μg/0.8 mL.

15. Azelastine nasal spray (Astelin; Meda Pharmaceuticals, Somerset, NJ) contains 0.1% w/v of azelastine hydrochloride. A container is capable of delivering 200 metered sprays of 0.137 mL each. How much azelastine hydrochloride would be contained in each spray?

    (A) 137 μg
    (B) 13.70 mg
    (C) 0.00137 g
    (D) 1.37 mg

16. Using the above problem data, how much nasal spray would be contained in the package?

    (A) 27.4 mL
    (B) 20.0 mL
    (C) 1.00 fl oz
    (D) 0.75 fl oz

17. Lantus (Sanofi, Bridgewater, NJ) contains 100 international units of insulin glargine, equivalent to 3.6378 mg/mL of injection. How many milligrams of insulin glargine would be present in each 0.8 mL of injection?

Specific Gravity

18. Calculate the following specific gravities:

    (A) 120 mL weigh 112 g
    (B) 96 mL weigh 104 g
    (C) 5 L of a syrup weighing 6.565 kg

19. Calculate the following weights:

    (A) 400 mL with a specific gravity of 1.25
    (B) 1 pt with a specific gravity of 0.90

20. Calculate the following volumes:

    (A) 30 g with a specific gravity of 0.90
    (B) 1 oz with a specific gravity of 1.11

21. A saturated solution contains, in each 100 mL, 100 g of a substance. If the solubility of the substance is 1 g in 0.7 mL of water, what is the specific gravity of the saturated solution?

    (A) 0.70
    (B) 1.00
    (C) 1.43
    (D) 1.70

Percentage Strength and Ratio Strength Expressions of Concentration

22. Calculate the percentage strength of the following:

    (A) 1 mg in 1 g
    (B) 2 μg in 50 mg
    (C) 0.25 g in 60 mL
    (D) 10 mg in 5 mL
    (E) 1:5000 w/v solution

23. Calculate the ratio strength of the following:

    (A) 1 mg in 1 g
    (B) 2 μg in 50 mg
    (C) 0.0025% v/v

24. Filgrastim (Neupogen) prefilled syringes contain 480 μg of drug in 0.8 mL of injection. Calculate the percentage of filgrastim in the injection.

25. Ipratropium bromide (Atrovent; Boehringer Ingelheim Pharmaceuticals, Ridgefield, CT) inhalation solution contains 0.02% w/v of drug per 2.5 mL. Calculate the equivalent concentration.

    (A) 2 mg/mL
    (B) 1 mg/5.0 mL
    (C) 100 μg/0.5 mL
    (D) 20 mg/2.5 mL

26. How many grams of active ingredient are present in a 60-g tube of a 0.005% w/w fluticasone propionate (Cutivate; PharmaDerm, Melville, NY) ointment?

27. If a solution contains 157 μg of fentanyl citrate in each 100 mL, calculate its percentage concentration.

28. If 78 mL of a 20% w/v solution of the surfactant Pluronic F-127 (Invitrogen, Eugene, OR) are used in preparing 100 mL of a product, calculate the percentage strength of the surfactant in the final product.

29. Mesalamine rectal suspension contains 4 g of mesalamine in each 60 mL of suspension. Calculate its percentage concentration.

30. If a 0.5-mL vial of levalbuterol hydrochloride (Xopenex; Sunovion Pharmaceuticals, Marlborough, MA) contains the equivalent of 1.25 mg of levalbuterol, calculate its percentage concentration.

31. If 15 g of a 5% w/w acyclovir ointment are used in preparing 60 g of a compound ointment, calculate the resultant concentration of acyclovir in the final product.

32. If an ophthalmic solution contains 0.02% w/v of mitomycin, how many milligrams of the drug were used in preparing each 100 mL of solution?

33. Zymar ophthalmic drops (Allergan, Irvine, CA) contain 0.3% w/v gatifloxacin. How many micrograms of the drug would be administered per drop from a dropper delivering 20 drops/mL?

34. How many milligrams of moxifloxacin (Vigamox; Alcon Laboratories, Fort Worth, TX) would be contained in a 3-mL container of a 0.5% w/v solution of the drug?

35. Travatan ophthalmic solution (Alcon Laboratories, Fort Worth, TX) contains 0.004% w/v of the drug travoprost and 0.015% w/v of the preservative benzalkonium chloride. Calculate (a) the micrograms of each agent in a 2.5-mL container and (b) the ratio strength of the benzalkonium chloride.

36. Ipratropium bromide (Atrovent) nasal spray packages contain 0.03% w/v drug in a 30-mL container and 0.06% w/v drug in a 15-mL container. Calculate the difference in the milligrams of drug present in the two packages.

37. If a solution of potassium permanganate is prepared by dissolving 16 0.2-g tablets in enough purified water to make 1600 mL, calculate (a) the percentage strength and (b) the ratio strength of the solution.

38. Calculate the percentage strength of misoprostol in the formula[1]:

Misoprostol	400 μg
Polyethylene Oxide	200 mg
Hydroxypropyl Methylcellulose ad	15 g

39. The cancer chemotherapy drug doxorubicin is available as an injection (2 mg/mL), which is diluted in 250 mL of 0.9% sodium chloride injection for intravenous infusion. For a particular patient, a dose of 16 mg of drug is to be infused. The concentration of doxorubicin in the infusion is

    (A) 6.2%.
    (B) 6.4%.
    (C) 0.0062%.
    (D) 0.0064%.

40. If the herb St. John's wort contains 0.3% w/w of pharmacologically active constituent, how many milligrams of active constituent would 900 mg of the herb provide?

41. Insulin injection is preserved with 0.25% w/v of metacresol. (a) Express this concentration as a ratio strength, and (b) calculate the quantity, in milligrams, of metacresol in a 20-mL vial of the injection.

Milliequivalents, Millimoles, and Milliosmoles

42. Express a patient's cholesterol level of 175 mg/dL in terms of millimoles per liter.

43. How many milliosmoles of sodium chloride are represented in 1 L of a 3% w/v hypertonic sodium chloride solution? Assume complete dissociation.

44. It is estimated that an adult with an average daily diet has a sodium chloride intake of 15 g/day. (a) How many milliequivalents of sodium and (b) how many millimoles of sodium chloride are represented in the daily salt intake?

45. What is the percentage concentration (w/v) of a solution containing 100 mEq of ammonium chloride per liter?

46. One liter of blood plasma contains 5 mEq of Ca^{++}. How many millimoles of calcium are represented in this concentration?

47. One hundred milliliters of blood plasma normally contain 3 mg of Mg^{++}. Express this concentration in milliequivalents per liter.

48. How many milliequivalents of potassium are in each 10 mL of a 5% w/v solution of potassium chloride?

49. Calculate the milliosmoles per liter of a sodium chloride solution containing 2.5 mEq of sodium chloride per milliliter.

Chemical and Physical Calculations

50. Calculate (a) the concentration of fentanyl (molecular weight [MW] 336) on a μg/mL basis in a solution containing 0.007% w/v fentanyl citrate (MW 528) and (b) the milligrams of erythromycin ethylsuccinate (MW 862) needed to provide 400 mg of erythromycin base (MW 734).

51. Sodium phosphates oral solution contains, in each 100 mL, 18 g of dibasic sodium phosphate ($Na_2HPO_4A7H_2O$, MW 268) and 48 g of monobasic sodium phosphate ($NaH_2PO_4AH_2O$, MW 138). How many grams of dried dibasic sodium phosphate (Na_2PO_4, MW 142) and of anhydrous monobasic sodium phosphate (NaH_2PO_4, MW 120) should be used in preparing 1 gal of the solution?

52. The dissociation constant of benzoic acid is 6.30×10^{-5}. Calculate its pK_a.

53. Calculate the pH of a buffer solution containing 0.8 mol of sodium acetate and 0.5 mol of acetic acid per liter. The pK_a value of acetic acid is 4.76.

54. What molar ratio of sodium acetate to acetic acid is required to prepare an acetate buffer solution with a pH of 5.0? The K_a value of acetic acid is 1.75×10^{-5}.

55. Calculate the molar ratio of dibasic sodium phosphate and monobasic sodium phosphate required to prepare a buffer system with a pH of 7.9. The pK_a value of monobasic sodium phosphate is 7.21.

56. What molar ratio of sodium borate to boric acid should be used in preparing a borate buffer with a pH of 8.8? The K_a value of boric acid is 6.4×10^{-10}.

57. Calculate the half-life (years) of ^{60}Co that has a disintegration constant of 0.01096 month^{-1}.

58. A sodium iodide I-131 solution has a labeled activity of 1 mCi/mL as of noon on November 17. How many milliliters of the solution should be administered at noon on December 1 to provide an activity of 250 μCi? The half-life of ^{131}I is 8.08 days.

59. Sodium phosphate P 32 solution is used intravenously in tumor localization in a dose range of 250 μCi to 1 mCi. Express this dose range of radioactivity in megabecquerel units.

60. A commercial product of thallous chloride TI-291 contains 244.2 MBq of radioactivity. Express this radioactivity in terms of millicuries.

B. PRESCRIPTIONS, FORMULATIONS, AND COMPOUNDING CALCULATIONS

Interpreting Prescription Notations and Prescription Calculations

61. Interpret the following prescription and medication order notations:

    (A) tab ii stat; i q4h prn pain
    (B) cap i w/gl H$_2$O qd A.M. for CHD
    (C) sig. 2 tsp qid
    (D) 20 mg/kg postop; rep q6h prn
    (E) 50,000 IU in 500 mL D$_5$W IV drip over 8 h

62. Identify any errors in the calculations for each of the following prescriptions and, when incorrect, correct the arithmetic error.

    (A) Rx Allopurinol   20 mg/mL
           Cherry Syrup   60 mL
           Methylcellulose Suspension ad 120 mL
           Sig: Take one teaspoonful daily in A.M.

    Having no allopurinol powder, the pharmacist used eight 300-mg tablets of allopurinol in compounding this prescription.

    (B) Rx Triamcinolone Acetonide Cream   0.1%
           Aquaphor Unibase aa   30 g
           M. ft. ungt.
           Sig: Apply to affected area on skin tid

The pharmacist used 15 g of a 0.1% triamcinolone acetonide cream and 15 g of Aquaphor Unibase in compounding this prescription.

    (C) Rx Ephedrine Sulfate   0.4% w/v
           Benzocaine   1:1000 w/v
           Cocoa Butter ad   2 g
           M. ft. suppos. DTD no. 24
           Sig: Insert one rectal suppository
           each night at bedtime.

In compounding this prescription, the pharmacist calculated for two extra suppositories to account for unavoidable loss in compounding (correct) and used a 10% w/w benzocaine ointment as the source of the benzocaine. Calculations then showed that 208 mg of ephedrine sulfate and 0.52 g of the benzocaine ointment would supply the proper amounts of these ingredients.

    (D) Rx Epinephrine   1% w/v
           Chlorobutanol   0.5%
           Sodium Chloride, qs
           Sterile Water for Injection ad 15 mL
           Make isotonic sol.
           Sig: Two drops in each eye at hs

The pharmacist calculated the need for 273 mg of epinephrine bitartrate (MW 333) to obtain the equivalent of epinephrine (MW 183), 75 mg of chlorobutanol, and 58 mg of sodium chloride to preparing this prescription.

    (E) Rx Potassium Permanganate, qs
           Purified Water ad 500 mL
           M. ft. solution. 5 mL added to a quart of
           water equals a 1:8000 solution
           Sig: Add one teaspoonful to a quart of
           warm water and soak toe as directed

The pharmacist used 59 0.2-g tablets of potassium permanganate in compounding this prescription.

63. Identify and correct any errors in the corresponding prescriptions or labels for the following:

    (A) Patient: John Smith   Weight: 165 lb
        Rx: Zithromax
        Disp: caps #16
        Sig: caps ii stat; cap i qA.M. with food × 4 days
        Label: Joan Smith
        Zithromax
        Take 2 capsules to start, then take 1 capsule every morning for 4 days

(B) Patient: Bob James   Weight: 180 lb
Rx: Lisinopril 20 mg
Disp: 30 tabs
Sig: tab i sid
Label: Bob James
Lisinopril 20 mg
Sig: Take 1 tablet several times a day

(C) Patient: Mary Jones   Weight: 132 lb
Rx: Leukeran   0.1 mg/kg/day
Disp: 2 mg tabs #50
Sig: Take _____ tablet(s) every day × 21 days
Label: Mary Jones
Leukeran 2 mg tablets
Sig: Take 3 tablets daily for 21 days

(D) Patient: Sara Smith   Height: 5′2″ Weight: 108 lb
Rx: Dexamethasone
Dose: 20 mg/m^2/day
Disp: 5-mg tablets
Sig: Take _____ tablets daily for treatment cycle
on days 1, 2, 3, 4, 9, 10, and 11
Label: Sara Smith
Dexamethasone 5-mg tablets
Take 6 tablets daily for treatment cycle on days 1,
2, 3, 4 and then on days 9, 10, and 11

64. Rx   Cyanocobalamin   10 μg/mL
Disp. 10-mL sterile vial
Sig: 1.5 mL every other week

(A) How many micrograms of cyanocobalamin will
be administered over 12 weeks?
(B) How many milligrams of cyanocobalamin are in
10 mL of this preparation?

65. Rx   Clindamycin Phosphate   0.6 g
Propylene Glycol   6 mL
Purified Water   8 mL
Isopropyl Alcohol ad   60 mL
Sig: Apply bid

(A) How many capsules, each containing 150 mg
of clindamycin phosphate, should be used in
preparing the prescription?
(B) What is the percentage concentration of
clindamycin phosphate in the prescription?

66. Rx   Codeine Sulfate   15 mg
Robitussin ad   120 mL
Sig: Two (2) teaspoonfuls q6h for cough

How many 30-mg tablets of codeine sulfate should be
used in preparing the prescription?

67. Rx   Hydrocortisone   1.5%
Neomycin Ointment
Emulsion Base aa ad 30 g
Sig: Apply

If the hydrocortisone is available in the form of 20-mg
scored tablets, how many tablets should be used to
obtain the hydrocortisone needed in preparing the
prescription?

68. Rx   Penicillin G Potassium   10,000 units/mL
Isotonic Sodium Chloride Solution ad   15 mL
Sig: For the nose. Store in the refrigerator

Only soluble penicillin tablets, each containing
400,000 units of penicillin G potassium, are available. Explain how to obtain the penicillin G potassium
needed to prepare the prescription.

69. Rx   Dextromethorphan   15 mg/5 mL
Guaifenesin Syrup ad   240 mL
Sig: 5 mL q4h prn cough

How many milligrams of dextromethorphan should
be used in preparing the prescription?

70. Rx^2 Noscapine   0.72 g
Guaifenesin   4.80 g
Alcohol   15 mL
Cherry Syrup ad   120 mL
Sig: 5 mL tid prn cough

How many milligrams each of noscapine and guaifenesin would be contained in each dose?

71. Rx^2 Cisapride   1 mg/mL
OraSweet ad 120 mL

(A) How many 10-mg tablets of cisapride may be
used in compounding the prescription?
(B) What is the percentage concentration of
cisapride in the prescription?

72. A commercial vial contains 20 million units of penicillin. The label directions state that when 32.4 mL
of sterile water for injection are added, an injection
containing 500,000 units of penicillin per milliliter
results. If a physician prescribes 1 million units of
penicillin per milliliter, how many milliliters of sterile
water for injection should be used to prepare the
product?

73. A physician prescribes 1.6 million units of penicillin G
potassium daily for 7 days. If 1 mg of penicillin G potassium is equal to 1595 penicillin G units, how many
250-mg tablets of penicillin G potassium should be
dispensed for the prescribed dosage regimen?

74. Rabies vaccine contains 1.25 international units per 0.5 mL. The postexposure dose is 2.5 international units administered the day of the exposure and an additional 2.5 international units on days 3, 7, 14, and 28 after exposure. How many milliliters of vaccine are needed for the full course of treatment?

    (A) 2.5 mL
    (B) 5 mL
    (C) 4 mL
    (D) 12.5 mL

75. If a physician prescribed penicillin V potassium, 500 mg qid for 10 days, how many milliliters of a suspension containing 500 mg of penicillin V potassium per 5 mL should be dispensed?

Formula and Admixture Calculations

76. The following is a formula for a diltiazem hydrochloride topical gel[2]:

Diltiazem Hydrochloride	2 g
Propylene Glycol	10 mL
Hydroxyethylcellulose	2 g
Preserved Water qs ad	100 mL

    If the specific gravity of propylene glycol is 1.04, how many grams of this agent may be used in the formula?

77. The following is a formula for a clotrimazole and gentamicin sulfate otic liquid[3]:

Clotrimazole	1 g
Gentamicin Sulfate	300 mg
Polyethylene Glycol ad	100 mL

    If the product is to be administered by drop, calculate the amount of gentamicin sulfate present in two drops from a dropper service delivering 20 drops/mL.

    (A) 3 mg
    (B) 30 μg
    (C) 0.03 mg
    (D) 300 μg

78. The following is a formula for a miconazole and tolnaftate topical liquid[3]:

Miconazole	2% w/v
Tolnaftate	1 g
Polyethylene Glycol 300 qs ad	100 mL

    How many grams each of (a) miconazole and (b) tolnaftate would be needed to prepare 1.5 L of the formulation?

79. The following is a formula for 30 antiemetic suppositories[4]:

Metoclopramide Hydrochloride	1.2 g
Haloperidol, powder	30 mg
Lorazepam	30 mg
Benztropine	30 mg
Fattibase	56 g

    If, in compounding the formula, 30 lorazepam 1-mg tablets, each weighing 200 mg, and 15 benztropine 2-mg tablets, each weighing 180 mg, are used as the sources of the two components, how much would each suppository weigh?

80. The following is a formula for acyclovir and chlorhexidine gel[4]:

Acyclovir	1 g
Chlorhexidine Digluconate	200 mg
Hydroxypropyl Methylcellulose	300 mg
Propylene Glycol	1 mL
Preserved Water ad	10 g

    How many milliliters of a 20% w/v aqueous solution of chlorhexidine digluconate may be used in the formula?

81. The following is a formula for a dexamethasone topical cream[4]:

Dexamethasone	0.1% w/w
Hydrophilic Ointment qs 100 g	

    If dexamethasone sodium phosphate (MW 516.41) rather than dexamethasone (MW 392.47) was used to prepare the formula, how many milligrams would be required?

82. The following is a formula for one sertraline hydrochloride capsule[5]:

Sertraline Hydrochloride	75 mg
Silica Gel	0.15 g
Calcium Citrate	0.10 g

    Calculate the quantities of each ingredient required to manufacture 100,000 such capsules.

83. The following is a formula for one verapamil hydrochloride suppository[4]:

Verapamil Hydrochloride	40 mg
Polyethylene Glycol 1450	65% w/w
Polyethylene Glycol 6000	28% w/w
Purified Water	7% w/w

    Calculate the quantities of each ingredient required for the preparation of 48 suppositories, each with 2 g of base.

84. The following is a formula for an interferon ophthalmic solution[6]:

Interferon Alpha-2a	100 million units
Ammonium Acetate	7.7 mg
Benzyl Alcohol	100 mg
Human Albumin	10 mg
Sterile Water for Injection ad	10 mL

Interferon alpha-2a is available in vials containing 18 million units or 66.7 μg in 3 mL of solution. Calculate (a) the milliliters of this solution required to prepare the prescription and (b) the number of micrograms and units of interferon alpha-2a in each 0.05 mL of the filled prescription.

85.
Coal Tar	10 g
Polysorbate 80	5 g
Zinc Oxide Paste	985 g

Calculate the quantity of each ingredient required to prepare 10 lb of the ointment.

86.
Menthol	0.2 g
Hexachlorophene	0.1 g
Glycerin	10 mL
Isopropyl Alcohol	35 mL
Purified Water ad	100 mL

Calculate the quantity of each ingredient required to prepare 1 gal of the lotion.

87. Set up a formula for 5 lb of glycerogelatin containing 10 parts by weight of zinc oxide, 15 parts by weight of gelatin, 40 parts by weight of glycerin, and 35 parts by weight of water.

88. The following formula for glycerin suppositories is sufficient to prepare 50 suppositories. Calculate the amount of each ingredient needed to prepare 300 suppositories.

Glycerin	91 g
Sodium Stearate	9 g
Purified Water	5 g

89. The formula for a potassium chloride elixir is as follows:

| Potassium Chloride | 5 mEq/tsp |
| Elixir Base qs | |

How many grams of potassium chloride are needed to prepare 5 gal of the elixir?

90. A vitamin liquid contains, in each 0.5 mL, the following:

Thiamine Hydrochloride	1 mg
Riboflavin	400 μg
Ascorbic Acid	50 mg
Nicotinamide	2 mg

Calculate the quantity, expressed in grams, of each ingredient in 30 mL of the liquid.

91. A formula for 200 g of an ointment contains 10 g of glycerin. How many milliliters of glycerin, with a specific gravity of 1.25, should be used in preparing 1 lb of the ointment?

92. Furosemide injection contains 10 mg of furosemide in each milliliter, packaged in prefilled 2-mL syringes. Calculate the amount, in grams, of furosemide required to manufacture 4000 such syringes.

93. How many milliliters of a 2.5% w/v solution of a drug and how many milliliters of water are required to prepare 500 mL of a 0.3% w/v solution of the drug?

94.
| Triethanolamine | 100 g |
| Purified Water ad | 100 mL |

Triethanolamine is a liquid with a specific gravity of 1.25. Calculate (a) the milliliters of triethanolamine needed to prepare the formula, (b) the percentage strength of triethanolamine in the formula on a v/v basis, and (c) the percentage strength of triethanolamine in the formula on a w/w basis (assume no contraction of volume on mixing the liquids).

95. How many fluid ounces of a commercially available 17% w/v solution of benzalkonium chloride should be used to prepare 1 gal of a 1:750 w/v solution?

96. How many grams of lidocaine should be added to 1 lb of a 1% lidocaine w/w ointment to increase the strength to 2% w/w?

97. How many grams of benzethonium chloride and how many milliliters of 95% v/v alcohol should be used in preparing 1 gal of a 1:1000 solution of benzethonium chloride in 70% v/v alcohol?

98. How many grams of talc should be added to 1 lb of a powder containing 20 g of zinc undecylenate per 100 g to reduce the concentration of zinc undecylenate to 3% w/w?

99. How many milliliters of 36% w/w hydrochloric acid, with a specific gravity of 1.18, are required to prepare 5 gal of 10% w/v hydrochloric acid?

100. A formula for an ophthalmic solution calls for 500 mL of a 0.02% w/v solution of benzalkonium chloride. How many milliliters of a 1:750 w/v solution should be used to obtain the amount of benzalkonium chloride needed in preparing the ophthalmic solution?

101. How many milliliters of each of two liquids with specific gravities of 0.950 and 0.875 should be used to prepare 12 L of a liquid with a specific gravity of 0.925?

102. A medication order calls for triamcinolone acetonide suspension to be diluted with normal saline solution to provide 3 mg/mL of triamcinolone acetonide for injection into a lesion. If each 5 mL of the suspension contains 125 mg of triamcinolone acetonide, how many milliliters should be used to prepare 10 mL of the prescribed dilution?

103. If a dry powder mixture of the antibiotic amoxicillin is diluted with water to 80 mL by a pharmacist to prepare a prescription containing 125 mg of amoxicillin per 5 mL, (a) how many grams of amoxicillin are in the dry mixture, and (b) what is the percentage strength of amoxicillin in the prepared prescription?

104. If 3 mL of diluent are added to a vial containing 1 g of a drug for injection, resulting in a final volume of 3.4 mL, what is the concentration, in milligrams per milliliter, of the drug in the injectable solution?

105. A medication order calls for the addition of 25 mEq of sodium bicarbonate to a hyperalimentation formula. How many milliliters of an 8.4% w/v solution should be added to the hyperalimentation formula? (You have on hand a 50-mL ampule of 8.4% w/v sodium bicarbonate solution.)

106. How many grams of calcium chloride ($CaCl_2 \cdot 2H_2O$, m.w. 147) are required to prepare half a liter of a solution containing 5 mEq of calcium chloride per milliliter?

107. A hospital medication order calls for the addition of 20 mEq of sodium chloride to a liter of mannitol injection. How many milliliters of a 14.5% w/v sodium chloride additive solution should be used?

C. DOSAGE CALCULATIONS AND OTHER PATIENT/CLINICAL PARAMETERS

Dosage Calculations Based on Weight

108. The initial dose of a drug is 0.25 mg/kg of body weight. How many milligrams should be prescribed for a person weighing 154 lb?

109. If a dosage table for a prefabricated drug product indicates the dose for a patient weighing 110 lb is 0.4 mg/kg of body weight, taken three times a day for 10 days, how many 10-mg tablets of the product should be dispensed?

110. The child's dose of gentamicin for a urinary tract infection is 1 mg/kg administered every 8 hours for 10 days. What would be (a) the single dose and (b) the total dose for a 15-year-old child weighing 110 lb?

111. The maintenance dose of oxtriphylline (Choledyl; Parke-Davis, Detroit, MI) is 13.2 mg/kg/day or 800 mg, whichever is less, in qid dosing. How many 100-mg tablets of the drug should a 200-lb patient take at each dosing interval?

112. A medication order calls for 6 μg/kg of body weight of pentagastrin to be administered subcutaneously to a patient weighing 154 lb. The source of the drug is an ampule containing 0.5 mg in each 2 mL of the solution. How many milliliters of the solution should be injected?

113. The rectal dose of sodium thiopental is 45 mg/kg of body weight. How many milliliters of a 10% w/v solution should be used for a person weighing 150 lb?

114. How many capsules, each containing 250 mg of drug, are needed to provide 25 mg/kg/day for 1 week for a person weighing 175 lb?

115. The dose of a drug is 50 mg/kg of body weight once daily for 7 consecutive days. How many milliliters of a syrup containing 500 mg of drug per teaspoonful should be prescribed for a child weighing 66 lb?

116. A physician prescribed 5 mg of a drug per kilogram of body weight once daily for a patient weighing 132 lb. How many 100-mg tablets of the drug are required for a dosage regimen of 2 weeks?

117. If the loading dose of kanamycin is 7 mg/kg of body weight, how many grams should be administered to a patient weighing 165 lb?

118. A medication order calls for 0.1 mg/kg of albuterol sulfate to be administered to a 23-lb child. The source of the drug is a solution containing 0.5 g of albuterol sulfate in 100 mL. How many milliliters of the solution should be used in filling the order?

119. If the recommended dose of gentamicin sulfate for a patient with normal kidney function is 3 mg/kg/day, divided into three equal doses given every 8 hours, how many milligrams should be administered per dose to a patient weighing 182 lb?

120. Plasma protein fraction (PPF) is available as a 5% w/v solution. If the dose of the solution for a child is given as 5 mL/lb, how many grams of PPF should be administered to a child weighing 20 kg?

121. The loading dose of Dilantin in children is 20 mg/kg administered at an infusion rate of 0.5 mg/kg/min.

    (A) What would be the dose for a child weighing 32 lb?
    (B) Over what period should the dose be administered?

122. If two patients, each weighing 110 lb, were given the drug amikacin sulfate, one at a regimen of 7.5 mg/kg every 12 hours and the other at 5 mg/kg every 8 hours, what is the difference in the total quantity of drug administered over a 24-hour period?

123. The loading dose of theophylline for a child is 5 mg/kg of body weight. For each milligram per kilogram of theophylline administered, the serum theophylline concentration increases by approximately 2 μg/mL. (a) Calculate the loading dose for a child weighing 44 lb, and (b) determine the approximate serum theophylline concentration.

Dosage Calculations Based on Body Surface Area

124. Using the equation below for the determination of body surface area (BSA), calculate the BSA for a patient 6 ft in height and weighing 185 lb.

$$BSA \ (m^2) = \sqrt{\frac{height \ (cm) \times weight \ (kg)}{3600}}$$

125. The dose of a drug is 15 mg/m^2 bid for 1 week. How many milligrams of the drug would be required for a full course of therapy for a child 42 in. tall and weighing 50 lb?

126. The dose of methotrexate for meningeal leukemia in children is 12 mg/m^2 by the intrathecal route. Calculate the dose, in milligrams, for a child 28 in. tall and weighing 52 lb.

127. If the dose of a drug is 17.5 mg/m^2/day, how many milligrams of the drug should be administered daily to a patient weighing 65 lb and measuring 3 ft 6 in. in height?

128. If the intravenous pediatric dose of dactinomycin is 2.5 mg/m^2/week, how many micrograms of the drug will a child having a BSA of 0.50 m^2 average per day of therapy?

129. The drug cyclophosphamide is administered for breast cancer at a daily dose of 100 mg/m^2 for up to 14 consecutive days. What would be the total quantity administered over the 2-week period for a patient measuring 5 ft 2 in. in height and weighing 102 lb?

130. The following is a 28-day cycle of a GC regimen for treating advanced non-small cell lung cancer[7]:

    Gemcitabine 1000 mg/m^2 IV, D-1, 8, 15
    Cisplatin 100 mg/m^2 IV, D-1 *or* 2 *or* 15
    Calculate the total quantity each of gemcitabine and cisplatin administered over the course of a single cycle to a patient determined to have a BSA of 1.6 m^2.

131. The following drugs are administered for metastatic colon cancer over a 4-week period, with the cycle repeating every 6 weeks[8]:

    Irinotecan 125 mg/m^2 IV, D-1, 8, 15, 22
    Fluorouracil 500 mg/m^2 IV, D-1, 8, 15, 22
    Leucovorin 20 mg/m^2 IV, D-1, 8, 15, 22

    If irinotecan is available in an injection containing 20 mg/mL, and fluorouracil is available in an injection containing 50 mg/mL, how many milliliters of each of the two injections would be used during a treatment cycle for a patient determined to have a BSA of 1.7 m^2?

132. Granulocyte macrophage colony stimulating factor (GM-CSF) is available as a lyophilized powder for injection in 250- and 500-μg vials. A dosage regimen is 250 μg/m^2/day intravenously over a 4-hour period.[9]

    (A) What would be the daily dose for a patient with a BSA of 1.59 m^2?
    (B) What would be the final drug concentration in μg/mL if the dose in (A) is diluted to 50 mL with 0.9% sodium chloride solution?
    (C) How many milligrams of human albumin should be added prior to diluting with the 0.9% w/v sodium chloride solution to achieve a concentration of 0.1% w/v human albumin in the 50-mL injection?
    (D) How many milliliters of 5% w/v human albumin can provide the required amount in (C)?

133. An anticancer drug is available in 30-mg vials costing $147 each. What would be the drug cost of administering 135 mg/m^2 once every 3 weeks during a 9-week period to a 1.9-m^2 patient?

134. The pediatric dose of a drug may be determined on the basis of (a) 8 mg/kg of body weight or (b) a pediatric dose of 250 mg/m². Calculate the dose on each basis for a child weighing 44 lb and measuring 36 in. in height.

Intravenous Infusions and Infusion Rate Calculations

135. A hospital pharmacy has available 2-mL prefilled syringes containing 80 mg of tobramycin and 1.5-mL prefilled syringes containing 60 mg of tobramycin. The syringes are calibrated in 0.25-mL units. Explain how you would prepare a medication order calling for 110 mg of tobramycin to be added to 100 mL of D_5W for intravenous infusion.

136. Using prefilled tobramycin syringes as described in the preceding problem and with a minimum of waste, explain how you would prepare a medication order calling for three piggyback infusions, each containing 110 mg of tobramycin in 100 mL of D_5W.

137. A liter of an intravenous solution of potassium chloride is to be administered over 5 hours, and the dropper in the venoclysis set calibrates 25 drops/mL. What is the required rate of flow in drops per minute?

138. A large-volume parenteral fluid contains 20 mg of a drug per liter. If the desired drug delivery rate is 1 mg/hr, and the venoclysis set calibrates 25 drops/mL, what should be the rate of flow in drops per minute?

139. A physician prescribes a 5-μg/kg/min IV drip of dopamine for a 175-lb patient, and the pharmacist adds an ampule of dopamine (200 mg/5 mL) to a 250-mL bottle of D_5W. What drip rate should be run, in drops per minute, using a minidrip set that delivers 60 drops/mL?

140. A medication order calls for 1 L of a TPN solution to be administered over 6 hours. If the venoclysis set calibrates 20 drops/mL, at what rate of flow, in drops per minute, should the set be adjusted to administer the solution in the designated interval?

141. A medication order calls for 20 mEq of potassium chloride in 500 mL of D_5W/0.45 NSS to be administered at the rate of 125 mL/hr. If the intravenous set is calibrated at 12 drops/mL, what should be the infusion rate in drops per minute?

142. The intravenous dose of ondansetron is three 0.15-mg/kg doses infused over 15 minutes.[10]

   (A) What would be the initial dose for a patient weighing 134 lb?
   (B) If the dose is diluted to 50 mL with 5% dextrose, what flow rate, in mL/hr, would be needed to administer the dose over 15 minutes?
   (C) What flow rate, in drops per minute, would be needed using an infusion set that delivers 20 drops/mL?

143. A drug is administered intravenously at a loading dose of 50 μg/kg over 10 minutes, followed by continuous intravenous infusion of 0.375 μg/kg/min.

   (A) How many micrograms of the drug would be administered to a 160-lb patient in the first hour of therapy?
   (B) If the drug is available in 10-mL vials containing the drug in a concentration of 1 mg/mL, how many vials would be needed for 4 hours of therapy?

144. A certain hyperalimentation solution contains 600 mL of a 5% w/v protein hydrolysate, 400 mL of 50% w/v dextrose injection, 35 mL of a 20% w/v sterile potassium chloride solution, 100 mL of sodium chloride injection, and 10 mL of a 10% calcium gluconate injection. The solution is to be administered over 6 hours. If the dropper in the venoclysis set calibrates 20 drops/mL, at what rate, in drops per minute, should the flow be adjusted to administer the solution during the designated interval?

145. A solution prepared by dissolving 500,000 units of polymyxin B sulfate in 10 mL of water for injection is added to 250 mL of 5% dextrose injection. The infusion is to be administered over 2 hours. If the dropper in the venoclysis set calibrates 25 drops/mL, at what rate, in drops per minute, should the flow be adjusted to administer the total volume over the designated interval?

146. A physician orders an intravenous solution to contain 10,000 units of heparin in 1 L of 5% w/v dextrose solution to be infused at such a rate that the patient will receive 500 units/hr. If the intravenous set delivers 10 drops/mL, how many drops per minute should be infused to deliver the desired dose?

147. A certain hyperalimentation solution measures 1 L. If the solution is to be administered over 6 hours and the administration set is calibrated at 25 drops/mL, at what rate should the set be adjusted to administer the solution during the designated interval?

148. If, in the previous problem, the patient was to receive nitroglycerin at the rate of 5 μg/min, at how many milliliters per hour should the infusion pump be set to deliver this dose?

149. If an infusion pump system is calibrated to deliver 15 microdrops per minute, equivalent to a delivery rate of 15 mL/hr, how many microdrops would be delivered per milliliter by the system?

150. A nitroglycerin concentrate solution contains 5 mg of nitroglycerin in each milliliter. A 10-mL ampule of the concentrate is added to 500 mL of D₅W and infused into a patient at a flow rate of 3 microdrops per minute. If the infusion pump system delivers 60 microdrops/mL, how many micrograms of nitroglycerin would the patient receive in the first hour of therapy?

151. The drug alprostadil is administered to infants by intravenous infusion following dilution in dextrose injection. If one ampule, containing 500 μg of alprostadil, is added to the indicated volume of dextrose injection, complete the table by calculating (a) the approximate concentration of the resulting solutions and (b) the infusion rates needed to provide 0.1 μg/kg/min of alprostadil.

500 μg Added to mL of Dextrose Injection	Approximate Concentration of Resulting Solution (μg/mL)	Infusion Rate (mL/kg/min)
250	_____	_____
100	_____	_____
50	_____	_____
25	_____	_____

Body Mass Index and Nutrition Calculations

152. Using the Harris-Benedict equation and assuming no stress factor, calculate (a) the daily calories required and (b) the daily protein needed for a 69-year-old man who is 5 ft 9 in. tall and weighs 165 lb.

153. Calculate the body mass index for a person 5 ft 4 in. tall and weighing 140 lb.

154. How many food calories would be provided by a daily diet of 50 g of fat, 600 g of carbohydrate, and 120 g of protein?

155. A hyperalimentation solution includes 500 mL of D₅W. If each gram of dextrose supplies 3.4 kcal, how many kilocalories would the hyperalimentation solution provide?

Other Dosage and Clinical Calculations

156. Calculate the creatinine clearance for a 30-year-old man weighing 80 kg with a serum creatinine of 2 mg/dL.

157. If 150 mg of a drug are administered intravenously and the resultant drug plasma concentration is determined to be 30 μg/mL, calculate the apparent volume of distribution.

158. In a neonatal intensive care unit, a 7.4-mg loading dose of aminophylline was ordered for a premature infant. Instead, by a tragic and fatal error, 7.4 mL of a 250-mg/10 mL solution were administered.[11] How many milligrams of aminophylline were administered rather than the prescribed amount?

159. The epidural dose of morphine sulfate should not exceed 10 mg/24 hours. A pharmacist needs to set up a patient-controlled analgesia epidural infusion that allows a patient to self-administer a dose every 30 minutes.[10]
   (A) If a solution with a morphine sulfate concentration of 0.5 mg/mL is used, what would be the maximum volume administered per dose that would not exceed 10 mg/24 hours?
   (B) How many days would a 50-mL cassette of the 0.5-mg/mL solution last a patient who administers the maximum dose?

160. A study of vancomycin dosing in neonates shows that average peak serum vancomycin concentrations of 30 μg/mL are achieved following doses of 10 mg/kg of body weight. On this basis, what would be the expected serum concentration of the drug if a 2500-g child received 20 mg of vancomycin?

161. Captopril is prescribed for an 11-lb dog at a dose of 1 mg/kg. How many drops of a suspension containing 50 mg/mL should be administered if a dropper delivers 20 drops/mL?

D. MISCELLANEOUS CALCULATIONS

162. Cefuroxime axetil for oral suspension should be constituted at the time of dispensing and stored in a refrigerator for maximum stability. If stored at room temperature, however, the half-life of the drug is only 10 days. If the original concentration of the constituted suspension was 250 mg/5 mL, how much cefuroxime axetil will remain per 5 mL after storage at room temperature for 25 days?

163. A transdermal patch contains 24.3 mg of testosterone and releases the drug at a rate of 5 mg/24 hours. The patch is intended to be worn for 24 hours, then removed and replaced by a new patch.

    (A) How many milligrams of testosterone would be released from the patch in 2 hours?
    (B) What percentage of total drug would have been released on removal of the patch?
    (C) Assuming that all of the drug would be released from the patch at a constant rate, how many hours would it take for the patch to be exhausted of drug?

164. The AUC for an oral dose of a drug is 4.5 μg/mL/hr and for an IV dose is 11.2 μg/mL/hr. What is the bioavailability of an oral dose of the drug?[12]

165. The half-life of warfarin is 1.0 to 2.5 days. What is the elimination rate constant?[13]

166. The elimination rate constant for a drug is 0.58 hour^{-1}. What is its half-life?[14]

167. The drug ranibizumab (Lucentis; Genentech, South San Francisco, CA) is administered by intravitreal injection in treating age-related macular degeneration. The recommended dose is 0.5 mg once a month for the first four treatments then an injection once every 3 months. The 0.2-mL vial for injection contains ranibizumab, 10 mg/mL. How many milliliters of injection should be administered per dose?

168. The antineoplastic drug decitabine is supplied in single-dose vials containing 50 mg of dry powdered drug. Immediately prior to use, the drug is reconstituted with 10 mL of sterile water for injection and then further diluted with 0.9% sodium chloride injection to a final drug concentration of 0.1 to 1.0 mg/mL for intravenous infusion. For the latter concentration, what would be the final volume of the infusion fluid?

    (A) 40 mL
    (B) 50 mL
    (C) 490 mL
    (D) 500 mL

169. If, in problem 174, the dose is 15 mg/m^2 and a drug concentration of 0.1 mg/mL is to be administered by continuous intravenous infusion over a 3-hour period, what should be the flow rate in mL/min for a patient with a BSA of 1.85 m^2?

170. If, in problem 175, the drop set used delivered 15 drops/mL, what should be the flow rate in drops per minute?

171. If the chemotherapy drug vinblastine is prescribed for intravenous administration at a dose of 4 mg/m^2, to be administered on days 1, 8, 15, 22, 29, and 36, what would be the (a) total dose per cycle for a patient with a BSA of 1.65 m^2 and (b) what would be the total dose per cycle on a mg/m^2 basis for that patient?

172. The anticancer drug melphalan may be administered orally at a dose of 8 mg/m^2 on days 1, 2, 3, and 4 during a 4-week cycle or intravenously at a dose of 15 mg/m^2 on day 1 of a 4-week cycle. Calculate the difference in total dose between the regimens on a mg/m^2 basis.

173. The starting pediatric dose of valsartan (Diovan; Novartis, East Hanover, NJ) is 1.3 mg/kg once daily to a maximum of 40 mg. On this basis, what would be the weight, in pounds, of a pediatric patient who received the maximum starting dose?

E. PHYSICIANS' MEDICATION ORDERS

174. Medication Order: Sirolimus Oral Solution (Rapamune; Pfizer, New York, NY), 1 mg/m^2/d
    Available: Sirolimus, 1 mg/mL oral solution with oral syringe
    Question: mL daily dose, patient, BSA 1.25 m^2?

175. Medication Order: Cefixime, 8 mg/kg/d in two divided doses
    Available: Cefixime oral suspension, 75 mL; cefixime, 200 mg/5 mL
    Question: mL dose, 36-lb child?

176. Medication Order: Heparin, 15 units/kg/hr
    Preparation: 25,000 heparin units in 500-mL normal saline solution
    Question: mL/hr infusion rate, 187-lb patient?

177. Medication Order: Zidovudine (Retrovir; GlaxoSmithKline, London, United Kingdom) 160 mg/m^2 q8h
    Available: Retrovir Syrup, 50 mg zidovudine/5 mL
    Question: Dose, mL, 12-year-old child, BSA 1.46 m^2?

178. Medication Order: Bevacizumab (Avastin; Genentech, South San Francisco, CA), 5 mg/kg
   Preparation: 16 mL vial (25 mg/mL), in sodium chloride injection to 100 mL
   Question (a): mL infusion, 135-lb patient?
   Question (b): 30-minute infusion rate, mL/min?

179. Medication Order: Lidocaine, 2 μg/kg/min
   Available: Lidocaine, 1 g in 500 mL infusion
   Question: Flow rate, mL/hr, 142-lb patient?

180. Medication Order: IV chlorothiazide sodium (Diuril sodium; Merck, Whitehouse Station, NJ), administer 500 mg
   Available: Reconstituted solution, chlorothiazide sodium, 28 mg/mL
   Question: mL, dose?

181. Medication Order: D_5W by infusion, 100 mL/hr
   Administration Set: 15 drops/mL
   Question: Infusion rate, drops per minute?

182. Medication Order: Augmentin, 45 mg q12h
   Available: Reconstituted oral suspension, 125 mg/5 mL
   Question: mL, dose?

183. Medication Order: 1.5% hydrocortisone cream, 30 g
   Available: 1% hydrocortisone cream and hydrocortisone powder
   Question: Grams each of hydrocortisone cream and hydrocortisone powder to use?

Answers to Review Problems

1. (A) 100 mg
   (B) 120 mg
   (C) 175 mg

2. (A) 5%
   (B) 8.7%

3. LWQ = 120 mg
   0.5 mg × 12 (caps) = 6 mg drug A needed
   6 mg × 20 (factor) = 120 mg drug A
   weigh 120 mg drug A
   dilute with 2280 mg lactose
   weigh 120 mg of the 2400 mg mixture

4. (A) 50 μg/mL
   (B) 18.2 mg/lb
   (C) 0.04 mg/mL
   (D) 0.5 kg
   (E) 354.84 mL
   (F) 709.5 mL
   (G) 4.44°C

5. 6.25 g levothyroxine sodium

6. 0.1 mL

7. 3.5 g codeine phosphate

8. (B) 0.075 g ibandronate sodium

9. 292.01 g, 728.59 g

10. (B) 2500 μg/mL

11. 3 mg/mL metoclopramide

12. 17.6 mg/kg cocaine

13. 100 mg/dL

14. zero

15. (A) 137 μg azelastine hydrochloride

16. (A) 27.4 mL

17. 2.9102 mg insulin glargine

18. (A) 0.93
    (B) 1.08
    (C) 1.31

19. (A) 500.0 g
    (B) 425.7 g

20. (A) 33.33 mL
    (B) 25.54 mL

21. (D) 1.70

22. (A) 0.10% w/w
(B) 0.004% w/w
(C) 0.42% w/v
(D) 0.2% w/v
(E) 0.02% w/v

23. (A) 1:1,000 w/w
(B) 1:25,000 w/w
(C) 1:40,000 v/v

24. 0.6% filgrastim

25. (B) 1 mg/5.0 mL ipratropium bromide

26. 0.003 g fluticasone propionate

27. 0.000157% w/v fentanyl citrate

28. 15.6% w/v Pluronic F-127

29. 6.67% w/v mesalamine

30. 0.25% w/v levalbuterol hydrochloride

31. 1.25% w/w acyclovir

32. 20 mg mitomycin

33. 150 μg gatifloxacin

34. 15 mg moxifloxacin

35. (A) 100 μg travoprost
375 μg benzalkonium chloride
(B) 1.6667 w/v benzalkonium chloride

36. zero

37. (A) 0.2% w/v potassium permanganate
(B) 1:500 w/v potassium permanganate

38. 0.0027% w/v misoprostol

39. (C) 0.0062%

40. 2.7 mg active constituent

41. (A) 1:400 w/v metacresol
(B) 50 mg metacresol

42. 4.52 mmol/L cholesterol

43. 1025.64 mOsm sodium chloride

44. (A) 256.41 mEq sodium
(B) 256.41 mOsm sodium chloride

45. 0.54% w/v ammonium chloride

46. 2.5 mmol calcium

47. 2.47 mEq magnesium

48. 6.71 mEq potassium

49. 5000 mOsm sodium chloride

50. (A) 44.5 μg/mL fentanyl
(B) 469.75 mg erythromycin ethylsuccinate

51. 360.99 g dibasic sodium phosphate
1579.83 g monobasic sodium phosphate

52. 4.2

53. 4.96

54. 1.7:1

55. 4.9:1

56. 0.4:1

57. 5.27 years

58. 0.83 mL sodium iodide I-131 solution

59. 9.25 to 37 MBq

60. 6.6 mCi

61. (A) Take 2 tablets to start, then 1 tablet every 4 hours as needed for pain.
(B) Take 1 capsule with a glass of water every morning for congestive heart disease.
(C) Take 2 teaspoonfuls four times a day.
(D) Give 20 mg/kg postoperatively. Repeat every 6 hours as needed.
(E) 50,000 international units in 500 mL of dextrose 5% in water. Administer by intravenous drip over 8 hours.

62. (A) correct
(B) incorrect; use 30 g of each
(C) correct
(D) incorrect quantity of sodium chloride; use 67.86 mg
(E) correct

63. **(A)** patient's name incorrect on label; drug strength missing; "with food" missing on label; incorrect number of capsules prescribed
(B) sid means "once a day"
(C) insufficient number of tablets prescribed; 63 tablets needed
(D) correct

64. (A) 90 μg
(B) 0.1 mg

65. (A) 4 capsules clindamycin phosphate
(B) 1% w/v clindamycin phosphate

66. 12 tablets codeine sulfate

67. 22.5 tablets hydrocortisone

68. ⅜ tablet needed; dissolve 1 tablet in enough isotonic sodium chloride solution to make 8 mL, and use 3 mL of the solution

69. 720 mg dextromethorphan

70. 30 mg noscapine
200 mg guaifenesin

71. **(A)** 12 tablets cisapride
(B) 0.1% w/v

72. 12.4 mL sterile water for injection

73. 128 tablets

74. **(B)** 5 mL rabies vaccine

75. 200 mL penicillin V potassium suspension

76. 10.4 g propylene glycol

77. **(D)** 300 μg gentamicin sulfate

78. **(A)** 30 g miconazole
(B) 15 g tolnaftate

79. 2.198 or 2.2 g

80. 1 mL chlorhexidine digluconate solution

81. 131.58 mg dexamethasone sodium phosphate

82. 7.5 kg sertraline hydrochloride
15 kg silica gel
10 kg calcium citrate

83. 1.92 g verapamil hydrochloride
62.4 g polyethylene glycol 1450
26.88 g polyethylene glycol 6000
6.72 g purified water

84. **(A)** 16.67 mL interferon solution
(B) 1.85 μg and 500,000 units interferon

85. 45.4 g coal tar
22.7 g polysorbate 80
4471.9 g zinc oxide paste

86. 7.57 g menthol
3.785 g hexachlorophene
378.5 mL glycerin
1324 mL isopropyl alcohol
ad 3785 mL with purified water

87. 227 g zinc oxide
340.5 g gelatin
908 g glycerin
795 g water

88. 546 g glycerin
54 g sodium stearate
30 g purified water

89. 1409.91 g potassium chloride

90. 0.06 g thiamine hydrochloride
0.024 g riboflavin
3 g ascorbic acid
0.12 g nicotinamide

91. 18.16 mL glycerin

92. 80 g furosemide

93. 60 mL drug solution
440 mL water

94. **(A)** 80 mL triethanolamine
(B) 80% v/v triethanolamine
(C) 83.3% w/w triethanolamine

95. 1 fluid ounce benzalkonium chloride solution

96. 4.633 g lidocaine

97. 3.785 g benzethonium chloride
2788.95 mL alcohol

98. 2572.7 g talc

99. 4455 mL hydrochloric acid, 36% w/w

100. 75 mL benzalkonium chloride solution

101. 8000 mL (sp gr 0.95) and 4000 mL (sp gr 0.875)

102. 1.2 mL triamcinolone acetonide suspension

103. (**A**) 2 g amoxicillin
     (**B**) 2.5% w/v amoxicillin

104. 294.12 mg/mL

105. 25 mL sodium bicarbonate solution

106. 183.75 g calcium chloride

107. 8.07 mL sodium chloride solution

108. 17.5 mg

109. 60 tablets

110. (**A**) 50 mg gentamicin
     (**B**) 1500 mg gentamicin

111. 2 tablets oxtriphylline

112. 1.68 mL pentagastrin solution

113. 30.68 mL or 31 mL sodium thiopental

114. 56 capsules

115. 105 mL

116. 42 tablets

117. 0.525 g kanamycin

118. 0.21 mL albuterol sulfate solution

119. 82.73 mg gentamicin sulfate

120. 11 g PPF

121. (**A**) 290.9 mg or 291 mg Dilantin
     (**B**) 40 minutes

122. zero

123. (**A**) 100 mg theophylline
     (**B**) 10 μg/mL theophylline

124. 2.067 or 2.07 m^2

125. 168 mg

126. 7.3 mg methotrexate

127. 15.58 mg

128. 178.6 μg dactinomycin

129. 2016 mg cyclophosphamide

130. 4800 mg gemcitabine
     160 mg cisplatin

131. 42.5 mL irinotecan injection
     68 mL fluorouracil injection

132. (**A**) 397.5 μg/day GM-CSF
     (**B**) 7.95 μg/mL GM-CSF
     (**C**) 50 mg human albumin
     (**D**) 1 mL human albumin (5%)

133. $3770.55

134. (**A**) 160 mg
     (**B**) 167.5 mg

135. use all of a 2-mL (80 mg) syringe and 0.75 mL (30 mg) of a 1.5-mL syringe

136. use two 2-mL syringes (160 mg) and three 1.5-mL syringes (180 mg)
     bottle 1: one 2-mL syringe (80 mL) + 0.75 mL (30 mg) of one 1.5-mL syringe
     bottle 2: one 2-mL syringe (80 mg) + the remaining 0.75 mL (30 mg) used in bottle 1
     bottle 3: one full 1.5-mL syringe (60 mg) + 1.25 mL (50 mg) of another 1.5-mL syringe

137. 83.3 or 83 drops/min

138. 20.8 or 21 drops/min

139. 30.45 or 30 drops/min

140. 55.6 or 56 drops/min

141. 25 drops/min

142. (**A**) 9.136 or 9.14 mg ondansetron
     (**B**) 200 mL/hr
     (**C**) 66.7 or 67 drops/min

143. (A) 5000 µg
     (B) 1 vial

144. 63.6 or 64 drops/min

145. 54.2 or 54 drops/min

146. 8.3 or 8 drops/min

147. 69.44 or 69 drops/min

148. 3.06 mL/hr

149. 60 microdrops/mL

150. 294.12 µg nitroglycerin

151. (A) 2 µg/mL
         5 µg/mL
         10 µg/mL
         20 µg/mL
     (B) 0.05 mL/kg/min
         0.02 mL/kg/min
         0.01 mL/kg/min
         0.005 mL/kg/min

152. (A) 1500.6 kcal
     (B) 56.25 g protein

153. 24.08 BMI

154. 3330 calories

155. 850 kcal

156. 61 mL/min

157. 5 L

158. 185 mg

159. (A) 0.417 or 0.42 mL
     (B) 2.5 days

160. 24 µg/mL

161. 2 drops

162. 44.19 mg/5 mL

163. (A) 0.42 mg
     (B) 20.6%
     (C) 116.64 hours

164. 0.4 or 40%

165. 0.69 day^{-1}

166. 1.19 hours

167. 0.05 mL ranibizumab injection

168. (B) 50 mL infusion fluid

169. 1.54 mL/min

170. 23 drops/min

171. (A) 39.6 mg vinblastine
     (B) 24 mg/m^2 vinblastine

172. 17 mg/m^2

173. 67.7 lb

174. 1.25 mL sirolimus oral solution

175. 1.6 mL cefixime oral suspension

176. 25.5 mL/hr

177. 23.4 mL zidovudine syrup

178. (A) 76.7 mL bevacizumab infusion
     (B) 2.6 mL/min

179. 3.87 mL/hr

180. 17.9 mL IV chlorothiazide sodium

181. 25 drops/min D_5W

182. 1.8 mL augmentin oral suspension

183. hydrocortisone cream, 29.85 g and hydrocortisone powder, 0.15 g

REFERENCES

1. Allen LV Jr. Misoprostol 0.0027% mucoadhesive powder. *Int J Pharm Compound*. 2000:4:212.
2. Allen LV Jr. Diltiazem HCl 2% topical gel. *Int J Pharm Compound*. 2002:6:43.
3. Paddock Laboratories. Compounding. Available at: http://paddocklabs.com/compounding.html. Accessed January 22, 2005.
4. Allen LV Jr. Allen's Compounded Formulations. 2nd ed. Washington DC: American Pharmacists Association, 2004.
5. Allen LV Jr. Sertraline 7.5 mg capsules. *Int J Pharm Compound*. 1998;2:443.
6. Allen LV Jr. Interferon ophthalmic solution. *Int J Pharm Compound*. 2000;4:380.
7. Waddell JA, Solimando DA Jr. Gemcitabine and cisplatin (GC) regimen for advanced non-small-cell lung cancer. *Hosp Pharm*. 2000;35:1169–1175.
8. Mayer MI, Solimando DA Jr, Waddell JA. Irinotecan, fluorouracil, and leucovorin for metastatic colorectal cancer. *Hosp Pharm*. 2000;35:1274–1279.
9. Prince SJ. Calculations. *Int J Pharm Compound*. 2000;4:393.
10. Prince SJ. Calculations. *Int J Pharm Compound*. 2000;4:314.
11. Cohen MR, Pacetti S. Infant's death reinforces need for adequate check systems and ready-to use medications forms. *Hosp Pharm*. 1998;33:1306.
12. Prince SJ. Basic pharmacokinetics. In: Ansel HC, Prince SJ, eds. *Pharmaceutical Calculations: The Pharmacist's Handbook*. Baltimore, MD: Lippincott Williams & Wilkins; 2004:156.
13. Prince SJ. Basic pharmacokinetics. In: Ansel HC, Prince SJ, eds. *Pharmaceutical Calculations: The Pharmacist's Handbook*. Baltimore, MD: Lippincott Williams & Wilkins; 2004:163–164.
14. Prince SJ. Basic pharmacokinetics. In: Ansel HC, Prince SJ, eds. *Pharmaceutical Calculations: The Pharmacist's Handbook*. Baltimore, MD: Lippincott Williams & Wilkins; 2004:163.

Common Prescription Drugs and Over-the-Counter Products

TOP OVER-THE-COUNTER (OTC) DRUGS*

	Generic Name	Trade Name	Drug Use
1	Docosanol	Abreva®	Cold sore medication
2	Ibuprofen and pseudoephedrine HCl	Advil Cold & Sinus®	Allergy and cold relief
3	Ibuprofen	Advil®	Analgesic
4	Oxymetazoline HCl	Afrin®	Nasal decongestant
5	Naproxen sodium	Aleve®	Analgesic
6	Orlistat	alli®	Weight management
7	Benzocaine, phenol	Anbesol®	Oral cavity analgesic
8	Phenazopyridine hydrochloride	Azo Standard®	UTI analgesic
9	Acetylsalicylic acid (ASA, aspirin), diphenhydramine, caffeine, calcium, phytosterols	Bayer® Aspirin	Analgesic
10	Diphenhydramine HCl, phenylephrine HCl	Benadryl® Oral	Allergy and cold relief
11	Diphenhydramine HCl, zinc acetate or camphor	Benadryl® Topical	Topical antipruritic
12	Methyl salicylate, menthol, and camphor	BENGAY®	Topical analgesic
13	Meclizine hydrochloride, cyclizine hydrochloride	Bonine®	Motion sickness medication
14	Acetylsalicylic acid (ASA, aspirin) with buffers	Bufferin®	Analgesic
15	Capsaicin	Capzasin-P	Topical analgesic
16	Menthol, camphor, alum, salicylic acid	Carmex® Lip Balm	Cold sore medication
17	Benzocaine, menthol, dextromethorphan	Cepacol®	Oral cavity analgesic
18	Benzocaine and menthol or phenol	Chloraseptic®	Oral cavity analgesic
19	Calcium citrate	Citracal®	Essential mineral
20	Loratadine and pseudoephedrine sulfate	Claritin-D®	Allergy and cold relief
21	Loratadine	Claritin®	Allergy and cold relief
22	Docusate sodium	Colace®	Stool softener
23	Zincum gluconicum	COLD-EEZE®	Cold relief
24	Salicylic acid	Compound W®	Keratolytic
25	Hydrocortisone	Cortaid®	Topical antipruritic
26	Acetaminophen, dextromethorphan HBr, phenylephrine HCl	DayQuil®	Allergy and cold relief
27	Carbamide peroxide solution	Debrox®	Ear wax removal aid
28	Dextromethorphan polistirex	Delsym®	Cough suppressant
29	Zinc oxide	Desitin®	Skin protectant
30	Brompheniramine maleate, phenylephrine hydrochloride, dextromethorphan hydrobromide, loratadine	Dimetapp®	Allergy and cold relief
31	Dimenhydrinate or meclizine HCl	Dramamine®	Motion sickness medication
32	Bisacodyl	Dulcolax®	Laxative
33		e.p.t.®	Pregnancy test
34	Acetylsalicylic acid (aspirin, ASA)	Ecotrin	Analgesic
35	Phosphorated carbohydrates	Emetrol®	Antiemetic

(Continued on next page)

TOP OVER-THE-COUNTER (OTC) DRUGS* (Continued)

	Generic Name	Trade Name	Drug Use
36	Soy, black cohosh	Estroven®	Menopause support
37		Eucerin®	Skin moisturizer
38	Acetaminophen, aspirin, caffeine, diphenhydramine citrate	Excedrin® & Excedrin® PM	Analgesic laxative
39	Polycarbophil calcium	FiberCon®	
40		First Response® Ovulation Test	Ovulation test
41	Undecylenic acid	Fungi-Nail®	Antifungal, topical
42	Simethicone, calcium carbonate	Gas-X®	Antiflatulent
43	Menthol or pectin	Halls® Cough Drops	Antitussive
44	Loperamide HCl	Imodium® A-D	Antidiarrheal
45	Ammonium lactate, urea, salicylic acid	Kerasal® Foot Cream	Skin moisturizer
46	Lactase enzyme	Lactaid®	Digestive aid
47	Terbinafine hydrochloride or tolnaftate	Lamisil® AT	Antifungal
48	Clotrimazole or miconazole nitrate	Lotrimin AF®	Antifungal, topical
49	Aluminum hydroxide, magnesium hydroxide, calcium carbonate, simethicone	Maalox® & Maalox® Max	Antacid
50	Psyllium hydrophilic mucilloid	Metamucil®	Laxative
51	Pamabrom, pyrilamine maleate, acetaminophen, caffeine, ibuprofen, naproxen sodium, diphenhydramine	Midol® Products	Analgesic
52	Polyethylene glycol 3350, NF	Miralax[a]	Laxative
53	Miconazole nitrate, tioconazole	Monistat® Vaginal	Vaginal antifungal
54	Ibuprofen	Motrin® IB	Analgesic
55	Guaifenesin, pseudoephedrine HCl, and dextromethorphan HBr	Mucinex® (Adult)	Expectorant
56	Aluminum hydroxide, magnesium (hydroxide and carbonate),calcium carbonate, simethicone	Mylanta®	Antacid
57	Simethicone	Mylicon® Drops	Antiflatulent
58	Pheniramine maleate, naphazoline HCl	Naphcon® A	Ophthalmic anti-allergy
59	Cromolyn sodium	Nasalcrom®	Allergy and cold relief
60	Polymyxin B sulfate, neomycin, bacitracin, pramoxine HCl	Neosporin®	Topical anti-infective
61	Nicotine transdermal	Nicoderm® CQ®	Smoking cessation aid
62	Nicotine polacrilex	Nicorette®	Smoking cessation aid
63	Permethrin	Nix®	Pediculicide
64	Ketoconazole	Nizoral® AD Shampoo	Antifungal, topical
65	Caffeine	NoDoz®	Analeptic
66	Chlorpheniramine maleate (CPH), dextromethorphan HBr (DXT), acetaminophen (APAP), doxylamine, succinate phenylephrine (PE)	NyQuil®	Cough and cold relief
67	Sodium chloride	Ocean® Nasal	Nasal decongestant
68	Benzocaine	Orabase®	Oral cavity analgesic
69	Benzocaine	Orajel®	Oral cavity anesthetic
70	Glucose oxidase, lactoperoxidase, lysozyme	OralBalance®	Oral moisturizer
71	Calcium carbonate	Os-Cal®	Essential mineral
72	Famotidine	Pepcid-AC®	Acid reducer
73	Famotidine, calcium carbonate, magnesium hydroxide	Pepcid® Complete	Acid reducer
74	Bismuth subsalicylate	Pepto Bismol®	Antidiarrheal
75	Docusate sodium and senna	Peri-Colace®	Stool softener plus laxative
76	Magnesium hydroxide	Phillips' MOM	Laxative/antacid
77	Pyrantel pamoate	Pin-X®	Anthelmintic
78	Shark liver oil, petrolatum, mineral oil, phenylephrine HCl	Preparation H® Products	Hemorrhoidal agent

TOP OVER-THE-COUNTER (OTC) DRUGS* (Continued)

	Generic Name	Trade Name	Drug Use
79	Lansoprazole	Prevacid® 24 Hour	Acid reducer
80	Omeprazole magnesium	Prilosec® OTC	Acid reducer
81	Epinephrine, ephedrine, guaifenesin	Primatene®	Bronchodilator
82	Pyrethrins	RID®	Pediculicide
83	Guaifenesin (GUA), dextromethorphan (DXT), chlorpheniramine, diphenhydramine, acetaminophen (APAP)	Robitussin® (Adult)	Cough relief
84	Minoxidil	Rogaine®	Hair growth stimulant
85	Synthetic saliva	Salivart®	Saliva substitute
86	Standardized senna concentrate with or without docusate	Senokot®	Laxative
87	Chamomilla, mercurius solubilis, and sulphur	Similasan Earache Relief®	Earache relief
88	Magnesium chloride and calcium	Slow-Mag®	Essential mineral
89	Pseudoephedrine HCl (PSE), phenylephrine (PE), dextromethorphan HBr (DXT), acetaminophen (APAP), chlorpheniramine HCl (CPH), guaifenesin (GUA), Diphenhydramine	Sudafed®	Allergy and cold relief
90	Polyethylene glycol 400, propylene glycol	Systane®	Artificial tears
91	Hydroxypropyl methylcellulose, dextran 70, white petrolatum, mineral oil	Tears Naturale®	Artificial tears
92	Calcium carbonate	TUMS®	Antacid
93	Acetaminophen (APAP)	Tylenol®	Analgesic
94	Pseudoephedrine HCl (PSE), chlorpheniramine maleate (CPH), acetaminophen (APAP), guaifenesin, Doxylamine succinate, diphenhydramine	Tylenol® Allergy & Sinus	Allergy and cold relief
95	Pseudoephedrine HCl (PSE), chlorpheniramine maleate (CPH), dextromethorphan HBr (DXT), acetaminophen (APAP), doxylamine succinate	Tylenol® Cold (Adult)	Allergy and cold relief
96	Acetaminophen and diphenhydramine HCl	Tylenol® PM	Analgesic/sleep aid
97	Doxylamine succinate or diphenhydramine HCl	Unisom®	Sleeping aid
98	Tetrahydrozoline HCl, oxymetazoline HCl, naphazoline HCl, pheniramine maleate, ketotifen	Visine®	Ophthalmic vasoconstrictor
99	Ketotifen fumarate	Zaditor®	Ophthalmic anti-allergy
100	Ranitidine hydrochloride	Zantac OTC	Acid reducer
101	Zincum gluconicum and zincum aceticum	Zicam® Cold Remedy	Cold relief
102	Benzyl alcohol and benzocaine	Zilactin®	Cold sore medication
103	Cetirizine hydrochloride with pseudoephedrine hydrochloride	Zyrtec-D®	Antiallergy agent
104	Cetirizine hydrochloride	Zyrtec®	Antiallergy agent

*Adapted with permission from SFI Medical Publishing, Copyright 2011.

TOP 300 PRESCRIPTION DRUGS BY TRADE NAME AND GENERIC NAME*

	Generic name	Trade name
1	Hydrocodone Bitartrate with Acetaminophen	Lortab®, Vicodin®, Lorcet®, Norco®
2	Levothyroxine Sodium	Synthroid®, Levoxyl®, Levothroid®
3	Simvastatin	Zocor®
4	Omeprazole	Prilosec®
5	Lisinopril	Prinivil®, Zestril®
6	Zolpidem Tartrate	Ambien® & Ambien CR®
7	Sertraline Hydrochloride	Zoloft®
8	Albuterol Sulfate (inhalation)	Proventil® HFA, Proair® HFA, Ventolin® HFA
9	Duloxetine Hydrochloride	Cymbalta®
10	Metformin	Hydrochloride Glucophage® (XR)
11	Amlodipine Besylate	Norvasc®
12	Bupropion Hydrochloride	Wellbutrin® (SR, XL), Zyban®
13	Prednisone	Deltasone®
14	Amoxicillin Trihydrate	Amoxil®, Moxatag®, Trimox®
15	Atorvastatin Calcium	Lipitor®
16	Alprazolam	Xanax® (XR)
17	Citalopram Hydrobromide	Celexa®
18	Azithromycin Dihydrate	Zithromax® & Zmax™
19	Hydrochlorothiazide	Microzide®
20	Clonazepam	Klonopin®
21	Fluticasone Propionate (nasal)	Flonase™
22	Escitalopram Oxalate	Lexapro®
23	Tramadol Hydrochloride	Ultram® (ER), Ryzolt®
24	Furosemide	Lasix®
25	Sulfamethoxazole with Trimethoprim	Bactrim®, Septra®
26	Esomeprazole Magnesium	Nexium®
27	Montelukast Sodium	Singulair®
28	Amoxicillin with Clavulanate Potassium	Augmentin® (XR)
29	Cyclobenzaprine Hydrochloride	Flexeril®, Amrix®, Fexmid®
30	Gabapentin	Neurontin®
31	Lorazepam	Ativan®
32	Fluticasone Propionate with Salmeterol Xinafoate (Inhalation)	Advair®
33	Metoprolol Succinate	Toprol-XL™
34	Meloxicam	Mobic®
35	Potassium Chloride (oral)	Klor-Con®, K-Dur®, Micro-K®
36	Warfarin Sodium (Crystalline)	Coumadin®, Jantoven®
37	Fluconazole	Diflucan®
38	Quetiapine Fumarate	Seroquel®
39	Naproxen	Naprosyn® & EC-Naprosyn®
40	Topiramate	Topamax®
41	Ciprofloxacin Hydrochloride	Cipro® (XR)
42	Acetaminophen with Codeine Phosphate	Tylenol®, (with Codeine)
43	Alendronate Sodium	Fosamax®
44	Rosuvastatin Calcium	Crestor®
45	Amitriptyline Hydrochloride	Elavil®
46	Fexofenadine Hydrochloride	Allegra®
47	Carvedilol	Coreg® & Coreg® CR
48	Risperidone	Risperdal®
49	Tolterodine Tartrate	Detrol® (LA)
50	Doxycycline Hyclate	Vibramycin®
51	Pantoprazole Sodium	Protonix®

TOP 300 PRESCRIPTION DRUGS BY TRADE NAME AND GENERIC NAME* (Continued)

	Generic name	Trade name
52	Pregabalin	Lyrica®
53	Amphetamine and Dextroamphetamine Salts	Adderall® (XR)
54	Ondansetron Hydrochloride	Zofran®
55	Lansoprazole	Prevacid®
56	Oxycodone Hydrochloride with Acetaminophen	Percocet®, Roxicet®, Endocet®
57	Atenolol	Tenormin®
58	Mometasone Furoate Monohydrate (intranasal)	Nasonex®
59	Divalproex Sodium	Depakote® (ER)
60	Metoprolol Tartrate	Lopressor®
61	Diclofenac Sodium (oral)	Voltaren® (XR)
62	Diltiazem Hydrochloride	Cardizem® (CD), Cartia®, Tiazac®
63	Lamotrigine	Lamictal® and Lamictal® XR
64	Venlafaxine Hydrochloride	Effexor® (XR)
65	Aspirin, enteric-coated	Aspirin, enteric-coated
66	Celecoxib	Celebrex®
67	Diazepam	Valium®
68	Eszopiclone	Lunesta®
69	Tamsulosin Hydrochloride	Flomax®
70	Donepezil Hydrochloride	Aricept™
71	Metoclopramide Hydrochloride	Reglan®
72	Allopurinol	Zyloprim®
73	Fluoxetine Hydrochloride	Prozac®
74	Insulin Glargine (rDNA origin)	Lantus®
75	Pioglitazone Hydrochloride	Actos®
76	Triamterene with Hydrochlorothiazide	Dyazide®, Maxzide®
77	Polyethylene Glycol 3350, NF	Miralax™, Glycolax®
78	Cefdinir	Omnicef®
79	Levofloxacin	Levaquin®
80	Niacin (extended-release)	Niaspan®
81	Lisinopril with Hydrochlorothiazide	Zestoretic®, Prinzide®
82	Fenofibrate (nanocrystallized)	TriCor®
83	Ziprasidone Hydrochloride	Geodon®
84	Olmesartan Medoxomil	Benicar®
85	Thyroid, desiccated	Armour® Thyroid
86	Aripiprazole	Abilify®
87	Ranitidine Hydrochloride	Zantac®
88	Oxycodone Hydrochloride (immediate-release)	Roxicodone®
89	Ramipril	Altace®
90	Clopidogrel Bisulfate	Plavix®
91	Ezetimibe	Zetia®
92	Spironolactone	Aldactone®
93	Tiotropium Bromide (inhalation)	Spiriva®
94	Famotidine	Pepcid®
95	Codeine Phosphate with Guaifenesin	Mytussin AC®, Robitussin® AC
96	Norgestimate with Ethinyl Estradiol (triphasic)	Ortho Tri-Cyclen®, TriSprintec®, Trinessa®
97	Ibuprofen	Motrin®
98	Memantine Hydrochloride	Namenda® (XR)
99	Folic Acid	Folic Acid
100	Cephalexin Monohydrate	Keflex®
101	Trazodone Hydrochloride	Desyrel®
102	Carisoprodol	Soma®

(Continued on next page)

TOP 300 PRESCRIPTION DRUGS BY TRADE NAME AND GENERIC NAME* (Continued)

	Generic name	Trade name
103	Norgestrel with Ethinyl Estradiol	Ovral®, Lo-Ovral®, Ogestrel®, Cryselle®
104	Glyburide	Micronase®, DiaBeta®
105	Olmesartan Medoxomil with Hydrochlorothiazide	Benicar-HCT®
106	Losartan Potassium	Cozaar®
107	Estrogens (Conjugated)	Premarin®
108	Valsartan	Diovan®
109	Lidocaine (Transdermal)	Lidoderm®
110	Enalapril Maleate	Vasotec®
111	Tadalafil	Cialis®
112	Glipizide	Glucotrol® (XL)
113	Mupirocin (topical)	Bactroban®
114	Ezetimibe with Simvastatin	Vytorin®
115	Vitamin D, Ergocalciferol	Drisdol®
116	Ferrous Sulfate	Slow FE®
117	Glimepiride	Amaryl®
118	Ibandronate Sodium	Boniva®
119	Drospirenone with Ethinyl Estradiol (21)	Yasmin®, Ocella®
120	Minocycline Hydrochloride	Minocin®
121	Norethindrone, Ethinyl Estradiol, Ferrous Fumarate	Loestrin FE®, Microgestin® FE, Junel® FE
122	Benazepril Hydrochloride	Lotensin®
123	Fentanyl (transdermal)	Duragesic®
124	Nitrofurantoin	Macrodantin® & Macrobid®
125	Norethindrone, Ethinyl Estradiol, Ferrous Fumarate	Loestrin® 24 FE
126	Norgestimate with Ethinyl Estradiol (triphasic)	Tri-Cyclen® Lo
127	Digoxin	Lanoxin®, Digitek®
128	Fluticasone Propionate (inhalation)	Flovent®
129	Levetiracetam	Keppra®
130	Terazosin Hydrochloride	Hytrin®
131	Acyclovir	Zovirax®
132	Irbesartan	Avapro®
133	Budesonide (inhalation)	Pulmicort®
134	Valacyclovir Hydrochloride	Valtrex®
135	Desvenlafaxine	Pristiq®
136	Carbamazepine	Tegretol®(XR), Carbatrol® ER, Equetrol® ER
137	Levonorgestrel with Ethinyl Estradiol	Alesse®, Aviane®
138	Lithium Carbonate	Lithonate®, Lithotabs®, Lithobid®
139	Etonogestrel with Ethinyl Estradiol (vaginal)	NuvaRing®
140	Lovastatin	Mevacor®
141	Pravastatin Sodium	Pravachol®
142	Benzonatate	Tessalon®
143	Insulin Aspart, (rDNA origin)	Novolog®
144	Paroxetine Hydrochloride	Paxil® (XR), Pexeva®
145	Promethazine HCl with Codeine Phosphate	Phenergan® with Codeine
146	Moxifloxacin Hydrochloride (oral)	Avelox®
147	Tizanidine Hydrochloride	Zanaflex®
148	Clonidine Hydrochloride	Catapres® and Catapres® TTS
149	Morphine Sulfate (extended release)	MS Contin®
150	Propranolol Hydrochloride	Inderal® (LA), Innopran® XL
151	Modafinil	Provigil®
152	Meclizine Hydrochloride	Antivert®
153	Hydroxyzine Hydrochloride	Atarax®

TOP 300 PRESCRIPTION DRUGS BY TRADE NAME AND GENERIC NAME* (Continued)

	Generic name	Trade name
154	Triamcinolone Acetonide (intranasal)	Nasacort® AQ
155	Oxybutynin Chloride (oral)	Ditropan®& Ditropan® XL
156	Diphenoxylate HCl with Atropine Sulfate	Lomotil®
157	Fluocinonide (topical)	Lidex®
158	Levalbuterol Hydrochloride	Xopenex®
159	Insulin Lispro (rDNA Origin)	Humalog®
160	Metronidazole	Flagyl®
161	Oxcarbazepine	Trileptal®
162	Levocetirizine Dihydrochloride	Xyzal®
163	Methylphenidate Hydrochloride (ER)	Concerta®
164	Buspirone Hydrochloride	BuSpar®
165	Lisdexamfetamine Dimesylate	Vyvanse
166	Carbidopa with Levodopa	Sinemet® (CR)
167	Clindamycin Hydrochloride (oral)	Cleocin®
168	Dipyridamole and Aspirin	Aggrenox®
169	Darifenacin Hydrobromide	Enablex®
170	Methylprednisolone	Medrol®
171	Baclofen	Lioresal®
172	Nystatin (topical)	Nystop®
173	Sumatriptan Succinate	Imitrex™
174	Phenytoin Sodium (Extended)	Dilantin® Kapseals®
175	Promethazine HCl	Phenergan®
176	Prednisolone Sodium Phosphate	Orapred®
177	Drospirenone with Ethinyl Estradiol (24)	Yaz®
178	Bumetanide	Bumex®
179	Mirtazapine	Remeron®
180	Gemfibrozil	Lopid®
181	Hydroxychloroquine Sulfate	Plaquenil®
182	Olopatadine Hydrochloride (Ophthalmic)	Patanol® & Pataday®
183	Budesonide and Formoterol Fumarate Dihydrate (Inhalation)	Symbicort
184	Norethindrone with Ethinyl Estradiol (1/35)	Necon® 1/35, Ortho Novum® 1/35
185	Testosterone Gel (topical)	Androgel
186	Clozapine	Clozaril®
187	Varenicline Tartrate	Chantix™
188	Insulin Detemir (Levemir®)	Levemir®
189	Phenazopyridine Hydrochloride	Pyridium®
190	Sildenafil Citrate	Viagra®
191	Sitagliptin Phosphate	Januvia®
192	Progesterone (oral)	Prometrium®
193	Atomoxetine Hydrochloride	Strattera®
194	Chlorhexidine Gluconate	Peridex®, Periogard®
195	Diclofenac Sodium (topical)	Voltaren Gel
196	Estradiol (oral)	Estrace®
197	Raloxifene Hydrochloride	Evista®
198	Insulin (Humulin®)	Humulin®
199	Hyoscyamine Sulfate	Levsin®, Levbid®
200	Telmisartan	Micardis®
201	Glyburide with Metformin Hydrochloride	Glucovance®
202	Isosorbide Mononitrate	Imdur®
203	Ropinirole Hydrochloride	Requip® (XL)
204	Fluticasone Furoate (nasal)	Veramyst®

(Continued on next page)

TOP 300 PRESCRIPTION DRUGS BY TRADE NAME AND GENERIC NAME* (Continued)

	Generic name	Trade name
205	Sucralfate	Carafate®
206	Solifenacin Succinate	Vesicare®
207	Moxifloxacin Hydrochloride (ophthalmic)	Vigamox®
208	Ipratropium Bromide with Albuterol Sulfate	DuoNeb®
209	Colchicine	Colcrys®
210	Nifedipine	Procardia®(XL),Nifedical® XL, Adalat CC®
211	Estrogens (Conjugated) with Medroxyprogesterone Acetate	Prempro™
212	Terbinafine Hydrochloride (oral)	Lamisil®
213	Temazepam	Restoril®
214	Ketoconazole	Nizoral®
215	Hydrocortisone (rectal)	Anusol-HC, Proctosol-HC
216	Triamcinolone Acetonide (topical)	Kenalog®
217	Cyclosporine Emulsion (ophthalmic)	Restasis®
218	Phentermine Hydrochloride	Adipex-P®, Ionamin®
219	Sitagliptin Phosphate and Metformin Hydrochloride	Janumet
220	Omega-3-Acid Ethyl Esters	Lovaza®
221	Methotrexate Sodium	Trexall®
222	Phenobarbital	Phenobarbital
223	Ciclopirox	Loprox
224	Quinine Sulfate	Qualaquin®
225	Valsartan with Hydrochlorothiazide	Diovan-HCT®
226	Metolazone	Zaroxolyn®
227	Efavirenz, Emtricitabine, and Tenofovir	Atripla®
228	Losartan Potassium with Hydrochlorothiazide	Hyzaar®
229	Quinapril Hydrochloride	Accupril®
230	Verapamil Hydrochloride	Isoptin®, Calan®, Verelan®
231	Anastrozole	Arimidex®
232	Dicyclomine Hydrochloride	Bentyl®
233	Finasteride	Proscar®
234	Methadone Hydrochloride	Methadone
235	Risedronate Sodium	Actonel®
236	Ipratropium Bromide with Albuterol Sulfate (MDI)	Combivent®
237	Conjugated Estrogens (Vaginal)	Premarin Vaginal®
238	Olanzapine	Zyprexa®
239	Chlorpheniramine with Hydrocodone	Tussionex®
240	Nebivolol Hydrochloride	Bystolic®
241	Oxycodone Hydrochloride (controlled-release)	OxyContin®
242	Scopolamine (topical)	Transderm Scop
243	Methylphenidate Hydrochloride (IR & ER)	Ritalin®, Methylin®, Metadate®
244	Clotrimazole with Betamethasone Dipropionate	Lotrisone®
245	Nitroglycerin (sublingual & injectable)	Nitrostat®, Nitroquick®
246	Estradiol (topical)	Vivelle-Dot®
247	Amlodipine Besylate with Benazepril Hydrochloride	Lotrel®
248	Nystatin with Triamcinolone Acetonide	Mycolog® II
249	Medroxyprogesterone Acetate	Provera®
250	Tramadol Hydrochloride with Acetaminophen	Ultracet®
251	Famciclovir	Famvir®
252	Penicillin V Potassium	Veetids, Pen-Vee K, V-Cillin
253	Ciprofloxacin with Dexamethasone (otic)	CiproDex®
254	Exenatide	Byetta®
255	Metaxalone	Skelaxin®

TOP 300 PRESCRIPTION DRUGS BY TRADE NAME AND GENERIC NAME* (Continued)

	Generic name	Trade name
256	Rabeprazole Sodium	Aciphex®
257	Doxepin Hydrochloride	Sinequan®
258	Timolol Maleate (ophthalmic)	Timoptic® (XR)
259	Latanoprost	Xalatan®
260	Irbesartan with Hydrochlorothiazide	Avalide®
261	Tetracycline Hydrochloride	Sumycin®, Panmycin®
262	Clobetasol Propionate (topical)	Temovate®
263	Torsemide	Demadex®
264	Candesartan Cilexetil	Atacand®
265	Fexofenadine HCl with Pseudoephedrine HCl	Allegra-D®
266	Norgestimate and Ethinyl Estradiol	Ortho-Cyclen®, Sprintec®
267	Pramipexole Dihydrochloride	Mirapex®
268	Desogestrel with Ethinyl Estradiol (.15/.03)	Desogen®, Ortho-Cept®, Apri®
269	Azelastine Hydrochloride	Astelin®
270	Hydrocodone Bitartrate with Ibuprofen	Vicoprofen®
271	Travoprost	Travatan® Z
272	Nystatin (oral)	Nystatin (oral)
273	Dexmethylphenidate Hydrochloride	Focalin® (XR)
274	Cefuroxime Axetil	Ceftin®
275	Doxazosin Mesylate	Cardura® (XL)
276	Benztropine Mesylate	Cogentin®
277	Levonorgestrel with Ethinyl Estradiol (triphasic)	Triphasil®, Trivora®, Enpresse®
278	Nortriptyline Hydrochloride	Pamelor®
279	Insulin (Novolin®)	Novolin®
280	Brimonidine Tartrate (ophthalmic)	Alphagan® P
281	Clarithromycin	Biaxin® (XL)
282	Indomethacin	Indocin®
283	Dexamethasone (oral)	Decadron®
284	Mometasone Furoate (topical)	Elocon®
285	Dutasteride	Avodart®
286	Fosinopril Sodium	Monopril®
287	Trandolapril	Mavik®
288	Oseltamivir Phosphate	Tamiflu®
289	Gatifloxacin (ophthalmic)	Zymaxid®
290	Tamoxifen Citrate	Nolvadex®
291	Sulindac	Clinoril®
292	Telmisartan with Hydrochlorothiazide	Micardis® HCT
293	Benazepril Hydrochloride with Hydrochlorothiazide	Lotensin HCT®
294	Methocarbamol	Robaxin®
295	Nabumetone	Relafen®
296	Prochlorperazine	Compazine®
297	Hydroxyzine Pamoate	Vistaril®
298	Butalbital, Acetaminophen and Caffeine	Fioricet®
299	Piroxicam	Feldene®
300	Buprenorphine HCl with Naloxone HCl	Suboxone®

*Adapted with permission from SFI Medical Publishing, Copyright 2011.

Prescription Dispensing Information and Metrology

Prescriptions

PARTS OF THE PRESCRIPTION

A prescription is an order for medication for use by a patient that is issued by a physician, dentist, veterinarian, or other licensed practitioner who is authorized to prescribe medication or by their agent via a collaborative practice agreement. A prescription is usually written on a single sheet of paper that is commonly imprinted with the prescriber's name, address, and telephone number. A medication order is similar to a prescription, but it is written on the patient chart and intended for use by a patient in an institutional setting.

All prescriptions should contain accurate and appropriate information about the patient and the medication that is being prescribed. In addition, a prescription order for a **controlled substance** must contain the following information:

1. Date of issue
2. Full name and address of the patient
3. Drug name, strength, dosage form, and quantity prescribed
4. Directions for use
5. Name, address, and Drug Enforcement Agency (DEA) number of the prescriber
6. Signature of the prescriber

A written prescription order is required for substances listed in **Schedule II.** Prescriptions for controlled substances listed in **Schedule II** are **never** refillable. Any other prescription that has no indication of refills is not refillable.

Prescriptions for medications that are listed in Schedules III, IV, and V may be issued either in writing or orally to the pharmacist. If authorized by the prescriber, these prescriptions may be refilled up to five times within 6 months of the date of issue. If the prescriber wishes the patient to continue to take the medication after 6 months or five refills, a new prescription order is required.

THE PRESCRIPTION LABEL

In addition to the name of the patient, the pharmacy, and the prescriber, the prescription label should accurately identify the medication and provide directions for its use.

The label for a prescription order for a controlled substance must contain the following information:

1. Name and address of the pharmacy
2. Serial number assigned to the prescription by the pharmacy
3. Date of the initial filling
4. Name of the patient
5. Name of the prescriber
6. Directions for use
7. Cautionary statements as required by law*

AUXILIARY LABELS

Auxiliary, or cautionary, labels provide additional important information about the proper use of the medication. Examples include "Shake Well" for suspensions or emulsions; "For External Use Only" for topical lotions, solutions, or creams; and "May Cause Drowsiness" for medications that depress the central nervous system. The information contained on auxiliary labels should be brought to the attention of the patient when the medication is dispensed. The pharmacist should place only appropriate auxiliary labels on the prescription container because too many labels may confuse the patient.

BEFORE DISPENSING THE PRESCRIPTION

Double-check the accuracy of the prescription.
Provide undivided attention when filling the prescription.

1. Check the patient information (e.g., name, address, date of birth, telephone number).
2. Check the patient profile (e.g., allergies, medical conditions, other drugs, including over-the-counter medications).
3. Check the drug (e.g., correct drug name, correct spelling, appropriate drug for the patient's condition), and verify that there are no known drug interactions. **Always verify**

---

*The label of any drug that is listed as a controlled substance in Schedule II, III, or IV of the Controlled Substances Act must contain the following warning: **CAUTION: Federal law prohibits the transfer of this drug to any person other than the patient for whom it was prescribed.**

the name of the drug. **Beware of drug names that look alike (see table).**

4. Check the dosage, including the drug strength, the dosage form (e.g., capsule, liquid, modified release), the individual dose, the total daily dose, the duration of treatment, and the units (e.g., mg, mL, tsp, tbsp).

5. Check the label. Compare the drug dispensed with the prescription. Verify the National Drug Code (NDC) number. Ensure that the information is accurate, that the patient directions are accurate and easily understood, and that the auxiliary labels are appropriate.

6. **Provide patient counseling. Be sure that the patient fully understands the drug treatment as well as any precautions.**

EXAMPLES OF DRUGS WITH SIMILAR NAMES

Brand name	Celebrex	Cerebyx	Celexa
Generic name	Celecoxib capsules	Fosphenytoin sodium injection	Citalopram HCl
Manufacturer	Searle	Parke-Davis	Forest
Indication	Osteoarthritis and rheumatoid arthritis	Prevention and treatment of seizures	Major depression

Dangerous or Confusing Abbreviations

Numerous common abbreviations and symbols have been associated with errors. Detailed lists of these can be found at the websites of the Institute for Safe Medication Practices (ISMP) and Joint Commission for the Accreditation of Healthcare Organizations (JCAHO) at :

http://www.ismp.org/Tools/abbreviationslist.pdf.
http://www.jcaho.org/accredited+organizations/patient+safety/06_dnu_list.pdf.

The JCAHO has created a "Do Not Use" list of abbreviations that its accredited organizations should not allow to be used.

- **"U" or "IU" for units**: the "U" has been misinterpreted as various numbers such as zero, four; serious harm has occurred with insulin and heparin as a result of confusion. For example, a patient received 66 units of insulin instead of 6 units. The order was written for "6u" of regular insulin but was misinterpreted. The word "units" should be written out in full.

- **"QD, Q.D, qd, q.d."**: common abbreviations for daily have been misinterpreted as "QID" or "qid" and overdoses have occurred. "Daily" should be written out in full.

- **"Q.O.D, QOD, qod"**: common abbreviations for every other day have been misinterpreted as QID (four times daily). This should be written out completely as "every other day."

- **Trailing zero**: when a dose is ordered and followed with a decimal point and a zero, such as 2.0 mg or 25.0 mg, errors can occur. The decimal point may be missed and an overdose can occur. For example, Warfarin 2.0 mg may be misinterpreted as 20 mg. Trailing zeros should be avoided and the dose written without the additional zero, for example Warfarin 2 mg rather than 2.0 mg.

- **Lack of leading zero**: a drug's dose may be less than 1 mg, such as Digoxin. Often the dose may be written without a leading zero, such as Digoxin .25 mg, rather than as Digoxin 0.25 mg. Errors have occurred because the decimal point is missed. For example, Warfarin .5 mg may be interpreted as Warfarin 5 mg. Leading zeroes should be included, so the dose is written as "Digoxin 0.25 mg or Warfarin 0.5 mg."

- **MS, MSO4, MgSO$_4$: Abbreviations for morphine sulfate (MS, MSO$_4$) have been confused with Magnesium sulfate (MgSO$_4$). It is recommend to write out each name in full rather than using abbreviations: morphine sulfate or magnesium sulfate.**

In addition to the above abbreviations, there are numerous other hazardous symbols and abbreviations which should be reviewed with caution when used on prescriptions. Examples include:

- **"cc"** : Often used instead of "mL." This has been misinterpreted as a "0" (zero). Use "mL."

- **"μg"** : Used for "micrograms," for example, Levothyroxine 250 μg. daily. The symbol has been mistaken for "mg." and overdoses have occurred. Best to use "mcg." Or write out "micrograms."

- **"<" or ">"** : Symbols for " less than" (<) or "greater than" (>) have been mistaken for each other or misinterpreted as numbers. Best to write out as "less than" or "greater than."

- **"HCT"** : An abbreviation for "hydrocortisone" has been misinterpreted as "hydrochlorothiazide. " Best to write name out completely.

- **"HCl"** : An abbreviation for "hydrochloric acid" has been misinterpreted as "KCl" (potassium chloride). Best to write out name completely.

COMMON ABBREVIATIONS

Considerable variation occurs in the use of capitalization, italicization, and punctuation in abbreviations. The following list shows the abbreviations that are most often encountered by pharmacists.

A, aa., or aa	of each
a.c.	before meals
ad	to, up to
a.d.	right ear
ad lib.	at pleasure, freely
a.m.	morning
amp.	ampule
ante	before
aq.	water
a.s.	left ear
asa	aspirin
a.u.	each ear, both ears
b.i.d.	twice a day
BP	British Pharmacopoeia
BSA	body surface area
c. or c	with
cap. or caps.	capsule
cp	chest pain
D.A.W.	dispense as written
cc or cc.	cubic centimeter
comp.	compound, compounded
dil.	dilute
D.C., dc, or disc.	discontinue
disp.	dispense
div.	divide, to be divided
dl or dL	deciliter
d.t.d.	give of such doses
DW	distilled water
D5W	dextrose 5% in water
elix.	elixir
e.m.p.	as directed
et	and
ex aq.	in water
fl or fld	fluid
fl oz	fluid ounce
ft.	make
g or Gm	gram
gal.	gallon
GI	gastrointestinal
gr or gr.	grain
gtt or gtt.	drop, drops
H	hypodermic
h. or hr.	hour
h.s.	at bedtime
IM	intramuscular
inj.	injection
IV	intravenous
IVP	intravenous push
IVPB	intravenous piggyback
K	potassium
l or L	liter

lb.	pound
μ	Greek mu
M	mix
m^2 or M^2	square meter
mcg, mcg., or μg	microgram
mEq	milliequivalent
mg or mg.	milligram
ml or mL	milliliter
μl or μL	microliter
℥	minim
N&V	nausea and vomiting
Na	sodium
N.F.	National Formulary
No.	number
noct.	night, in the night
non rep.	do not repeat
NPO	nothing by mouth
N.S., NS, or N/S	normal saline
1/2 NS	half-strength normal saline
O	pint
o.d.	right eye, every day
o.l. or o.s.	left eye
OTC	over the counter
o.u.	each eye, both eyes
oz.	ounce
p.c.	after meals
PDR	*Physicians' Desk Reference*
p.m.	afternoon, evening
p.o.	by mouth
Ppt	precipitated
pr	for the rectum
prn or p.r.n.	as needed
pt.	pint
pulv.	powder
pv	for vaginal use
q.	every
q.d.	every day
q.h.	every hour
q. 4 hr.	every four hours
q.i.d.	four times a day
q.o.d.	every other day
q.s.	a sufficient quantity
q.s. ad	a sufficient quantity to make
R	rectal
R.L. or R/L	Ringer's lactate
℞	prescription
s. or s	without
Sig.	write on label
sol.	solution
S.O.B.	shortness of breath
s.o.s.	if there is need (once only)

ss. or ss	one-half	**t.i.d.**	three times a day
stat.	immediately	**tr. or tinct.**	tincture
subc, subq, or s.c.	subcutaneously	**tsp. or t.**	teaspoonful
sup. or supp	suppository	**TT**	tablet triturates
susp.	suspension	**U or u.**	unit
syr.	syrup	**u.d. or ut dict.**	as directed
tab.	tablet	**ung.**	ointment
tal.	such, such a one	**U.S.P. or USP**	United States Pharmacopoeia
tal. dos.	such doses	**w/v**	weight/volume
tbsp. or T	tablespoonful		

Metrology

THE METRIC, APOTHECARY, AND AVOIRDUPOIS SYSTEMS

Metric system

1. **Basic units**

    Mass = g or gram
    Length = m or meter
    Volume = L or liter
        1 cc (cubic centimeter) of water is approximately equal to 1 mL and weighs 1 g.

2. **Prefixes**

    kilo- 10^3, or 1000 times the basic unit
    hekto- 10^2, or 100 times the basic unit
    deka- 10^1, or 10 times the basic unit
    deci- 10^{-1}, or 0.1 times the basic unit
    centi- 10^{-2}, or 0.01 times the basic unit
    milli- 10^{-3}, or 0.001 times the basic unit
    micro- 10^{-6}, or one-millionth of the basic unit
    nano- 10^{-9}, or one-billionth of the basic unit
    pico- 10^{-12}, or one-trillionth of the basic unit

    Examples of these prefixes include milligram (mg), which equals one-thousandth of a gram, and deciliter (dL), which equals 100 mL, or 0.1 L.

Apothecary system

1. **Volume (fluids or liquid)**

                60 minims (♏) = 1 fluidrachm or fluidram (f ʒ)
                            or (ʒ)
    8 fluidrachms (480 minims) = 1 fluid ounce (f ℥ or ℥)
            16 fluid ounces = 1 pint (pt or 0)
    2 pints (32 fluid ounces) = 1 quart (qt)
            4 quarts (8 pints) = 1 gallon (gal or C)

2. **Mass (weight)**

                20 grains (gr) = 1 scruple (Ә)
     3 scruples (60 grains) = 1 drachm or dram (ʒ)
    8 drachms (480 grains) = 1 ounce (℥)
    12 ounces (5760 grains) = 1 pound (lb)

Avoirdupois system

1. **Volume**

    1 fluidrachm = 60 min.
    1 fluid ounce = 8 fl. dr.
                = 480 min.
        1 pint = 16 fl. oz.
                = 7680 min.
        1 quart = 2 pt.
                = 32 fl. oz.
        1 gallon = 4 qt.
                = 128 fl. oz.

2. **Mass (weight)**

    The grain is common to both the apothecary and the avoirdupois systems.

    437.5 grains (gr) = 1 ounce (oz)
    16 ounces (7000 grains) = 1 pound (lb)

CONVERSION

Exact equivalents

Exact equivalents are used for the conversion of specific quantities in pharmaceutical formulas and prescription compounding.

1. **Length**

    1 meter (m) = 39.37 in.
        1 inch (in) = 2.54 cm.

2. **Volume**

            1 ml = 16.23 minims (♏)
            1 ♏ = 0.06 mL
            1 f ʒ = 3.69 mL
            1 f ℥ = 29.57 mL
            1 pt = 473 mL
        1 gal (U.S.) = 3785 mL

3. **Mass**

$$1 \text{ g} = 15.432 \text{ gr}$$
$$1 \text{ kg} = 2.20 \text{ lb (avoir.)}$$
$$1 \text{ gr} = 0.065 \text{ g or } 65 \text{ mg}$$
$$1 \text{ oz (avoir.)} = 28.35 \text{ g}$$
$$1 \text{ ℥ (apoth.)} = 31.1 \text{ g}$$
$$1 \text{ lb (avoir.)} = 454 \text{ g}$$
$$1 \text{ lb (apoth.)} = 373.2 \text{ g}$$

4. **Other equivalents**

$$1 \text{ oz (avoir.)} = 437.5 \text{ gr}$$
$$1 \text{ ℥ (apoth.)} = 480 \text{ gr}$$
$$1 \text{ gal (U.S.)} = 128 \text{ fl ℥}$$
$$1 \text{ fl ℥ (water)} = 455 \text{ gr}$$
$$1 \text{ gr (apoth.)} = 1 \text{ gr (avoir.)}$$

Approximate equivalents

Physicians may use approximate equivalents to prescribe the dose quantities using the metric and apothecary systems of weights and measures, respectively. Household units are often used to inform the patient of the size of the dose. In view of the almost universal practice of using an ordinary household teaspoon to administer medication, a teaspoon may be considered 5 mL. However, when accurate measurement of a liquid dose is required, the USP recommends the use of a calibrated oral syringe or dropper.

$$1 \text{ fluid dram} = 1 \text{ teaspoonful}$$
$$= 5 \text{ mL}$$
$$4 \text{ fluid ounces} = 120 \text{ mL}$$
$$8 \text{ fluid ounces} = 1 \text{ cup}$$
$$= 240 \text{ mL}$$
$$1 \text{ grain} = 65 \text{ mg}$$
$$1 \text{ kg} = 2.2 \text{ pounds (lb)}$$

Reference Charts For Patient Counseling

DRUGS THAT SHOULD NOT BE CRUSHED

Listed below are various slow-release as well as enteric-coated products that should not be crushed or chewed. Slow-release (sr) represents products that are controlled-release, extended-release, long-acting, or timed-release. Enteric-coated (ec) represents products that are delayed-release.

In general, capsules containing slow-release or enteric-coated particles may be opened and their contents administered on a spoonful of soft food. Instruct patients not to chew the particles, though. (Patients should, in fact, be discouraged from chewing any medication unless it is specifically formulated for that purpose.)

This list should not be considered all-inclusive. Generic and alternate brands of some products may exist. Tablets intended for sublingual or buccal administration (not included in this list) should also be administered only as intended, in an intact form.

Drug	Manufacturer	Form
Aciphex	Eisai	ec
Adalat CC	Schering Plough	sr
Adderall XR	Shire US	sr
Advicor	KOS	sr
Aerohist	Aero	sr
Aerohist Plus	Aero	sr
Afeditab CR	Watson	sr
Aggrenox	Boehr, Ingelheim	sr
Aldex	Zyber	sr
Aldex-G	Zyber	sr
Aleve Cold & Sinus	Bayer Healthcare	sr
Aleve Sinus & Headache	Bayer Healthcare	sr
Allegra-D 12 Hour	Sanofi-Aventis	sr
Allegra-D 24 Hour	Sanofi-Aventis	sr
Allerx	Cornerstone	sr
Allerx-D	Cornerstone	sr
Allfen	MCR American	sr
Allfen-DM	MCR American	sr
Alophen	Numark	ec
Altex-PSE	Alphagen	sr
Altoprev	First Horizon	sr
Ambi 1000/55	Ambi	sr
Ambi 45/800	Ambi	sr
Ambi 45/800/30	Ambi	sr
Ambi 60/580	Ambi	sr
Ambi 60/580/30	Ambi	sr
Ambi 80/700	Ambi	sr

(Continued on next page)

Drug	Manufacturer	Form
Ambi 80/700/40	Ambi	sr
Ambien CR	Sanofi-Aventis	sr
Ambifed-G	Ambi	sr
Ambifed-G DM	Ambi	sr
Amdry-C	Prasco	sr
Amdry-D	Prasco	sr
Amibid DM	Amide	sr
Amibid LA	Amide	sr
Amidal	Amide	sr
Aminoxin	Tyson Neutraceuticals	ec
Ami-Tex PSE	Amide	sr
Anextuss	Cypress	sr
Aquabid-DM	Alphagen	sr
Aquatab C	Adams	sr
Aquatab D	Adams	sr
Aquatab DM	Adams	sr
Arthrotec	Pharmacia	ec
Asacol	Procter & Gamble	ec
Ascocid-1000	Key	sr
Ascocid-500-D	Key	sr
Ascriptin Enteric	Novartis Consumer	ec
ATP	Tyson Neutraceuticals	ec
Atrohist Pediatric	Celltech	sr
Augmentin XR	GlaxoSmithKline	sr
Avinza	Ligand	sr
Azulfidine Entabs	Pharmacia	ec
Bayer Aspirin Regimen	Bayer Healthcare	ec
Bellahist-D LA	Cypress	sr
Bellatal ER	Qualitest	sr
Biaxin XL	Abbott	sr
Bidex-DM	Stewart-Jackson	sr
Bidhist	Cypress	sr
Bidhist-D	Cypress	sr
Biohist LA	Ivax	sr
Bisac-Evac	G & W	ec
Biscolax	Global Source	ec
Blanex-A	Blansett	sr
Bontril Slow-Release	Valeant	sr
Bromfed	Victory	sr
Bromfed-PD	Victory	sr
Bromfenex	Ethex	sr
Bromfenex PD	Ethex	sr
Bromfenex PE	Ethex	sr
Bromfenex PE Pediatric	Ethex	sr
Budeprion SR	Teva	sr
Buproban	Teva	sr
Calan SR	Pharmacia	sr
Campral	Forest	ec
Carbatrol	Shire US	sr
Cardene SR	Roche	sr
Cardizem CD	Biovail	sr
Cardizem LA	KOS	sr
Cardura XL	Pfizer	sr

Drug	Manufacturer	Form
Carox Plus	Seneca	sr
Cartia XT	Andrx	sr
Catemine	Tyson Neutraceuticals	ec
Cemill 1000	Miller	sr
Cemill 500	Miller	sr
Certuss-D	Capellon	sr
Cevi-Bid	Lee	sr
Chlorex-A	Cypress	sr
Chlor-Phen	Truxton	sr
Chlor-Trimeton Allergy	Schering Plough	sr
Chlor-Trimeton Allergy Decongestant	Schering Plough	sr
Cipro XR	Schering Plough	sr
Clarinex-D 24 Hour	Schering Plough	sr
Coldamine	Breckenridge	sr
Coldec D	Breckenridge	sr
Coldec TR	Breckenridge	sr
Coldex-A	United Research	sr
ColdMist DM	Breckenridge	sr
ColdMist Jr	Breckenridge	sr
ColdMist LA	Breckenridge	sr
Colfed-A	Breckenridge	sr
Concerta	McNeil Consumer	sr
Contac 12-Hour	GlaxoSmithKline	sr
Correctol	Schering Plough	ec
Cotazym-S	Organon	ec
Covera-HS	Pfizer	sr
CPM 8/PE 20/MSC 1.25	Cypress	sr
Crantex ER	Breckenridge	sr
Crantex LA	Breckenridge	sr
Crantex Lac	Breckenridge	sr
Creon 10	Solvay	ec
Creon 20	Solvay	ec
Creon 5	Solvay	ec
Cymbalta	Eli Lilly	ec
Cypex-LA	Cypress	sr
Dacex-PE	Cypress	sr
Dairycare	Plainview	ec
Dallergy	Laser	sr
Dallergy-Jr	Laser	sr
D-Amine-SR	Alphagen	sr
Deconamine SR	Kenwood Therapeutics	sr
Deconex	Poly	sr
Decongest II	Qualitest	sr
De-Congestine	Qualitest	sr
Deconsal II	Cornerstone	sr
Depakote	Abbott	ec
Depakote ER	Abbott	sr
Depakote Sprinkles	Abbott	ec
Despec SR	Int'l Ethical	sr
Detrol LA	Pharmacia	sr
Dexaphen SA	Major	sr
Dexcon-PE	Cypress	sr
Dexedrine Spansules	GlaxoSmithKline	sr

(Continued on next page)

Drug	Manufacturer	Form
D-Feda II	WE Pharm.	sr
Diabetes Trio	Mason Vitamins	sr
Diamox Sequels	Duramed	sr
Dilacor XR	Watson	sr
Dilantin Kapseals	Pfizer	sr
Dilatrate-SR	Schwarz Pharma	sr
Diltia XT	Andrx	sr
Dilt-XR	Apotex	sr
Dimetane Extentabs	Wyeth	sr
Disophrol Chronotab	Schering Plough	sr
Ditropan XL	Ortho-McNeil	sr
Donnatal Extentabs	PBM	sr
Doryx	Warner Chilcott	ec
Drexophed SR	Qualitest	sr
Drihist SR	Prasco	sr
Drixomed	Iopharm	sr
Drixoral	Schering Plough	sr
Drixoral Plus	Schering Plough	sr
Drixoral Sinus	Schering Plough	sr
Drize-R	Monarch	sr
Drysec	A. G. Marin	sr
Dulcolax	Boehr, Ingelheim	ec
Duomax	Capellon	sr
Duradex	Proethic	sr
Duradryl Jr	Breckenridge	sr
Durahist	Proethic	sr
Durahist D	Proethic	sr
Durahist PE	Proethic	sr
Duraphen DM	Proethic	sr
Duraphen Forte	Proethic	sr
Duraphen II	Proethic	sr
Duraphen II DM	Proethic	sr
Duratuss	Victory	sr
Duratuss GP	Victory	sr
Dynabac	Muro	ec
Dynabac D5-Pak	Muro	ec
Dynacirc CR	Reliant	sr
Dynahist-ER Pediatric	Breckenridge	sr
Dynex	Athlon	sr
Dytan-CS	Hawthorn	sr
Easprin	Harvest	ec
EC Naprosyn	Roche	ec
Ecotrin	GlaxoSmithKline	ec
Ecotrin Adult Low Strength	GlaxoSmithKline	ec
Ecotrin Maximum Strength	GlaxoSmithKline	ec
Ecpirin	Prime Marketing	ec
Ed A-Hist	Edwards	sr
Ed-Chlor-Tan	Edwards	sr
Effexor-XR	Wyeth	sr
Efidac 24 Chlorpheniramine	Novartis Consumer	sr
Efidac 24 Pseudoephedrine	Novartis Consumer	sr
Enablex	Novartis	sr
Endal	Pediamed	sr

Drug	Manufacturer	Form
Entab-DM	Rising	sr
Entercote	Global Source	ec
Entex ER	Andrx	sr
Entex LA	Andrx	sr
Entex PSE	Andrx	sr
Entocort EC	Prometheus	ec
Equetro	Shire US	sr
ERYC	Warner Chilcott	ec
Ery-Tab	Abbott	ec
Eskalith-CR	GlaxoSmithKline	sr
Exefen-DM	Larken	sr
Exefen-PD	Larken	sr
Extendryl Jr	Fleming	sr
Extendryl SR	Fleming	sr
Extress-30	Key	sr
Extuss LA	Cypress	sr
Feen-A-Mint	Schering Plough	ec
Femilax	G & W	ec
Fero-Folic-500	Abbott	sr
Fero-Grad-500	Abbott	sr
Ferro-Sequels	Inverness Medical	sr
Ferro-Time	Time-Cap	sr
Ferrous Fumarate DS	Vita-Rx	sr
Fetrin	Lunsco	sr
Flagyl ER	Pharmacia	sr
Fleet Bisacodyl	Fleet, C. B.	ec
Focalin XR	Novartis	sr
Folitab 500	Rising	sr
Fortamet	First Horizon	sr
Fumatinic	Laser	sr
G/P 1200/75	Cypress	sr
Genacote	Ivax	ec
GFN 1000/DM 50	Cypress	sr
GFN 1200/DM 20/PE 40	Cypress	sr
GFN 1200/DM 60/PSE 60	Cypress	sr
GFN 1200/Phenylephrine 40	Cypress	sr
GFN 1200/PSE 50	Cypress	sr
GFN 500/DM 30	Cypress	sr
GFN 550/PSE 60	Cypress	sr
GFN 550/PSE 60/DM 30	Cypress	sr
GFN 595/PSE 48	Cypress	sr
GFN 595/PSE 48/DM 32	Cypress	sr
GFN 795/PSE 85	Cypress	sr
GFN 800/DM 30	Cypress	sr
GFN 800/PE 25	Cypress	sr
GFN 800/PSE 60	Cypress	sr
Gilphex TR	Gil	sr
Giltuss TR	Gil	sr
Glucophage XR	Bristol-Myers Squibb	sr
Glucotrol XL	Pfizer	sr
GP-1200	Iopharm	sr
Guaifed	Victory	sr
Guaifed-PD	Victory	sr

(Continued on next page)

Drug	Manufacturer	Form
Guaifenex DM	Ethex	sr
Guaifenex GP	Ethex	sr
Guaifenex PSE 120	Ethex	sr
Guaifenex PSE 60	Ethex	sr
Guaifenex PSE 80	Ethex	sr
Guaimax-D	Schwarz Pharma	sr
Gua-SR	Seatrace	sr
Guia-D	Breckenridge	sr
Guiadex D	Breckenridge	sr
Guiadex PD	Breckenridge	sr
Guiadrine DM	Breckenridge	sr
Guiadrine G-1200	Breckenridge	sr
Guiadrine GP	Breckenridge	sr
Guiadrine PSE	Breckenridge	sr
H 9600 SR	Hawthorn	sr
Halfprin	Kramer	ec
Hemax	Pronova	sr
Histacol LA	Breckenridge	sr
Histade	Breckenridge	sr
Histade MX	Breckenridge	sr
Hista-Vent DA	Ethex	sr
Hista-Vent PSE	Ethex	sr
Histex CT	Teamm	sr
Histex I/E	Teamm	sr
Histex SR	Teamm	sr
Humavent LA	WE Pharm.	sr
Humibid DM	Carolina	sr
Humibid L.A.	Carolina	sr
Hydro Pro DM SR	Breckenridge	sr
Hyoscyamine TR	Breckenridge	sr
Iberet-500	Abbott	sr
Iberet-Folic-500	Abbott	sr
Icar-C Plus SR	Hawthorn	sr
Imdur	Schering Plough	sr
Inderal LA	Wyeth	sr
Indocin SR	Forte Pharma	sr
Innopran XL	Reliant	sr
Iobid DM	Iopharm	sr
Ionamin	Celltech	sr
Iosal II	Iopharm	sr
Iotex PSE	Iopharm	sr
Isochron	Forest	sr
Isoptin SR	FSC	sr
Kadian	Alphagen	sr
Kaon-Cl 10	Savage	sr
K-Dur 10	Schering Plough	sr
K-Dur 20	Schering Plough	sr
Klor-Con 10	Upsher-Smith	sr
Klor-Con 8	Upsher-Smith	sr
Klor-Con M10	Upsher-Smith	sr
Klor-Con M15	Upsher-Smith	sr
Klor-Con M20	Upsher-Smith	sr
Klotrix	Bristol-Myers Squibb	sr

Drug	Manufacturer	Form
Kronofed-A	Ferndale	sr
Kronofed-A-Jr	Ferndale	sr
K-Tab	Abbott	sr
K-Tan	Prasco	sr
Lescol XL	Novartis	sr
Levall G	Athlon	sr
Levbid	Schwarz Pharma	sr
Levsinex	Schwarz Pharma	sr
Lexxel	Astra Zeneca	sr
Lipram 4500	Global	ec
Lipram-CR10	Global	ec
Lipram-CR20	Global	ec
Lipram-CR5	Global	ec
Lipram-PN10	Global	ec
Lipram-PN16	Global	ec
Lipram-PN20	Global	ec
Lipram-UL12	Global	ec
Lipram-UL18	Global	ec
Lipram-UL20	Global	ec
Liquibid-D	Capellon	sr
Liquibid-D 1200	Capellon	sr
Liquibid-PD	Capellon	sr
Lithobid	JDS Pharm.	sr
Lodine XL	Wyeth	sr
Lodrane 12 Hour	ECR	sr
Lodrane 12D	ECR	sr
Lodrane 24	ECR	sr
Lohist-12	Larken	sr
Lohist-12D	Larken	sr
Lusonex	Wraser	sr
Mag Delay	Major	ec
Mag64	Rising	ec
Mag-SR	Cypress	sr
Mag-SR Plus Calcium	Cypress	sr
Mag-Tab SR	Niche	sr
Maxifed	MCR American	sr
Maxifed DM	MCR American	sr
Maxifed DMX	MCR American	sr
Maxifed-G	MCR American	sr
Maxiphen DM	Ambi	sr
Maxovite	Tyson Neutraceuticals	sr
Medent DM	Stewart-Jackson	sr
Medent LD	Stewart-Jackson	sr
Mega-C	Merit	sr
Melfiat	Numark	sr
Menopause Trio	Mason Vitamins	sr
Mestinon Timespan	Valeant	sr
Metadate CD	Celltech	sr
Metadate ER	Celltech	sr
Methylin ER	Mallinckrodt	sr
Micro-K	Ther-Rx	sr
Micro-K 10	Ther-Rx	sr
Mild-C	Carlson, J. R.	sr

(Continued on next page)

Drug	Manufacturer	Form
Mindal	Breckenridge	sr
Mindal DM	Breckenridge	sr
Mintab C	Breckenridge	sr
Mintab D	Breckenridge	sr
Mintab DM	Breckenridge	sr
Miraphen PSE	Caraco	sr
Modane	Savage	ec
MS Contin	Purdue	sr
MSP-BLU	Cypress	ec
Mucinex	Adams	sr
Mucinex D	Adams	sr
Muco-Fen DM	Ivax	sr
Multi-Ferrous Folic	United Research	sr
Multiret Folic-500	Amide	sr
Myfortic	Novartis	ec
Nacon	Cypress	sr
Nalex-A	Blansett	sr
Naprelan	Blansett	sr
Nasatab LA	ECR	sr
Nasex	Cypress	sr
Nd Clear	Seatrace	sr
Nescon-PD	Cypress	sr
New Ami-Tex LA	Amide	sr
Nexium	Astra Zeneca	ec
Niaspan	KOS	sr
Nicomide	Sirius	sr
Nifediac CC	Teva	sr
Nifedical XL	Teva	sr
Nitrocot	Truxton	sr
Nitro-Time	Time-Cap	sr
Nohist	Larken	sr
Norel SR	U.S. Pharm. Corp.	sr
Norpace CR	Pharmacia	sr
Obstetrix EC	Seyer Pharmatec	ec
Omnihist L.A.	WE Pharm.	sr
Opana ER	Endo	sr
Oramorph SR	AAI Pharma	sr
Oracea	Collagenex	sr
Oruvail	Wyeth	sr
Oxycontin	Purdue	sr
Palcaps 10	Breckenridge	ec
Palcaps 20	Breckenridge	ec
Palgic-D	Pamlab	sr
Pancrease	McNeil Consumer	ec
Pancrease MT 10	McNeil Consumer	ec
Pancrease MT 16	McNeil Consumer	ec
Pancrease MT 20	McNeil Consumer	ec
Pancrecarb MS-16	Digestive Care	ec
Pancrecarb MS-4	Digestive Care	ec
Pancrecarb MS-8	Digestive Care	ec
Pangestyme CN-10	Ethex	ec
Pangestyme CN-20	Ethex	ec
Pangestyme EC	Ethex	ec

Drug	Manufacturer	Form
Pangestyme MT16	Ethex	ec
Pangestyme UL12	Ethex	ec
Pangestyme UL18	Ethex	ec
Pangestyme UL20	Ethex	ec
Panmist DM	Pamlab	sr
Panmist Jr	Pamlab	sr
Panmist LA	Pamlab	sr
Pannaz	Pamlab	sr
Panocaps	Breckenridge	ec
Panocaps MT 16	Breckenridge	ec
Panocaps MT 20	Breckenridge	ec
Papacon	Consolidated Midland	sr
Para-Time SR	Time-Cap	sr
Paser	Jacobus	sr
Pavacot	Truxton	sr
Paxil CR	GlaxoSmithKline	sr
PCE Dispertab	Abbott	sr
PCM LA	Cypress	sr
Pendex	Cypress	sr
Pentasa	Shire US	sr
Pentopak	Zoetica	sr
Pentoxil	Upsher-Smith	sr
Pharmadrine	Breckenridge	sr
Phenabid	Gil	sr
Phenabid DM	Gil	sr
Phenavent	Ethex	sr
Phenavent D	Ethex	sr
Phenavent LA	Ethex	sr
Phenavent PED	Ethex	sr
Phendiet-105	Truxton	sr
Phenytek	Mylan Bertek	sr
Plendil	Astra Zeneca	sr
Poly Hist Forte	Poly	sr
Poly-Vent	Poly	sr
Poly-Vent Jr	Poly	sr
Prehist D	Marnel	sr
Prelu-2	Roxane	sr
Prevacid	Tap	ec
Prilosec	Astra Zeneca	ec
Prilosec OTC	Procter & Gamble	sr
Procanbid	Monarch	sr
Procardia XL	Pfizer	sr
Profen Forte	Ivax	sr
Profen Forte DM	Ivax	sr
Profen II	Ivax	sr
Profen II DM	Ivax	sr
Prolex PD	Blansett	sr
Prolex-D	Blansett	sr
Pronestyl-SR	Bristol-Myers Squibb	sr
Proquin XR	Esprit	sr
Prosed EC	Star	ec
Proset-D	Blansett	sr
Protid	Lunsco	sr

(Continued on next page)

Drug	Manufacturer	Form
Protonix	Wyeth	ec
Prozac Weekly	Eli Lilly	ec
Pseubrom	Alphagen	sr
Pseubrom-PD	Alphagen	sr
Pseudatex	Breckenridge	sr
Pseudocot-C	Truxton	sr
Pseudocot-G	Truxton	sr
Pseudovent	Ethex	sr
Pseudovent 400	Ethex	sr
Pseudovent DM	Ethex	sr
Pseudovent PED	Ethex	sr
P-Tuss DM	Prasco	sr
Qdall	Atley	sr
Quibron-T/SR	Monarch	sr
Quindal	Qualitest	sr
Ralix	Cypress	sr
Ranaxa	CV Therapeutics	sr
Razadyne ER	Ortho-McNeil	sr
Reliable Gentle Laxative	Ivax	ec
Rescon-Jr	Capellon	sr
Rescon-MX	Capellon	sr
Respa-1ST	Respa	sr
Respa-AR	Respa	sr
Respa-DM	Respa	sr
Respahist	Respa	sr
Respaire-120 SR	Laser	sr
Respaire-60 SR	Laser	sr
Respa-PE	Respa	sr
Rhinabid	Breckenridge	sr
Rhinabid PD	Breckenridge	sr
Rhinacon A	Breckenridge	sr
Ribo-2	Tyson Neutraceuticals	ec
Risperdal Consta	Janssen	sr
Ritalin LA	Novartis	sr
Ritalin-SR	Novartis	sr
Rodex Forte	Legere	sr
Rondec-TR	Biovail	sr
Ru-Tuss 800	Sage	sr
Ru-Tuss 800 DM	Sage	sr
Ru-Tuss Jr	Sage	sr
Ryneze	Stewart-Jackson	sr
Rythmol SR	Reliant	sr
Sam-E	Pharmavite	ec
Sinemet CR	Bristol-Myers Squibb	sr
Sinutuss DM	WE Pharm.	sr
Sinuvent PE	WE Pharm.	sr
Sitrex	Vindex	sr
Slo-Niacin	Upsher-Smith	sr
Slow Fe	Novartis Consumer	sr
Slow Fe With Folic Acid	Novartis Consumer	sr
Slow-Mag	Purdue	ec
Solodyn	Medicis	sr
Spacol T/S	Dayton	sr

Drug	Manufacturer	Form
St. Joseph Pain Reliever	McNeil Consumer	ec
Sta-D	Magna	sr
Stahist	Magna	sr
Stamoist E	Magna	sr
Sudafed 12 Hour	Pfizer	sr
Sudafed 24 Hour	Pfizer	sr
Sudal DM	Atley	sr
Sudal SR	Atley	sr
Sular	First Horizon	sr
Sulfazine EC	Qualitest	ec
Symax Duotab	Capellon	sr
Symax-SR	Capellon	sr
Tarka	Abbott	sr
Taztia XT	Andrx	sr
Tegretol-XR	Novartis	sr
Tenuate Dospan	Sanofi-Aventis	sr
Theo-24	UCB	sr
Theocap	Forest	sr
Theochron	Forest	sr
Theo-Time	Major	sr
Thiamilate	Tyson Neutraceuticals	ec
Tiazac	Forest	sr
Time-Hist	MCR American	sr
Toprol XL	Astra Zeneca	sr
TotalDay	Nat'l Vitamin Co.	sr
Touro Allergy	Dartmouth	sr
Touro CC	Dartmouth	sr
Touro CC-LD	Dartmouth	sr
Touro DM	Dartmouth	sr
Touro HC	Dartmouth	sr
Touro LA	Dartmouth	sr
Touro LA-LD	Dartmouth	sr
Tranxene-SD	Ovation	sr
Trental	Sanofi-Aventis	sr
Trikof-D	Respa	sr
Trinalin Repetabs	Schering Plough	sr
Trituss-ER	Everett	sr
Tussafed-LA	Everett	sr
Tussall-ER	Everett	sr
Tussbid	Breckenridge	sr
Tussi-Bid	Capellon	sr
Tussitab	Iopharm	sr
Tylenol Arthritis	McNeil Consumer	sr
Ultrabrom	WE Pharm.	sr
Ultrabrom PD	WE Pharm.	sr
Ultracaps MT 20	Breckenridge	ec
Ultram ER	Ortho-McNeil	sr
Ultrase	Axcan Scandipharm	ec
Ultrase MT12	Axcan Scandipharm	ec
Ultrase MT18	Axcan Scandipharm	ec
Ultrase MT20	Axcan Scandipharm	ec
Uniphyl	Purdue	sr
Uni-Tex	United Research	sr

(Continued on next page)

Drug	Manufacturer	Form
Urimax	Xanodyne	ec
Uritact-EC	Cypress	ec
Urocit-K 10	Mission	sr
Urocit-K 5	Mission	sr
Uroxatral	Sanofi-Aventis	sr
Utira	Hawthorn	sr
V-Dec-M	Seatrace	sr
Veracolate	Numark	ec
Verelan	Schwarz Pharma	sr
Verelan PM	Schwarz Pharma	sr
Versacaps	Seatrace	sr
Videx EC	Bristol-Myers Squibb	ec
Vivotif Berna	Berna Products	ec
Voltaren	Novartis	ec
Voltaren-XR	Novartis	sr
Vospire	Dava	sr
Vospire ER	Odyssey	sr
We Mist II LA	WE Pharm.	sr
We Mist LA	WE Pharm.	sr
Wellbid-D	Prasco	sr
Wellbid-D 1200	Prasco	sr
Wellbutrin SR	GlaxoSmithKline	sr
Wellbutrin XL	GlaxoSmithKline	sr
Wobenzym N	Marlyn	ec
Xanax XR	Pharmacia	sr
Xiral	Hawthorn	sr
XpeCT-At	Hawthorn	sr
XpeCT-HC	Hawthorn	sr
Z-Cof LA	Zyber	sr
Z-Cof LAX	Zyber	sr
Zephrex LA	Sanofi-Aventis	sr
Zmax	Pfizer	sr
Zorprin	Par	sr
Zyban	GlaxoSmithKline	sr
Zymase	Organon	ec
Zyrtec-D	Pfizer	sr

Reprinted with permission from *The Drug Topics Red Book*. Montvale NJ: Thomson Medical Economics, 2007.

SUGAR-FREE PRODUCTS

Listed below, by therapeutic category, is a selection of drug products that contain no sugar. When recommending these products to diabetic patients, keep in mind that many may contain sorbitol, alcohol, or other sources of carbohydrates. This list should not be considered all-inclusive. Generics and alternate brands of some products may be available. Check product labeling for a current listing of inactive ingredients.

Analgesics	Manufacturer
Actamin Maximum Strength Liquid	Cypress
Addaprin Tablet	Dover
Aminofen Tablet	Dover
Aminofen Max Tablet	Dover
Aspirtab Tablet	Dover

Back Pain-Off Tablet	Textilease Medique
Backprin Tablet	Hart Health and Safety
Buffasal Tablet	Dover
Dyspel Tablet	Dover
Febrol Liquid	Scot-Tussin
I-Prin Tablet	Textilease Medique
Medi-Seltzer Effervescent Tablet	Textilease Medique
Ms.-Aid Tablet	Textilease Medique
PMS Relief Tablet	Textilease Medique
Silapap Children's Elixir	Silarx

Antacids/Antiflatulents

Almag Chewable Tablet	Textilease Medique
Alcalak Chewable Tablet	Textilease Medique
Aldroxicon I Suspension	Textilease Medique
Aldroxicon II Suspension	Textilease Medique
Baby Gasz Drops	Lee
Dimacid Chewable Tablet	Otis Clapp & Son
Diotame Chewable Tablet	Textilease Medique
Diotame Suspension	Textilease Medique
Gas-Ban Chewable	Textilease Medique
Mallamint Chewable	Textilease Medique
Mylanta Gelcaplet	Johnson & Johnson/Merck
Neutralin Tablet	Dover
Tums E-X Chewable Tablet	GlaxoSmithKline Consumer

Antiasthmatic/Respiratory Agents

Jay-Phyl Syrup	Pharmakon

Antidiarrheals

Diarrest Tablet	Dover
Di-Gon II Tablet	Textilease Medique
Imogen Liquid	Pharmaceutical Generic

Blood Modifiers/Iron Preparations

I.L.X. B-12 Elixir	Kenwood
Irofel Liquid	Dayton
Nephro-Fer Tablet	R & D

Corticosteroids

Pediapred Solution	Celltech

Cough/Cold/Allergy Preparations

Accuhist DM Pediatric Drops	Pediamed
Accuhist Pediatric Drops	Pediamed
Alacol DM Syrup	Ballay
Amerifed DM Liquid	MCR American
Amerifed Liquid	Ambi
Amerituss AD Solution	Ambi
Anaplex DM Syrup	ECR
Anaplex DMX Syrup	ECR
Anaplex HD Syrup	ECR

(Continued on next page)

Andehist DM Liquid	Cypress
Andehist DM NR Liquid	Cypress
Andehist DM NR Syrup	Cypress
Andehist DM Syrup	Cypress
Andehist Liquid	Cypress
Andehist NR Liquid	Cypress
Andehist NR Syrup	Cypress
Andehist Syrup	Cypress
Aridex Solution	Gentex
Atuss EX Liquid	Atley
Atuss NX Solution	Atley
Baltussin Solution	Ballay
Bellahist-D LA Tablet	Cypress
Benadryl Allergy/Sinus Children's Solution	Warner-Lambert Consumer
Biodec DM Drops	Bio-Pharm
Bromaxefed DM RF Syrup	Morton Grove
Bromaxefed RF Syrup	Morton Grove
Bromdec Solution	Scientific Laboratories
Bromdec DM Solution	Scientific Laboratories
Bromhist-DM Solution	Cypress
Bromhist Pediatric Solution	Cypress
Bromophed DX Syrup	Qualitest
Bromphenex DM Solution	Breckenridge
Bromphenex HD Solution	Breckenridge
Bromplex DM Solution	Prasco
Bromplex HD Solution	Prasco
Bromluss DM Solution	Breckenridge
Broncotron Liquid	Seyer Pharmatec
Broncotron-D Suspension	Seyer Pharmatec
Brovex HC Solution	Athlon
B-Tuss Liquid	Blansett
Carbaphen 12 Ped Suspension	Gil
Carbaphen 12 Suspension	Gil
Carbatuss-CL Solution	GM
Carbetaplex Solution	Breckenridge
Carbihist Solution	Boca Pharmacal
Carbinoxamine PSE Solution	Boca Pharmacal
Carbofed DM Liquid	Hi-Tech
Carbofed DM Syrup	Hi-Tech
Carbofed DM Drops	Hi-Tech
Carboxine Solution	Cypress
Carboxine-PSE Solution	Cypress
Cardec DM Syrup	Qualitest
Cetafen Cold Tablet	Hart Health and Safety
Cheratussin DAC Liquid	Qualitest
Chlordex GP Syrup	Cypress
Codal-DM Syrup	Cypress
Colace Solution	Purdue Pharma
ColdCough EXP Solution	Breckenridge
ColdCough HC Solution	Breckenridge
ColdCough PD Solution	Breckenridge
ColdCough Solution	Breckenridge
ColdCough XP Solution	Breckenridge
Coldec DS Solution	Breckenridge
ColdMist DM Syrup	Breckenridge

Coldonyl Tablet	Dover
Colidrops Pediatric Liquid	A.G. Marin
Cordron-D Solution	Cypress
Cordron-DM Solution	Cypress
Cordron-HC Solution	Cypress
Corfen DM Solution	Cypress
Co-Tussin Liquid	American Generics
Cotuss-V Syrup	Alphagen
Coughtuss Solution	Breckenridge
Crantex HC Syrup	Breckenridge
Crantex Syrup	Breckenridge
Cypex-LA Tablet	Cypress
Cytuss HC Syrup	Cypress
Dacex-A Solution	Cypress
Dacex-DM Solution	Cypress
Dacex-PE Solution	Cypress
Decahist-DM Solution	Cypress
De-Chlor DM Solution	Cypress
De-Chlor DR Solution	Cypress
De-Chlor G Solution	Cypress
De-Chlor HC Solution	Cypress
De-Chlor HD Solution	Cypress
De-Chlor MR Solution	Cypress
De-Chlor NX Solution	Cypress
Decorel Forte Tablet	Textilease Medique
Denaze Solution	Cypress
Despec Liquid	International Ethical
Despec-SF Liquid	International Ethical
Dexcon-DM Solution	Cypress
Diabetic Tussin Allergy Relief Liquid	Health Care Products
Diabetic Tussin Allergy Relief Gelcaplet	Health Care Products
Diabetic Tussin C Expectorant Liquid	Health Care Products
Diabetic Tussin Cold & Flu Gelcaplet	Health Care Products
Diabetic Tussin DM Liquid	Health Care Products
Diabetic Tussin EX Liquid	Health Care Products
Dimetapp Allergy Children's Elixir	Wyeth Consumer
Diphen Capsule	Textilease Medique
Double-Tussin DM Liquid	Reese
Drocon-CS Solution	Cypress
Duratuss DM Solution	Victory
Dynatuss Syrup	Breckenridge
Dynatuss HC Solution	Breckenridge
Dynatuss HCG Solution	Breckenridge
Dytan-CS Tablet	Hawthorn
Emagrin Forte Tablet	Otis Clapp & Son
Endacof DM Solution	Larken Laboratories
Endacof HC Solution	Larken Laboratories
Endacof XP Solution	Larken Laboratories
Endacof-PD Solution	Larken Laboratories
Endal HD Liquid	Pediamed
Endal HD Plus Liquid	Pediamed
Endotuss-HD Syrup	American Generics
Enplus-HD Syrup	Alphagen
Entex Syrup	Andrx
Entex HC Syrup	Andrx

(Continued on next page)

Exo-Tuss Syrup	American Generics
Ganidin NR Liquid	Cypress
Gani-Tuss NR Liquid	Cypress
Gani-Tuss-DM NR Liquid	Cypress
Genebronco-D Liquid	Pharm Generic Developers
Genecof-HC Liquid	Pharmaceutical Generic
Genecof-XP Liquid	Pharmaceutical Generic
Genedel Syrup	Pharmaceutical Generic
Genedotuss-DM Liquid	Pharmaceutical Generic
Genelan Liquid	Pharm Generic Developers
Genetuss-2 Liquid	Pharm Generic Developers
Genexpect DM Liquid	Pharmaceutical Generic
Genexpect-PE Liquid	Pharmaceutical Generic
Genexpect-SF Liquid	Pharmaceutical Generic
Gilphex TR Tablet	Gil
Giltuss Liquid	Gil
Giltuss HC Syrup	Gil
Giltuss Pediatric Liquid	Gil
Giltuss TR Tablet	Gil
Guai-Co Liquid	Alphagen
Guaicon DMS Liquid	Textilease Medique
Guai-DEX Liquid	Alphagen
Guaitussin AC Solution	Scientific Laboratories
Guaitussin DAC Solution	Scientific Laboratories
Guapetex HC Solution	Scientific Laboratories
Guapetex Syrup	Scientific Laboratories
Guiatuss AC Syrup	Alpharma
Guiatuss AC Syrup	Ivax
Halotussin AC Liquid	Watson
Hayfebrol Liquid	Scot-Tussin
Histacol DM Pediatric Solution	Breckenridge
Histex PD Liquid	TEAMM
Histex PD 12 Suspension	Teamm
Histinex HC Syrup	Ethex
Histinex PV Syrup	Ethex
Histuss HC Solution	Scientific Laboratories
Histuss PD Solution	Scientific Laboratories
Hydex-PD Solution	Cypress
Hydone Liquid	Hyrex
Hydro-DP Solution	Cypress
Hydro GP Syrup	Cypress
Hydro PC Syrup	Cypress
Hydro PC II Plus Solution	Cypress
Hydro Pro Solution	Breckenridge
Hydrocof-HC Solution	Morton Grove
Hydron CP Syrup	Cypress
Hydron EX Syrup	Cypress
Hydron KGS Liquid	Cypress
Hydron PSC Liquid	Cypress
Hydro-Tussin CBX Solution	Ethex
Hydro-Tussin DM Elixir	Ethex
Hydro-Tussin HC Syrup	Ethex
Hydro-Tussin HD Liquid	Ethex
Hydro-Tussin XP Syrup	Ethex
Hytuss Tablet	Hyrex

Hytuss 2X Capsule	Hyrex
Jaycof Expectorant Syrup	Pharmakon
Jaycof-HC Liquid	Pharmakon
Jaycof-XP Liquid	Pharmakon
Kita LA Tos Liquid	R.I.D.
Lodrane Liquid	ECR
Lodrane D Suspension	ECR
Lodrane XR Suspension	ECR
Lohist-LQ Solution	Larken
Lortuss DM Solution	Proethic Laboratories
Lortuss HC Solution	Proethic Laboratories
Marcof Expectorant Syrup	Marnel
Maxi-Tuss HCX Solution	MCR American
M-Clear Syrup	McNeil, R.A.
M-Clear Jr Solution	McNeil, R.A.
Metanx Tablet	Pamlab
Mintex PD Liquid	Breckenridge
Mintuss NX Solution Syrup	Breckenridge
Mytussin DAC Syrup	Morton Grove
Nalex DH Liquid	Blansett
Nalex-A Liquid	Blansett
Nasop Suspension	Hawthorn
Neotuss S/F Liquid	A.G. Marin
Nescon-PD Tablet	Cypress
Niferex Elixir	Ther-Rx
Norel DM Liquid	U.S. Corp
Nycoff Tablet	Dover
Onset Forte Tablet	Textilease Medique
Orgadin Liquid	American Generics
Orgadin-Tuss Liquid	American Generics
Orgadin-Tuss DM Liquid	American Generics
Organidin NR Liquid	Wallace
Organidin NR Tablet	Wallace
Palgic-DS Syrup	Pamlab
Pancof Syrup	Pamlab
Pancof EXP Syrup	Pamlab
Pancof HC Solution	Pamlab
Pancof XP Liquid	Pamlab
Pancof XP Solution	Pamlab
Panmist DM Syrup	Pamlab
Pediatex Solution	Zyber
Pediatex D	Zyber
Pediatex DM Liquid	Zyber
Pediatex DM Solution	Zyber
Pediatex HC Solution	Zyber
Phanasin Syrup	Pharmakon
Phanasin Diabetic Choice Syrup	Pharmakon
Phanatuss Syrup	Pharmakon
Phanatuss DM Diabetic Choice Syrup	Pharmakon
Phanatuss-HC Diabetic Choice Solution	Pharmakon
Phena-HC Solution	GM
Phenabid DM Tablet	Gil
Phenydryl Solution	Scientific Laboratories
Pneumotussin 2.5 Syrup	ECR
Poly Hist DM Solution	Poly

(Continued on next page)

Poly Hist PD Solution	Poly
Poly-Tussin Syrup	Poly
Poly-Tussin DM Syrup	Poly
Poly-Tussin HD Syrup	Poly
Poly-Tussin XP Syrup	Poly
Pro-Clear Solution	Pro-Pharma
Pro-Cof D Liquid	Qualitest
Pro-Red Solution	Pro-Pharma
Protex DH Liquid	Blansett
Protex DM Liquid	Blansett
Protex Solution	Scientific Laboratories
Protex D Solution	Scientific Laboratories
Protuss Liquid	First Horizon
Quintex Syrup	Qualitest
Quintex HC Syrup	Qualitest
Relacon-DM Solution	Cypress
Relacon-HC Solution	Cypress
Rescon-DM Liquid	Capellon
Rhinacon A Solution	Breckenridge
Rhinacon DH Solution	Breckenridge
Rindal HD Liquid	Breckenridge
Rindal HD Plus Solution	Breckenridge
Rindal HPD Solution	Breckenridge
Romilar AC Liquid	Scot-Tussin
Romilar DM Liquid	Scot-Tussin
Rondamine DM Liquid	Major
Rondec Syrup	Biovail
Rondec DM Syrup	Biovail
Rondec DM Drops	Biovail
Ru-Tuss A Syrup	Sage
Ru-Tuss DM Syrup	Sage
Scot-Tussin Allergy Relief Formula Liquid	Scot-Tussin
Scot-Tussin DM Cough Chasers Lozenge	Scot-Tussin
Scot-Tussin Original Liquid	Scot-Tussin
Siladryl Allergy Liquid	Silarx
Siladryl DAS Liquid	Silarx
Sildec Syrup	Silarx
Sildec Drops	Silarx
Sildec-DM Syrup	Silarx
Silexin Syrup	Otis Clapp & Son
Silexin Tablet	Otis Clapp & Son
Sil-Tex Liquid Liquid	Silarx
Siltussin DM DAS Cough Formula Syrup	Silarx
S-T Forte 2 Liquid	Scot-Tussin
Statuss Green Liquid	Magna
Sudodrin Tablet	Textilease Medique
Sudafed Children's Cold & Cough Solution	Pfizer
Sudafed Children's Solution	Pfizer
Sudafed Children's Tablet	Pfizer
Sudanyl Tablet	Dover
Sudatuss-SF Liquid	Pharm Generic Developers
Sudodrin Tablet	Textilease Medique
Supress DX Pediatric Drops	Kramer-Novis
Suttar-SF Syrup	Gil
Triant-HC Solution	Hawthorn

Tricodene Syrup	Pfeiffer
Trispec-PE Liquid	Deliz
Trituss DM Solution	Breckenridge
Trituss Solution	Everett
Tri-Vent DM Solution	Ethex
Tusdec-DM Solution	Cypress
Tusdec-HC Solution	Cypress
Tusnel Solution	Llorens
Tussafed Syrup	Everett
Tussafed-EX Pediatric Drops	Everett
Tussafed-HC Syrup	Everett
Tussafed-HCG Solution	Everett
Tussall Solution	Everett
Tuss-DM Liquid	Seatrace
Tuss-ES Syrup	Seatrace
Tussi-Organidin DM NR Liquid	Wallace
Tussi-Organidin NR Liquid	Wallace
Tussi-Organidin-S NR Liquid	Wallace
Tussi-Pres Liquid	Kramer-Novis
Tussirex Liquid	Scot-Tussin
Uni Cof EXP Solution	United Research Labs
Uni Cof Solution	United Research Labs
Uni-Lev 5.0 Solution	United Research Labs
Vazol Solution	Wraser
Vi-Q-Tuss Syrup	Qualitest
Vitussin Expectorant Syrup	Cypress
Welltuss EXP Solution	Prasco
Welltuss HC Solution	Prasco
Z-Cof HC Solution	Zyber
Z-Cof HC Syrup	Zyber
Ztuss Expectorant Solution	Magna
Zyrtec Syrup	Pfizer

Fluoride Preparations

Ethedent Chewable Tablet	Ethex
Fluor-A-Day Tablet	Pharmascience
Fluor-A-Day Lozenge	Pharmascience
Flura-Loz Tablet	Kirkman
Lozi-Flur Lozenge	Dreir
Sensodyne w/Fluoride Gel	GlaxoSmithKline Consumer
Sensodyne w/Fluoride Tartar Control Toothpaste	GlaxoSmithKline Consumer
Sensodyne w/Fluoride Toothpaste	GlaxoSmithKline Consumer

Laxatives

Citrucel Powder	GlaxoSmithKline Consumer
Colace Solution	Purdue Pharma
Fiber Ease Liquid	Plainview
Fibro-XL Capsule	Key
Genfiber Powder	Ivax
Konsyl Easy Mix Formula Powder	Konsyl
Konsyl-Orange Powder	Konsyl
Metamucil Smooth Texture Powder	Procter & Gamble
Reguloid Powder	Rugby
Senokot Wheat Bran	Purdue Products

(Continued on next page)

Miscellaneous

Acidoll Capsule	Key
Alka-Gest Tablet	Key
Bicitra Solution	Ortho-McNeil
Colidrops Pediatric Drops	A.G. Marin
Cytra-2 Solution	Cypress
Cytra-K Solution	Cypress
Cytra-K Crystals	Cypress
Melatin Tablet	Mason Vitamins
Methadose Solution	Mallinckrodt
Neutra-Phos Powder	Ortho-McNeil
Neutra-Phos-K Powder	Ortho-McNeil
Polycitra-K Solution	Ortho-McNeil
Polycitra-LC Solution	Ortho-McNeil
Questran Light Powder	Par

Mouth/Throat Preparations

Aquafresh Triple Protection Gum	GlaxoSmithKline Consumer
Cepacol Maximum Strength Spray	J.B. Williams
Cepacol Sore Throat Lozenges	J.B. Williams
Cheracol Sore Throat Spray	Lee
Cylex Lozenges	Pharmakon
Fisherman's Friend Lozenges	Mentholatum
Fresh N Free Liquid	Geritrex
Isodettes Sore Throat Spray	GlaxoSmithKline Consumer
Larynex Lozenges	Dover
Listerine Pocketpaks Film	Pfizer Consumer
Medikoff Drops	Textilease Medique
Oragesic Solution	Parnell
Orasept Mouthwash/Gargle Liquid	Pharmakon
Robitussin Lozenges	Wyeth Consumer
Sepasoothe Lozenges	Textilease Medique
Thorets Maximum Strength Lozenges	Otis Clapp & Son
Throto-Ceptic Spray	S.S.S.
Vademecum Mouthwash & Gargle Concentrate	Dermatone

Potassium Supplements

Cena K Liquid	Century
Kaon Elixir	Savage
Kaon-Cl 20% Liquid	Savage
Rum-K Liquid	Fleming

Vitamins/Minerals/Supplements

Action-Tabs Made For Men	Action Labs
Adaptosode For Stress Liquid	HVS
Adaptosode R+R For Acute Stress Liquid	HVS
Alamag Tablet	Textilease Medique
Alcalak Tablet	Textilease Medique
Aldroxicon I Suspension	Textilease Medique
Aldroxicon II Suspension	Textilease Medique
Aminoplex Powder	Tyson
Aminostasis Powder	Tyson
Aminotate Powder	Tyson

Apetigen Elixir	Kramer-Novis
Apptrim Capsule	Physician Therapeutics
Apptrim-D Capsule	Physician Therapeutics
B-C-Bid Caplet	Lee
Bevitamel Tablet	Westlake
Biosode Liquid	HVS
Biotect Plus Caplet	Gil
C & M Caps-375 Capsule	Key
Calbon Tablet	Emrex/Economed
Cal-Cee Tablet	Key
Calcet Plus Tablet	Mission Pharmacal
Calcimin-300 Tablet	Key
Cal-Mint Chewable Tablet	Freeda Vitamins
Cena K Solution	Century
Cerefolin Tablet	Pamlab
Cevi-Bid Tablet	Lee
Choice DM Liquid	Bristol-Myers Squibb
Cholestratin Tablet	Key
Chromacaps Tablet	Key
Chromium K6 Tablet	Rexall Consumer
Citrimax 500 Plus Tablet	Mason Vitamins
Combi-Cart Tablet	Atrium Bio-Tech
Delta D3 Tablet	Freeda Vitamins
Detoxosode Liquids	HVS
Dexfol Tablet	Rising
DHEA Capsule	ADH Health Products
Diabeze Tablet	Key
Diatx Tablet	Pamlab
Diatx ZN Tablet	Pamlab
Diet System 6 Gum	Applied Nutrition
Dimacid Tablet	Otis Clapp & Son
Diucaps Capsule	Legere
Dl-Phen-500 Capsule	Key
Electrolab Tablet	Hart Health And Safety
Endorphenyl Capsule	Tyson
Ensure Nutra Shake Pudding	Ross Products
Enterex Diabetic Liquid	Victus
Essential Nutrients Plus Silica Tablet	Action Labs
Evening Primrose Oil Capsule	National Vitamin
Evolve Softgel	Bionutrics Health Products
Ex-L Tablet	Key
Extress Tablet	Key
Eyetamins Tablet	Rexall Consumer
Fem-Cal Tablet	Freeda Vitamins
Fem-Cal Plus Tablet	Freeda Vitamins
Ferrocite F Tablet	Breckenridge
Folacin-800 Tablet	Key
Folbee Plus Tablet	Breckenridge
Folplex 2.2 Tablet	Breckenridge
Foltx Tablet	Pamlab
Gabadone Capsule	Physician Therapeutics
Gram-O-Leci Tablet	Freeda Vitamins
Hemovit Tablet	Dayton
Herbal Slim Complex Capsule	ADH Health Products
Irofol Liquid	Dayton

(Continued on next page)

Lynae Calcium/Vitamin C Chewable Tablet	Boscogen
Lynae Chondroitin/Glucosamine Capsule	Boscogen
Lynae Ginse-Cool Chewable Tablet	Boscogen
Mag-Caps Capsule	Rising
Mag-Ox 400 Tablet	Blaine
Mag-SR Tablet	Cypress
Magimin Tablet	Key Company
Magnacaps Capsule	Key Company
Mangimin Capsule	Key Company
Mangimin Tablet	Key Company
Medi-Lyte Tablet	Textilease Medique
Metanx Tablet	Pamlab
Multi-Delyn w/Iron Liquid	Silarx
Natelle C Tablet	Pharmelle
Nephro-Fer Tablet	Watson
Neutra-Phos Powder	Ortho-Mcneil
Neutra-Phos-K Powder	Ortho-Mcneil
New Life Hair Tablet	Rexall Consumer
Niferex Elixir	Ther-Rx
Nutrisure OTC Tablet	Westlake
O-Cal Fa Tablet	Pharmics
Plenamins Plus Tablet	Rexall Consumer
Powervites Tablet	Green Turtle Bay Vitamin
Prostaplex Herbal Complex Capsule	ADH Health Products
Prostatonin Capsule	Pharmaton Natural Health
Protect Plus Liquid	Gil
Protect Plus NR Softgel	Gil
Pulmona Capsule	Physician T
Quintabs-M Tablet	Freeda Vitamins
Re/Neph Liquid	Ross Products
Replace Capsule	Key
Replace w/o Iron Capsule	Key
Resource Arginaid Powder	Novartis Nutrition
Ribo-100 T.D. Capsule	Key
Samolinic Softgel	Key
Sea Omega 30 Softgel	Rugby
Sea Omega 50 Softgel	Rugby
Sentra AM Capsule	Physician Therapeutics
Sentra PM Capsule	Physician Therapeutics
Soy Care for Bone Health Tablet	Inverness Medical
Soy Care for Menopause Capsule	Inverness Medical
Span C Tablet	Freeda Vitamins
Strovite Forte Syrup	Everett
Sunnie Tablet	Green Turtle Bay Vitamin
Sunvite Tablet	Rexall Consumer
Super Dec B100 Tablet	Freeda Vitamins
Super Quints-50 Tablet	Freeda Vitamins
Supervite Liquid	Seyer Pharmatec
Suplevit Liquid	Gil
Theramine Capsule	Physician Therapeutics
Triamin Tablet	Key
Triamino Tablet	Freeda Vitamins
Ultramino Powder	Freeda Vitamins
Uro-Mag Capsule	Blaine
Vinatal 600 Kit	Breckenridge

Vitalize Liquid	Scot-Tussin
Vitamin C/Rose Hips Tablet	ADH Health Products
Vitrum Jr Chewable Tablet	Mason Vitamins
Xtramins Tablet	Key
Yohimbe Power Max 1500 For Women Tablet	Action Labs
Yohimbized 1000 Capsule	Action Labs
Ze-Plus Softgel	Everett

Reprinted with permission from *The Drug Topics Red Book.* Montvale NJ: Thomson Medical Economics, 2007.

ALCOHOL-FREE PRODUCTS

The following is a selection of alcohol-free products by therapeutic category. The list is not comprehensive.

Generic and alternate brands may exist. Always check product labeling for definitive information on specific ingredients.

Analgesics	Manufacturer
Acetaminophen Infants Drops	Ivax
Actamin Maximum Strength Liquid	Cypress
Addaprin Tablet	Dover
Advil Children's Suspension	Wyeth Consumer
Aminofen Tablet	Dover
Aminofen Max Tablet	Dover
APAP Elixir	Bio-Pharm
Aspirtab Tablet	Dover
Buffasal Tablet	Dover
Demerol Hydrochloride Syrup	Sanofi-Aventis
Dolono Elixir	R.I.D.
Dyspel Tablet	Dover
Genapap Children Elixir	Ivax
Genapap Infant's Drops	Ivax
Motrin Children's Suspension	McNeil Consumer
Motrin Infants' Suspension	McNeil Consumer
Silapap Children's Elixir	Silarx
Silapap Infant's Drops	Silarx
Tylenol Children's Suspension	McNeil Consumer
Tylenol Extra Strength Solution	McNeil Consumer
Tylenol Infant's Drops	McNeil Consumer
Tylenol Infant's Suspension	McNeil Consumer

Antiasthmatic Agents

Dilor-G Liquid	Savage
Dy-G Liquid	Cypress
Elixophyllin-GG Liquid	Forest

Anticonvulsants

Zarontin Syrup	Pfizer

Antiviral Agents

Epivir Oral Solution	GlaxoSmithKline

(Continued on next page)

Cough/Cold/Allergy Preparations

Accuhist Pediatric Drops	Propst
Alacol DM Syrup	Ballay
Allergy Relief Medicine Children's Elixir	Hi-Tech Pharmacal
Altarussin Syrup	Altaire
Amerifed DM Liquid	MCR American
Amerifed Liquid	Ambi
Anaplex DM Syrup	ECR
Anaplex DMX Suspension	ECR
Anaplex HD Syrup	ECR
Andehist DM Drops	Cypress
Andehist DM Syrup	Cypress
Andehist DM NR Liquid	Cypress
Andehist DM NR Syrup	Cypress
Andehist NR Syrup	Cypress
Andehist Syrup	Cypress
Aquatab DM Syrup	Adams
Aridex Solution	Gentex
Atuss DR Syrup	Atley
Atuss EX Liquid	Atley
Atuss G Liquid	Atley
Atuss HC Syrup	Atley
Atuss MS Syrup	Atley
Baltussin Solution	Ballay Pharm
Benadryl Allergy Solution	Pfizer Consumer
Benadryl Allergy/Sinus Children's Solution	Pfizer
Biodec DM Drops	Bio-Pharm
Bromaline Solution	Rugby
Bromaline DM Elixir	Rugby
Bromanate Elixir	Alpharma USPD
Bromatan-DM Suspension	Cypress
Bromaxefed DM RF Syrup	Morton Grove
Bromaxefed RF Syrup	Morton Grove
Broncotron Liquid	Seyer Pharmatec
Bromdec Solution	Scientific Laboratories
Bromdec DM Solution	Scientific Laboratories
Bromhist Pediatric Solution	Cypress
Bromhist-DM Pediatric Syrup	Cypress
Bromhist-DM Solution	Cypress
Bromphenex HD Solution	Breckenridge
Bromplex DM Solution	Prasco Laboratories
Bromplex HD Solution	Prasco Laboratories
Broncotron-D Suspension	Seyer Pharmatec
Bron-Tuss Liquid	American Generics
Brovex HC Solution	Athlon
B-Tuss Liquid	Blansett
Carbaphen 12 Ped Suspension	Gil
Carbaphen 12 Suspension	Gil
Carbatuss Liquid	GM
Carbatuss-CL Solution	GM
Carbaxefed DM RF Liquid	Morton Grove
Carbetaplex Solution	Breckenridge
Carbihist Solution	Boca Pharmacal
Carbofed DM Drops	Hi-Tech Pharmacal

Carbofed DM Syrup	Hi-Tech Pharmacal
Carboxine Solution	Cypress
Carboxine-PSE Solution	Cypress
Cardec Syrup	Qualitest
Cardec DM Syrup	Qualitest
Cepacol Sore Throat Liquid	J. B. Williams
Chlordex GP Syrup	Cypress
Chlor-Mes D Solution	Cypress
Chlor-Trimeton Allergy Syrup	Schering Plough
Codal-DH Syrup	Cypress
Codal-DM Syrup	Cypress
Codotuss Liquid	Major
Coldec DS Solution	Breckenridge
Coldec-DM Syrup	United Research Labs
Coldmist DM Solution	Breckenridge
Coldmist DM Syrup	Breckenridge
Coldmist S Syrup	Breckenridge
Coldonyl Tablet	Dover
Coldtuss DR Syrup	United Research Labs
Colidrops Pediatric Liquid	A. G. Marin
Complete Allergy Elixir	Cardinal Health
Cordron-D Solution	Cypress
Cordron-DM Solution	Cypress
Cordron-HC Solution	Cypress
Corfen DM Solution	Cypress
Co-Tussin Liquid	American Generics
Cotuss-V Syrup	Alphagen
Crantex HC Syrup	Breckenridge
Crantex Syrup	Breckenridge
Creomulsion Complete Syrup	Summit Industries
Creomulsion Cough Syrup	Summit Industries
Creomulsion For Children Syrup	Summit Industries
Creomulsion Pediatric Syrup	Summit Industries
Cytuss HC Syrup	Cypress
Dacex-A Solution	Cypress
Dacex-DM Solution	Cypress
Decahist-DM Solution	Cypress
De-Chlor DM Solution	Cypress
De-Chlor DR Solution	Cypress
Dehistine Syrup	Cypress
Deka Liquid	Dayton
Deka Pediatric Drops Solution	Dayton
Deltuss Liquid	Deliz
Denaze Solution	Cypress
Despec Liquid Labs	International Ethical
Dex PC Syrup	Boca Pharmacal
Dexcon-DM Solution	Cypress
Diabetic Tussin Allergy Relief Liquid	Healthcare Products
Diabetic Tussin C Expectorant Liquid	Healthcare Products
Diabetic Tussin Cold & Flu Tablet	Healthcare Products
Diabetic Tussin DM Liquid	Healthcare Products
Diabetic Tussin DM Maximum Strength Liquid	Healthcare Products
Diabetic Tussin DM Maximum Strength Capsule	Healthcare Products
Diabetic Tussin EX Liquid	Healthcare Products
Dimetapp Allergy Children's Elixir	Whitehall-Robins

(Continued on next page)

Dimetapp Cold & Fever Children's Suspension	Wyeth Consumer
Dimetapp Decongestant Pediatric Drops	Wyeth Consumer
Double-Tussin DM Liquid	Rease
Drocon-CS Solution	Cypress
Duradal HD Plus Syrup	Prasco Laboratories
Duratan DM Suspension	Proethic Laboratories
Duratuss DM Solution	Victory
Dynatuss Syrup	Breckenridge
Dynatuss EX Syrup	Breckenridge
Dynatuss HC Solution	Breckenridge
Dynatuss HCG Solution	Breckenridge
Endacof DM Solution	Larken Laboratories
Endacof HC Solution	Larken Laboratories
Endacof XP Solution	Larken Laboratories
Endagen-HD Syrup	Monarch
Endal HD Solution	Pediamed
Endal HD Syrup	Propst
Endal HD Plus Syrup	Propst
Endotuss-HD Syrup	American Generics
Enplus-HD Syrup	Alphagen
Entex Syrup	Andrx
Entex HC Syrup	Andrx
Exo-Tuss	American Generics
Father John's Medicine Plus Drops	Oakhurst
Friallergia DM Liquid	R.I.D.
Friallergia Liquid	R.I.D.
Ganidin NR Liquid	Cypress
Gani-Tuss NR Liquid	Cypress
Gani-Tuss-DM NR Liquid	Cypress
Genahist Elixir	Ivax
Genebronco-D Liquid	Pharm Generic
Genecof-HC Liquid	Pharm Generic
Genecof-XP Liquid	Pharm Generic
Genecof-XP Syrup	Pharm Generic
Genedel Syrup	Pharm Generic
Genedotuss-DM Liquid	Pharm Generic
Genepatuss Liquid	Pharm Generic
Genetuss-2 Liquid	Pharm Generic
Genexpect DM Liquid	Pharm Generic
Genexpect-PE Liquid	Pharm Generic
Genexpect-SF Liquid	Pharm Generic
Giltuss HC Syrup	Gil
Giltuss Liquid	Gil
Giltuss Pediatric Liquid	Gil
Guai-Co Liquid	Alphagen
Guaicon DMS Liquid	Textilease Medique
Guai-Dex Liquid	Alphagen
Guaifed Syrup	Muro
Guaitussin AC Solution	Scientific Laboratories
Guaitussin DAC Solution	Scientific Laboratories
Guapetex HC Solution	Scientific Laboratories
Guapetex Syrup	Scientific Laboratories
Halotussin AC Liquid	Watson Pharma
Hayfebrol Liquid	Scot-Tussin
H-C Tussive Syrup	Vintage

Histacol DM Pediatric Solution	Breckenridge
Histacol DM Pediatric Syrup	Breckenridge
Histex HC Syrup	TEAMM
Histex Liquid	TEAMM
Histex PD Drops	TEAMM
Histex PD Liquid	TEAMM
Histinex HC Syrup	Ethex
Histinex PV Syrup	Ethex
Histuss HC Solution	Scientific Laboratories
Hi-Tuss Syrup	Hi-Tech Pharmacal
Hycomal DH Liquid	Alphagen
Hydex-PD Solution	Cypress
Hydone Liquid	Hyrex
Hydramine Elixir	Ivax
Hydro PC Syrup	Cypress
Hydro PC II Plus Solution	Cypress
Hydro Pro Solution	Breckenridge
Hydrocol-HC Solution	Morton Grove
Hydro-DP Solution	Cypress
Hydron CP Syrup	Cypress
Hydron EX Syrup	Cypress
Hydron KGS Liquid	Cypress
Hydron PSC Liquid	Cypress
Hydro-Tussin DM Elixir	Ethex
Hydro-Tussin HC Syrup	Ethex
Hydro-Tussin HD Liquid	Ethex
Hydro-Tussin XP Syrup	Ethex
Hyphen-HD Syrup	Alphagen
Jaycof Expectorant Syrup	Pharmakon
Jaycof-HC Liquid	Pharmakon
Jaycof-XP Liquid	Pharmakon
Kita La Tos Liquid	R.I.D.
Levall Liquid	Andrx
Levall 5.0 Liquid	Andrx
Lodrane Liquid	ECR
Lodrane D Suspension	ECR
Lodrane XR Suspension	ECR
Lohist D Syrup	Larken Laboratories
Lohist-LQ Solution	Larken
Lortuss DM Solution	Proethic
Lortuss HC Solution	Proethic
Marcof Expectorant Syrup	Marnel
Maxi-Tuss HCX Solution	MCR American
M-Clear Jr Solution	McNeil, R.A.
M-Clear Syrup	McNeil, R.A.
Medi-Brom Elixir	Medicine Shoppe
Mintex Liquid	Breckenridge
Mintex PD Liquid	Breckenridge
Mintuss DM Syrup	Breckenridge
Mintuss EX Syrup	Breckenridge
Mintuss G Syrup	Breckenridge
Mintuss HD Syrup	Breckenridge
Mintuss MR Syrup	Breckenridge
Mintuss MS Syrup	Breckenridge
Mintuss NX Solution	Breckenridge

(Continued on next page)

Motrin Cold Children's Suspension	McNeil Consumer
Mytussin-PE Liquid	Morton Grove
Nalex DH Liquid	Blansett Pharmacal
Nalex-A Liquid	Blansett Pharmacal
Nalspan Senior DX Liquid	Morton Grove
Nasop Suspension	Hawthorn
Neotuss S/F Liquid	A.G. Marin
Neotuss-D Liquid	A.G. Marin
Norel DM Liquid	U.S. Pharmaceutical
Nucofed Syrup	Monarch
Nycoff Tablet	Dover
Orgadin Liquid	American Generics
Orgadin-Tuss Liquid	American Generics
Orgadin-Tuss DM Liquid	American Generics
Organidin NR Liquid	Wallace
Palgic-DS Syrup	Pamlab
Pancof Syrup	Pamlab
Pancof EXP Syrup	Pamlab
Pancof HC Liquid	Pamlab
Pancof HC Solution	Pamlab
Pancof XP Liquid	Pamlab
Pancof XP Solution	Pamlab
Panmist DM Syrup	Pamlab
Panmist-S Syrup	Pamlab
PediaCare Cold + Allergy Children's Liquid	Pharmacia
PediaCare Cough + Cold Children's Liquid	Pharmacia
PediaCare Decongestant Infants Drops	Pharmacia
PediaCare Decongestant Plus Cough Drops	Pharmacia
PediaCare Multi-Symptom Liquid	Pharmacia
PediaCare Nightrest Liquid	Pharmacia
Pediahist DM Syrup	Boca Pharmacal
Pedia-Relief Liquid	Major
Pediatex Liquid	Zyber
Pediatex Solution	Zyber
Pediatex-D Liquid	Zyber
Pediatex D Solution	Zyber
Pediatex DM Solution	Zyber
Pediox Liquid	Atley
Phanasin Syrup	Pharmakon Labs
Phanatuss Syrup	Pharmakon Labs
Phanatuss-HC Diabetic Choice Solution	Pharmakon Labs
Phena-HC Solution	GM
Phena-S Liquid	GM
Phena-S 12 Suspension	GM
Pneumotussin 2.5 Syrup	ECR
Poly Hist DM Solution	Poly
Poly Hist PD Solution	Poly
Poly-Tussin Syrup	Poly
Poly-Tussin DM Syrup	Poly
Poly-Tussin HD Syrup	Poly
Poly-Tussin XP Syrup	Poly
Primsol Solution	Medicis
Pro-Clear Solution	Pro-Pharma
Pro-Cof Liquid	Qualitest
Pro-Cof D Liquid	Qualitest

Prolex DH Liquid	Blansett Pharmacal
Prolex DM Liquid	Blansett Pharmacal
Pro-Red Solution	Pro-Pharma
Protex Solution	Scientific Laboratories
Protex D Solution	Scientific Laboratories
Protuss Liquid	First Horizon
Protuss-D Liquid	First Horizon
Pyrroxate Extra Strength Tablet	Lee
Q-Tussin PE Liquid	Qualitest
Qual-Tussin DC Syrup	Pharm. Associates
Quintex Syrup	Qualitest
Quintex HC Syrup	Qualitest
Relacon-DM Solution	Cypress
Relacon-HC Solution	Cypress
Relasin DM Solution	Cypress
Rescon-DM Liquid	Capellon
Rescon-GG Liquid	Capellon
Rhinacon A Solution	Breckenridge
Rhinacon DH Solution	Breckenridge
Rindal HD Liquid	Breckenridge
Rindal HD Plus Solution	Breckenridge
Rindal HPD Solution	Breckenridge
Robitussin Cough & Congestion Liquid	Wyeth Consumer
Robitussin DM Syrup	Wyeth Consumer
Robitussin PE Syrup	Wyeth Consumer
Robitussin Pediatric Drops	Wyeth Consumer
Robitussin Pediatric Cough Syrup	Wyeth Consumer
Robitussin Pediatric Night Relief Liquid	Wyeth Consumer
Romilar AC Liquid	Scot-Tussin
Romilar DM Liquid	Scot-Tussin
Rondamine DM Liquid	Major
Rondec Syrup	Biovail
Rondec DM Drops	Biovail
Rondec DM Syrup	Biovail
Ru-Tuss A Syrup	Sage
Ru-Tuss DM Syrup	Sage
Scot-Tussin Allergy Relief Formula Liquid	Scot-Tussin
Scot-Tussin DM Liquid	Scot-Tussin
Scot-Tussin Expectorant Liquid	Scot-Tussin
Scot-Tussin Original Syrup	Scot-Tussin
Scot-Tussin Senior Liquid	Scot-Tussin
Siladryl Allergy Liquid	Silarx
Siladryl DAS Liquid	Silarx
Sildec Liquid	Silarx
Sildec Syrup	Silarx
Sildec-DM Drops	Silarx
Sildec-DM Syrup	Silarx
Sil-Tex Liquiduid Liquid	Silarx
Siltussin DAS Liquid	Silarx
Siltussin DM Syrup	Silarx
Siltussin DM DAS Cough Formula Syrup	Silarx
Siltussin SA Syrup	Silarx
Simply Cough Liquid	McNeil Consumer
Simply Stuffy Liquid	McNeil Consumer
S-T Forte 2 Liquid	Scot-Tussin

(Continued on next page)

Statuss DM Syrup	Magna
Sudafed Children's Cold & Cough Solution	Pfizer
Sudafed Children's Solution	Pfizer
Sudafed Children's Tablet	Pfizer
Sudanyl Tablet	Dover
Sudatuss DM Syrup	Pharmaceutical Generic
Sudatuss-2 Liquid	Pharmaceutical Generic
Sudatuss-SF Liquid	Pharmaceutical Generic
Triaminic Infant Decongestant Drops	Novartis Consumer
Triant-HC Solution	Hawthorn
Trispec-PE Liquid	Deliz
Trituss DM Solution	Breckenridge
Trituss Solution	Everett
Tri-Vent DM Solution	Ethex
Tri-Vent DPC Syrup	Ethex
Tusdec-DM Solution	Cypress
Tusdec-HC Solution	Cypress
Tusnel Pediatric Solution	Llorens Pharma
Tusnel Solution	Llorens Pharma
Tussafed Syrup	Everett
Tussafed-EX Syrup	Everett
Tussafed-EX Pediatric Liquid	Everett
Tussafed-HC Syrup	Everett
Tussafed-HCG Solution	Everett
Tussall Solution	Everett
Tussbid Capsule	Breckenridge
Tuss-DM Liquid	Seatrace
Tuss-ES Syrup	Seatrace
Tussex Syrup	H. L. Moore
Tussinate Syrup	Pediamed
Tussi-Organidin DM NR Liquid	Wallace
Tussi-Organidin NR Liquid	Wallace
Tussi-Pres Liquid	Kramer-Novis
Tussirex Liquid	Scot-Tussin
Tussirex Syrup	Scot-Tussin
Tylenol Allergy-D Children's Liquid	McNeil Consumer
Tylenol Cold Children's Liquid	McNeil Consumer
Tylenol Cold Children's Suspension	McNeil Consumer
Tylenol Cold Infants' Drops	McNeil Consumer
Tylenol Cold Plus Cough Children's Liquid	McNeil Consumer
Tylenol Cold Plus Cough Infants' Suspension	McNeil Consumer
Tylenol Flu Children's Suspension	McNeil Consumer
Tylenol Flu Night Time Max Strength Liquid	McNeil Consumer
Tylenol Sinus Children's Liquid	McNeil Consumer
Uni-Lev 5.0 Solution	United Research
Vanex-HD Syrup	Monarch
Vazol Solution	Wraser Pharm
Vicks 44E Pediatric Liquid	Procter & Gamble
Vicks 44M Pediatric Liquid	Procter & Gamble
Vicks Dayquil Multi-Symptom Liquicap	Procter & Gamble
Vicks Dayquil Multi-Symptom Liquid	Procter & Gamble
Vicks 44 Liquid Capsules Cold, Flu, Cough	Procter & Gamble
Vicks Nyquil Children's Liquid	Procter & Gamble
Vicks Sinex 12 Hour Spray	Procter & Gamble
Vicks Sinex Spray	Procter & Gamble

Vi-Q Tuss Syrup	Vintage
V-Tann Suspension	Breckenridge
Vitussin Expectorant Syrup	Cypress
Vortex Syrup	Superior
Welltuss EXP Solution	Prasco Laboratories
Welltuss HC Solution	Prasco Laboratories
Z-Cof DM Syrup	Zyber
Z-Cof DMX Solution	Zyber
Z-Cof HC Syrup	Zyber
Ztuss Expectorant Solution	Magna

Ear/Nose/Throat Products

4-Way Saline Moisturizing Mist Spray	Bristol-Myers
Ayr Baby Saline Spray	B. F. Ascher
Bucalcide Solution	Seyer Pharmatec
Bucalcide Spray	Seyer Pharmatec
Bucalsep Solution	Gil
Bucalsep Spray	Gil
Cepacol Sore Throat Liquid	Combe
Cheracol Sore Throat Spray	Lee
Fresh N Free Liquid	Geritrex
Gly-Oxide Liquid	GlaxoSmithKline
Isodettes Sore Throat Spray	GlaxoSmithKline
Lacrosse Mouthwash Liquid	Aplicare
Larynex Lozenges	Dover
Listermint Liquid	Pfizer Consumer
Nasal Moist Gel	Blairex
Orajel Baby Liquid	Del
Orajel Baby Nighttime Gel	Del
Oramagic Oral Wound Rinse Powder for Suspension	MPM Medical
Orasept Mouthwash/Gargle Liquid	Pharmakon Labs
Tanac Liquid	Del
Tech 2000 Dental Rinse Liquid	Care-Tech
Throto-Ceptic Spray	S.S.S.
Zilactin Baby Extra Strength Gel	Zila Consumer

Gastrointestinal Agents

Axid	Pediamed Pharm
Axid Solution	Reliant
Baby Gasz Drops	Lee
Colidrops Pediatric Drops	A.G. Marin
Colace Solution	Purdue Pharma
Diarrest Tablet	Dover
Imogen Liquid	Pharmacon Labs
Kaodene NN Suspension	Pfeiffer
Liqui-Doss Liquid	Ferndale
Mylicon Infants' Suspension	J&J-Merck
Neoloid Liquid	Kenwood
Neutralin Tablet	Dover
Senokot Children's Syrup	Purdue Frederick

Hematinics

Irofol Liquid	Dayton

(Continued on next page)

Miscellaneous

Cytra-2 Solution	Cypress
Cytra-K Solution	Cypress
Emetrol Solution	Pharmacia
Fluorinse Solution	Oral B
Primsol Solution	FSC
Rum-K Liquid	Fleming

Psychotropics

Thorazine Syrup	GlaxoSmithKline

Topical Products

Aloe Vesta 2-N-1 Antifungal Ointment	Convatec
Blistex Complete Moisture Stick	Blistex
Blistex Fruit Smoothies Stick	Blistex
Blistex Herbal Answer Gel	Blistex
Blistex Herbal Answer Stick	Blistex
Dermatone Lips N Face Protector Ointment	Dermatone
Dermatone Moisturizing Sunblock Cream	Dermatone
Dermatone Outdoor Skin Protection Cream	Dermatone
Dermatone Skin Protector Cream	Dermatone
Eucapsulein Facial Lotion	Beiersdorf, Inc.
Evoclin Foam	Connetics
Fleet Pain Relief Pads	Fleet
Fresh & Pure Douche Solution	Unico
Handclens Solution	Woodward
Joint-Ritis Maximum Strength Ointment	Naturopathic Laboratories
Neutrogena Acne Wash Liquid	Neutrogena
Neutrogena Antiseptic Liquid	Neutrogena
Neutrogena Clear Pore Gel	Neutrogena
Neutrogena T/Derm Liquid	Neutrogena
Neutrogena Toner Liquid	Neutrogena
Podiciens Spray	Woodward
Propa pH Foaming Face Wash Liquid	Del
Sea Breeze Foaming Face Wash Gel	Clairol
Shade Uvaguard Lotion	Schering Plough
Sportz Bloc Cream	Med-Derm
Stri-Dex Maximum Strength Pad	Blistex
Stri-Dex Sensitive Skin Pad	Blistex
Stri-Dex Super Scrub Pad	Blistex
Therasoft Anti-Acne Cream	SFC/Solvent Free
Therasoft Skin Protectant Cream	SFC/Solvent Free
Tiger Balm Arthritis Rub Lotion	Prince of Peace Enterprises

Vitamins/Minerals/Supplements

Adaptosode For Stress Liquid	HVS
Adaptosode R+R For Acute Stress Liquid	HVS
Apetigen Elixir	Kramer-Novis
Biosode Liquid	HVS
Detoxosode Products Liquid	HVS
Folbic Tablet	Breckenridge
Folplex 2.2 Gel	Breckenridge
Genesupp-500 Liquid	Pharmaceutical

Genetect Plus Liquid	Pharmaceutical
Multi-Delyn w/Iron Liquid	Silarx
Poly-Vi-Sol Drops	Mead Johnson
Poly-Vi-Sol w/Iron Drops	Mead Johnson
Poly-Vi-Solution Liquid	Mead Johnson
Poly-Vi-Solution w/Iron Liquid	Mead Johnson
Protect Plus Liquid	Gil
Soluvite-F Drops	Pharmics
Strovite Forte Syrup	Everett
Supervite Liquid	Seyer Pharmatec
Suplevit Liquid	Gil
Tri-Vi-Sol Drops	Mead Johnson
Tri-Vi-Sol w/Iron Drops	Mead Johnson
Vitafol Syrup	Everett
Vitalize Liquid	Scot-Tussin
Vitamin C/Rose Hips Tablet, Extended Release	ADH Health Products

Reprinted with permission from *The Drug Topics Red Book*. Montvale NJ: Thomson Medical Economics, 2007.

DRUGS THAT MAY CAUSE PHOTOSENSITIVITY

The drugs in this table are known to cause photosensitivity in some individuals. Effects can range from itching, scaling, rash, and swelling to skin cancer, premature skin aging, skin and eye burns, cataracts, reduced immunity, blood vessel damage, and allergic reactions.

The list is not all-inclusive, and shows only representative brands of each generic. When in doubt, always check specific product labeling. Individuals should be advised to wear protective clothing and to apply sunscreens while taking the medications listed below.

Generic	Brand
Acamprosate	Campral
Acetazolamide	Diamox
Acitretin	Soriatane
Acyclovir	Zovirax
Alendronate	Fosamax
Alitretinoin	Panretin
Almotriptan	Axert
Amiloride/hydrochlorothiazide	Moduretic
Aminolevulinic acid	Levulan Kerastick
Amiodarone	Cordarone, Pacerone
Amitriptyline	Elavil
Amitriptyline/chlordiazepoxide	Limbitro
Amitriptyline/perphenazine	Triavil
Amlodipine/atorvastatin	Caduet
Amoxapine	
Anagrelide	Agrylin
Apripiprazole	Abilify
Atazanavir	Reyataz
Atenolol/chlorthalidone	Tenoretic
Atorvastatin	Lipitor
Atovaquone/proguanil	Malarone
Azatadine/pseudoephedrine	Rynatan, Trinalin
Azithromycin	Zithromax

(Continued on next page)

Generic	Brand
Benazepril	Lotensin
Benazepril/hydrochlorothiazide	Lotensin HCT
Bendroflumethiazide/nadolol	Corzide
Bexarotene	Targretin
Bismuth/metronidazole/tetracycline	Helidac
Bisoprolol/hydrochlorothiazide	Ziac
Brompheniramine/dextromethorphan/phenylephrine	Alacol DM
Brompheniramine/dextromethorphan/pseudoephedrine	Bromfed-DM
Buffered aspirin/pravastatin	Pravigard PAC
Bupropion	Wallbutrin, Zyban
Candesartan/hydrochlorothiazide	Atacand HCT
Capecitabine	Xeloda
Captopril	Capoten
Captopril/hydrochlorothiazide	Capozide
Carbamazepine	Carbatrol, Tegretol, Tegretol-XR
Carbinoxamine/pseudoephedrine	Palgic-D, Palgic-DS, Pediatex-D
Carvedilol	Coreg
Celecoxib	Celebrex
Cetirizine	Zyrtec
Cetirizine/pseudoephedrine	Zyrtec-D
Cevimeline	Evoxac
Chlorhexidine gluconate	Hibistat
Chloroquine	Aralen
Chlorothiazide	Diuril
Chlorphenirmine/hydrocodone/pseudoephedrine	Tussend
Chlorpheniramine/phenylephrine/pyrilamine	Rynatan
Chlorpromazine	Thorazine
Chlorpropamide	Diabinese
Chlorthalidone	Thalitone
Chlorthalidone/clonidine	Clorpres
Cidofovir	Vislide
Ciprofloxacin	Cipro
Citalopram	Celexa
Clemastine	Tavist
Clonidine/chlorthalidone	Clorpres
Clozapine	Clozaril, Fazacio
Cromolyn sodium	Gastrocrom
Cyclobenzaprine	Flexeril
Cyproheptadine	Cyproheptadine
Dacarbazine	DTIC-Dome
Dantrolene	Dantrium
Demeclocycline	Declomycin
Desipramine	Norpramin
Diclofenac potassium	Catalfam
Diclofenac sodium	Voltaren
Diclofenac sodium/misoprostol	Arthrotec
Diflunisal	Dolobid
Dihydroergotamine	D.H.E. 45
Diltiazem	Cardizem, Tiazac
Diphenhydramine	Benadryl
Divalproex	Depakote
Doxepin	Sinequan
Doxycycline hyclate	Doryx, Periostat, Vibra-Tabs, Vibramycin

Generic	Brand
Doxycycline monohydrate	Monodox
Duloxetine	Cymbalta
Enalapril	Vasotec
Enalapril/felodipine	Lexxel
Enalapril/hydrochlorothiazide	Vaseretic
Enalaprilat	Vasotec I.V.
Epirubicin	Ellence
Eprosartan mesylate/hydrochlorothiazide	Teveten HCT
Erythromycin/sulfisoxazole	Pediazole
Estazolam	ProSom
Estradiol	Gynodiol, Estrogel
Eszopiclone	Lunesta
Ethionamide	Trecator-SC
Etodolac	Lodine
Felbamate	Felbatol
Fenofibrate	Tricor, Lofibra
Floxuridine	Sterile FUDR
Flucytosine	Ancobon
Fluorouracil	Efudex
Fluoxetine	Prozac, Sarafem
Fluphenazine	Prolixin
Flutamide	Eulexin
Fluvastatin	Lescol
Fluvoxamine	Luvox
Fosinopril	Monopril
Fosphenytoin	Cerebyx
Furosemide	Lasix
Gabapentin	Neurontin
Gatifloxacin	Tequin
Gemfibrozil	Lopid
Gemifloxacin mesylate	Factive
Gentamicin	Garamycin
Glatiramer	Copaxone
Glimepiride	Amaryl
Glipizide	Glucotrol
Glyburide	DiaBeta, Glynase, Micronase
Glyburide/metformin HCl	Glucovance
Griseofulvin	Fulvicin P/G, Grifulvin, Gris-PEG
Haloperidol	Haldol
Hexachlorophene	pHisoHex
Hydralazine/hydrochlorothiazide	Hydra-zide
Hydrochlorothiazide	HydroDIURIL, Microzide, Oretic
Hydrochlorothiazide/fosinopril	Monopril HCT
Hydrochlorothiazide/Irbesartan	Avalide
Hydrochlorothiazide/lisinopril	Prinzide, Zestoretic
Hydrochlorothiazide/losartan potassium	Hyzaar
Hydrochlorothiazide/methyldopa	Aldoril
Hydrochlorothiazide/moexipril	Uniretic
Hydrochlorothiazide/propranolol	Inderide
Hydrochlorothiazide/quinapril	Accuretic
Hydrochlorothiazide/spironolactone	Aldactazide
Hydrochlorothiazide/telmisartan	Micardis HCT
Hydrochlorothiazide/timolol	Timolide

(Continued on next page)

Generic	Brand
Hydrochlorothiazide/triamterene	Dyazide, Maxzide
Hydrochlorothiazide/valsartan	Diovan HCT
Hydroflumethiazide	Hydroflumethiazide
Hydroxychloroquine	Plaquenil
Hypericum	Kira, St. John's wort
Hypericum/vitamin B_1/vitamin C/kava-kava	One-A-Day Tension & Mood
Ibuprofen	Motrin
Imatinib Mesylate	Gleevec
Imipramine	Tofranil
Imiquimod	Aldara
Indapamide	Lozol
Interferon alfa-2b, recombinant	Intron A
Interferon alfa-n3 (human leukocyte derived)	Alferon-N
Interferon beta-1a	Avonex
Interferon beta-1b	Betaseron
Irbesartan/hydrochlorothiazide	Avalide
Isoniazid/pyrazinamide/rifampin	Rifater
Isotretinoin	Accutane, Amnesteem
Itraconazole	Sporanox
Ketoprofen	Orudis, Oruvail
Lamotrigine	Lamictal
Leuprolide	Lupron
Levamisole	Levamisole
Lisinopril	Prinivil, Zestril
Lisinorpil/hydrochlorothiazide	Prinivil, Zestoretic
Lomefloxacin	Maxaquin
Loratadine	Claritin
Loratadine/pseudoephedrine	Claritin-D
Losartan	Cozaar
Losartan/hydrochlorothiazide	Hyzaar
Lovastatin	Altoprev, Mevacor
Lovastatin/niacin	Advicor
Maprotiline	Maprotiline
Mefenamic acid	Ponstel
Meloxicam	Mobic
Mesalamine	Pentasa
Methazolamide	
Methotrexate	Trexall
Methoxsalen	Uvadex, Oxsoralen, 8-MOP
Methyclothiazide	Enduron
Methyldopa/hydrochlorothiazide	Aldoril
Metolazone	Mykrox, Zaroxolyn
Minocycline	Dynacin, Minocin
Mirtazapine	Remeron
Moexipril	Univasc
Moexipril/hydrochlorothiazide	Uniretic
Moxifloxacin	Avelox
Nabumetone	Relafen
Nadolol/bendroflumethiazide	Corzide
Nalidixic acid	Nalidixic acid
Naproxen	Naprosyn, EC-Naprosyn
Naproxen sodium	Anaprox, Naprelan
Naratriptan	Amerge

Generic	Brand
Nefazodone	Serzone
Nifedipine	Adalat CC, Procardia
Nisoldipine	Sular
Norfloxacin	Noroxin
Nortriptyline	Pamelor
Ofloxacin	Floxin
Olanzapine	Zyprexa
Olanzapine/fluoxetine	Symbyax
Olmesartan medoxomil/hydrochlorothiazide	Benicar HCT
Olsalazine	Dipentum
Oxaprozin	Daypro
Oxcarbazepine	Trileptal
Oxycodone	Roxicodone
Oxytetracycline	Terramycin
Pantoprazole	Protonix
Paroxetine	Paxil
Pastinaca sativa	Parsnip
Pentosan polysulfate	Elmiron
Pentostatin	Nipent
Perphenazine	Perphenazine
Pilocarpine	Salagen
Piroxicam	Feldene
Polythiazide	Renese
Polythiazide/prazosin	Minizide
Porfimer sodium	Photofrin
Pravastatin	Pravachol
Prochlorperazine	Compazine, Compro
Promethazine	Phenergan
Protriptyline	Vivactil
Pyrazinamide	Pyrazinamide
Quetiapine	Seroquel
Quinapril	Accupril
Quinapril/hydrochlorethiazide	Accuretic
Quinidine gluconate	Quinidine
Quinidine sulfate	Quinidex
Rabeprazole sodium	Aciphex
Ramipril	Altace
Riluzole	Rilutek
Risperidone	Risperdal, Risperdal Consta
Ritonavir	Norvir
Rizatriptan	Maxalt
Ropinirole	Requip
Rosuvastatin	Crestor
Ruta graveolens	Rue
Saquinavir	Fortovase
Saquinavir mesylate	Invirase
Selegiline	Eldepryl
Sertraline	Zoloft
Sibutramine	Meridia
Sildenafil	Viagra
Simvastatin	Zocor
Simvastatin/ezetimibe	Vytorin
Somatropin	Serostim

(Continued on next page)

Generic	Brand
Sotalol	Betapace, Betapace
Sulfamethoxazole/trimethoprim	Bactrim, Septra
Sulfasalazine	Azulfidine
Sulindac	Clinoril
Sumatriptan	Imitrex
Tacrolimus	Prograf, Protopic
Tazarotene	Tazorac
Telmisartan/hydrochlorothiazide	Micardis HCT
Tetracycline	Sumycin
Thalidomide	Thalomid
Thioridazine hydrochloride	Mellaril
Thiothixene	Navane
Tiagabine	Gabitril
Tolazamide	Tolazamide
Tolbutamide	Tolbutamide
Topiramate	Topamax
Tretinoin	Retin-A
Triamcinolone	Azmacort
Triamterene	Dyrenium
Triamterene/hydrochlorothiazide	Dyazide, Maxzide
Trifluoperazine	Trifluoperazine
Trimipramine	Surmontil
Trovafloxacin	Trovan
Valacyclovir	Valtrex
Valdecoxib	Bextra
Valproate	Depacon
Valproic acid	Depakene
Valsartan/hydrochlorothiazide	Diovan HCT
Vardenafil	Levitra
Venlafaxine	Effexor
Verteporfin	Visudyne
Vinblastine	Vinblastine
Voriconazole	Vfend
Zalcitabine	Hivid
Zaleplon	Sonata
Ziprasidone	Geodon
Zolmitriptan	Zomig
Zolpidem	Ambien

DRUG/ALCOHOL INTERACTIONS

Product	Interaction	Onset	Severity
ACETAMINOPHEN	ETHANOL	2	2
	Concurrent use of ACETAMINOPHEN and ETHANOL may result in an increased risk of hepatotoxicity.		
ACETOPHENAZINE	ETHANOL	1	2
	Concurrent use of ACETOPHENAZINE and ETHANOL may result in increased CNS depression and an increased risk of extrapyramidal reactions.		
ACITRETIN	ETHANOL	2	1
	Concurrent use of ACITRETIN and ETHANOL may result in a prolonged risk of teratogenicity.		
ALFENTANIL	ETHANOL	2	2
	Concurrent use of ALFENTANOL and ETHANOL may result in decreased therapeutic effects for alfentanil.		
ALPRAZOLAM	ETHANOL	1	2
	Concurrent use of ALPRAZOLAM and ETHANOL may result in increased sedation.		
AMITRIPTYLINE	ETHANOL	1	2
	Concurrent use of AMITRIPTYLINE and ETHANOL may result in enhanced CNS depression and impairment of motor skills.		
AMOBARBITAL	ETHANOL	1	2
	Concurrent use of AMOBARBITAL and ETHANOL may result in excessive CNS depression.		
AMOXAPINE	ETHANOL	1	2
	Concurrent use of AMOXAPINE and ETHANOL may result in enhanced drowsiness and impairment of motor skills.		
AMPRENAVIR	ETHANOL	2	1
	Concurrent use of AMPRENAVIR and ETHANOL may result in an increased risk of propylene glycol toxicity (seizures, tachycardia, lactic acidosis, renal toxicity, and hemolysis).		
APROBARBITAL	ETHANOL	1	2
	Concurrent use of APROBARBITAL and ETHANOL may result in excessive CNS depression.		
ASPIRIN	ETHANOL	1	2
	Concurrent use of ASPIRIN and ETHANOL may result in increased gastrointestinal blood loss.		
BUPROPION	ETHANOL	2	1
	Concurrent use of BUPROPION and ETHANOL may result in an increased risk of seizures.		
BUTABARBITAL	ETHANOL	1	2
	Concurrent use of BUTABARBITAL and ETHANOL may result in excessive CNS depression.		
BUTALBITAL	ETHANOL	1	2
	Concurrent use of BUTALBITAL and ETHANOL may result in excessive CNS depression.		
CALAMUS	ETHANOL	1	2
	Concurrent use of CALAMUS and ETHANOL may result in increased sedation.		
CANNABIS	ETHANOL	1	2
	Concurrent use of CANNABIS and ETHANOL may result in increased intoxication.		
CARVEDILOL, PHOSPHATE	ETHANOL	1	2
	Concurrent use of CARVEDILOL, PHOSPHATE and ETHANOL may result in faster than normal rate of release of carvedilol phosphate.		

(Continued on next page)

Product	Interaction	Onset	Severity
CEFAMANDOLE	ETHANOL Concurrent use of CEFAMANDOLE and ETHANOL may result in disulfiram-like reactions.	2	1
CEFMENOXINE	ETHANOL Concurrent use of CEFMENOXINE and ETHANOL may result in disulfiram-like reactions.	1	1
CEFOPERAZONE	ETHANOL Concurrent use of CEFOPERAZONE and ETHANOL may result in disulfiram-like reactions.	2	1
CEFOTETAN	ETHANOL Concurrent use of CEFOTETAN and ETHANOL may result in disulfiram-like reactions.	2	1
CHAPARRAL	ETHANOL Concurrent use of CHAPARRAL and ETHANOL may result in elevated liver transaminases with or without concomitant hepatic damage.	1	2
CHLORAL HYDRATE	ETHANOL Concurrent use of CHLORAL HYDRATE and ETHANOL may result in increased sedation.	1	3
CHLORDIAZEPOXIDE	ETHANOL Concurrent use of CHLORDIAZEPOXIDE and ETHANOL may result in increased sedation.	1	2
CHLORPROMAZINE	ETHANOL Concurrent use of CHLORPROMAZINE and ETHANOL may result in increased sedation.	1	2
CHLORPROPAMIDE	ETHANOL Concurrent use of CHLORPROPAMIDE and ETHANOL may result in disulfiram-like reactions.	1	1
CIMETIDINE	ETHANOL Concurrent use of CIMETIDINE and ETHANOL may result in increased ethanol concentrations.	1	3
CISAPRIDE	ETHANOL Concurrent use of CISAPRIDE and ETHANOL may result in increased blood levels of ethanol.	1	2
CITALOPRAM	ETHANOL Concurrent use of CITALOPRAM and ETHANOL may result in potentiation of the cognitive and motor effects of alcohol.	0	2
CLOMIPRAMINE	ETHANOL Concurrent use of CLOMIPRAMINE and ETHANOL may result in enhanced drowsiness and impairment of motor skills.	1	2
CLORAZEPATE	ETHANOL Concurrent use of CLORAZEPATE and ETHANOL may result in increased sedation.	1	2
COCAINE	ETHANOL Concurrent use of COCAINE and ETHANOL may result in increased heart rate and blood pressure.	1	2
CODEINE	ETHANOL Concurrent use of CODEINE and ETHANOL may result in increased sedation.	1	2
COMFREY	ETHANOL Concurrent use of COMFREY and ETHANOL may result in elevated inner transaminases with or without concomitant hepatic damage.	1	1
CYCLOSERINE	ETHANOL Concurrent use of CYCLOSERINE and ETHANOL may result in an increased risk of seizures.	1	1

Product	Interaction	Onset	Severity
DESIPRAMINE	ETHANOL Concurrent use of DESIPRAMINE and ETHANOL may result in enhanced drowsiness and impairment of motor skills.	1	2
DIAZEPAM	ETHANOL Concurrent use of DIAZEPAM and ETHANOL may result in increased sedation.	1	2
DIMETHINDENE	ETHANOL Concurrent use of DIMETHINDENE and ETHANOL may result in increased sedation.	1	2
DIPHENHYDRAMINE	ETHANOL Concurrent use of DIPHENHYDRAMINE and ETHANOL may result in increased sedation.	1	2
DISULFIRAM	ETHANOL Concurrent use of DISULFIRAM and ETHANOL may result in ethanol intolerance.	1	1
DOTHIEPIN	ETHANOL Concurrent use of ETHANOL and DOTHIEPIN may result in enhanced drowsiness and impairment of motor skills.	1	2
DOXEPIN	ETHANOL Concurrent use of DOXEPIN and ETHANOL may result in enhanced drowsiness and impairment of motor skills.	1	2
ESCITALOPRAM	ETHANOL Concurrent use of ESCITALOPRAM and ETHANOL may result in potentiation of the cognitive and motor effects of alcohol.	0	2
ESZOPICLONE	ETHANOL Concurrent use of ESZOPICLONE and ETHANOL may result in impaired psychomotor functions and risk of increased sedation.	1	2
ETEROBARB	ETHANOL Concurrent use of ETEROBARB and ETHANOL may result in excessive CNS depression.	1	2
ETHOPROPAZINE	ETHANOL Concurrent use of ETHOPROPAZINE and ETHANOL may result in increased CNS depression and an increased risk of extrapyramidal reactions.	1	2
FLUNITRAZEPAM	ETHANOL Concurrent use of FLUNITRAZEPAM and ETHANOL may result in excessive sedation and psychomotor impairment.	1	2
FLUPHENAZINE	ETHANOL Concurrent use of FLUPHENAZINE and ETHANOL may result in increased CNS depression and an increased risk of extrapyramidal reactions.	1	2
FOMEPIZOLE	ETHANOL Concurrent use of FOMEPIZOLE and ETHANOL may result in the reduced elimination of both drugs.	2	2
FOSPHENYTOIN	ETHANOL Concurrent use of FOSPHENYTOIN and ETHANOL may result in decreased phenytoin serum concentrations, increased seizure potential, and additive CNS depressant effects.	1	2
FURAZOLIDONE	ETHANOL Concurrent use of FURAZOLIDONE and ETHANOL may result in disulfiram-like reactions.	1	1
GERMANDER	ETHANOL Concurrent use of GERMANDER and ETHANOL may result in elevated liver transaminases with or without concomitant hepatic damage.	2	1
GLIPIZIDE	ETHANOL Concurrent use of GLIPIZIDE and ETHANOL may result in prolonged hypoglycemia and disulfiram-like reactions.	1	1

(Continued on next page)

Product	Interaction	Onset	Severity
GLICLAZIDE	ETHANOL Concurrent use of ETHANOL and GLICLAZIDE may result in prolonged hypoglycemia and disulfiram-like reactions.	1	1
GLUTETHIMIDE	ETHANOL Concurrent use of GLUTETHIMIDE and ETHANOL may result in increased sedation.	1	2
GLYBURIDE	ETHANOL Concurrent use of GLYBURIDE and ETHANOL may result in prolonged hypoglycemia and disulfiram-like reactions.	1	2
GOSSYPOL	ETHANOL Concurrent use of GOSSYPOL and ETHANOL may result in delayed effects of gossypol and/or increased toxic effects of ethanol.	1	2
GRISEOFULVIN	ETHANOL Concurrent use of GRISEOFULVIN and ETHANOL may result in disulfiram-like reactions.	1	1
GUAR GUM	ETHANOL Concurrent use of GUAR GUM and ETHANOL may result in increased intoxication effects of ethanol.	2	2
GUARANA	ETHANOL Concurrent use of GUARANA and ETHANOL may result in increased risk of ethanol intoxication.	1	3
HYDROCODONE	ETHANOL Concurrent use of HYDROCODONE and ETHANOL may result in increased sedation.	1	2
HYDROMORPHONE	ETHANOL Concurrent use of HYDROMORPHONE and ETHANOL may result in increased sedation.	1	2
IMIPRAMINE	ETHANOL Concurrent use of IMIPRAMINE and ETHANOL may result in enhanced drowsiness and impairment of motor skills.	1	2
INSULIN	ETHANOL Concurrent use of INSULIN and ETHANOL may result in increased hypoglycemia.	1	2
INSULIN LISPRO, HUMAN	ETHANOL Concurrent use of INSULIN LISPRO, HUMAN and ETHANOL and may result in increased hypoglycemia.	1	2
ISONIAZID	ETHANOL Concurrent use of ISONIAZID and ETHANOL may result in decreased isoniazid concentrations and disulfiram-like reactions.	2	1
ISOTRETINOIN	ETHANOL Concurrent use of ISOTRETINOIN and ETHANOL may result in disulfiram-like reactions.	1	1
KAVA	ETHANOL Concurrent use of KAVA and ETHANOL may result in increased CNS depression and/or increased risk of hepatotoxicity.	1	2
KETOCONAZOLE	ETHANOL Concurrent use of KETOCONAZOLE and ETHANOL may result in disulfiram-like reactions (flushing, vomiting, increased respiratory rate, tachycardia).	1	1
LOFEPRAMINE	ETHANOL Concurrent use of LOFEPRAMINE and ETHANOL may result in enhanced drowsiness and impairment of motor skills.	1	2
LORAZEPAM	ETHANOL Concurrent use of LORAZEPAM and ETHANOL may result in increased sedation.	1	2

Product	Interaction	Onset	Severity
MA HUANG	ETHANOL	1	1
	Concurrent use of MA HUANG and ETHANOL may result in effects on mental status.		
MATE	ETHANOL	1	3
	Concurrent use of MATE and ETHANOL may result in increased risk of ethanol intoxication.		
MEPERIDINE	ETHANOL	1	2
	Concurrent use of MEPERIDINE and ETHANOL may result in increased sedation.		
MEPHOBARBITAL	ETHANOL	1	2
	Concurrent use of MEPHOBARBITAL and ETHANOL may result in excessive CNS depression.		
MEPROBAMATE	ETHANOL	1	2
	Concurrent use of MEPROBAMATE and ETHANOL may result in increased sedation.		
MESORIDAZINE	ETHANOL	1	2
	Concurrent use of MESORIDAZINE and ETHANOL may result in increased CNS depression and an increased risk of extrapyramidal reactions.		
METFORMIN	ETHANOL	2	2
	Concurrent use of METFORMIN and ETHANOL may result in an increased risk of lactic acidosis.		
METHADONE	ETHANOL	1	2
	Concurrent use of METHADONE and ETHANOL may result in increased sedation.		
METHOHEXITAL	ETHANOL	1	2
	Concurrent use of METHOHEXITAL and ETHANOL may result in excessive CNS depression.		
METHOTREXATE	ETHANOL	2	2
	Concurrent use of METHOTREXATE and ETHANOL may result in increased hepatotoxicity.		
METHOTRIMEPRAZINE	ETHANOL	1	2
	Concurrent use of METHOTRIMEPRAZINE and ETHANOL may result in increased CNS depression and an increased risk of extrapyramidal reactions.		
METRONIDAZOLE	ETHANOL	1	1
	Concurrent use of METRONIDAZOLE and ETHANOL may result in disulfiram-like reactions (flushing, increased respiratory rate, tachycardia) or sudden death.		
MIRTAZAPINE	ETHANOL	1	2
	Concurrent use of MIRTAZAPINE and ETHANOL may result in psychomotor impairment.		
MORPHINE	ETHANOL	1	2
	Concurrent use of MORPHINE and ETHANOL may result in increased risk of respiratory depression, hypotension, profound sedation, or coma.		
MORPHINE SULFATE LIPOSOME	ETHANOL	1	1
	Concurrent use of MORPHINE SULFATE LIPOSOME and ETHANOL may result in increased risk of respiratory depression, hypotension, profound sedation, or coma.		
MOXALACTAM	ETHANOL	2	1
	Concurrent use of ETHANOL and MOXALACTAM may result in disulfiram-like reactions.		
NEFAZODONE	ETHANOL	1	3
	Concurrent use of NEFAZODONE and ETHANOL may result in an increased risk of CNS side effects.		

(Continued on next page)

Product	Interaction	Onset	Severity
NIACIN	ETHANOL	0	2
	Concurrent use of NIACIN and ETHANOL may result in increased side effects of flushing and pruritus.		
NILUTAMIDE	ETHANOL	1	3
	Concurrent use of NILUTAMIDE and ETHANOL may result in an increased risk of ethanol intolerance (facial flushing, malaise, and hypotension).		
NITROGLYCERIN	ETHANOL	1	2
	Concurrent use of NITROGLYCERIN and ETHANOL may result in hypotension.		
NORTRIPTYLINE	ETHANOL	1	2
	Concurrent use of NORTRIPTYLINE and ETHANOL may result in enhanced drowsiness and impairment of motor skills.		
OLANZAPINE	ETHANOL	1	2
	Concurrent use of OLANZAPINE and ETHANOL may result in excessive CNS depression.		
OXYCODONE	ETHANOL	1	2
	Concurrent use of OXYCODONE and ETHANOL may result in increased sedation.		
OXYMORPHONE	ETHANOL	0	1
	Concurrent use of OXYMORPHONE and ETHANOL may result in increased oxymorphone plasma levels (extended-release formulation) and additive CNS/ respiratory depression.		
PARALDEHYDE	ETHANOL	2	2
	Concurrent use of PARALDEHYDE and ETHANOL may result in metabolic acidosis.		
PAROXETINE	ETHANOL	1	3
	Concurrent use of PAROXETINE and ETHANOL may increase the risk of mental and motor-skill impairment.		
PENNYROYAL	ETHANOL	1	1
	Concurrent use of PENNYROYAL and ETHANOL may result in elevated liver transaminases with or without concomitant hepatic damage.		
PENTAZOCINE	ETHANOL	1	2
	Concurrent use of PENTAZOCINE and ETHANOL may result in increased sedation.		
PERPHENAZINE	ETHANOL	1	2
	Concurrent use of PERPHENAZINE and ETHANOL may result in increased CNS depression and an increased risk of extrapyramidal reactions.		
PHENELZINE	ETHANOL	1	2
	Concurrent use of PHENELZINE and ETHANOL may result in hypertension urgency or emergency.		
PHENOBARBITAL	ETHANOL	1	2
	Concurrent use of PHENOBARBITAL and ETHANOL may result in excessive CNS depression.		
PHENYTOIN	ETHANOL	1	2
	Concurrent use of PHENYTOIN and ETHANOL may result in decreased phenytoin serum concentrations, increased seizure potential, and additive CNS depressant effects.		
PIPOTIAZINE	ETHANOL	1	2
	Concurrent use of PIPOTIAZINE and ETHANOL may result in increased CNS depression and an increased risk of extrapyramidal reactions.		
PRIMIDONE	ETHANOL	1	2
	Concurrent use of PRIMIDONE and ETHANOL may result in excessive CNS depression.		

Product	Interaction	Onset	Severity
PROCARBAZINE	ETHANOL	1	1
	Concurrent use of PROCARBAZINE and ETHANOL may result in disulfiram-like reactions and increased sedation.		
PROCHLORPERAZINE	ETHANOL	1	2
	Concurrent use of PROCHLORPERAZINE and ETHANOL may result in increased CNS depression and an increased risk of extrapyramidal reactions.		
PROMAZINE	ETHANOL	1	2
	Concurrent use of PROMAZINE and ETHANOL may result in increased CNS depression and an increased risk of extrapyramidal reactions.		
PROPIOMAZINE	ETHANOL	1	2
	Concurrent use of PROPIOMAZINE and ETHANOL may result in increased CNS depression and an increased risk of extrapyramidal reactions.		
PROTRIPTYLINE	ETHANOL	1	2
	Concurrent use of PROTRIPTYLINE and ETHANOL may result in enhanced drowsiness and impairment of motor skills.		
QUETIAPINE	ETHANOL	1	2
	Concurrent use of QUETIAPINE and ETHANOL may result in potentiation of the cognitive and motor effects of alcohol.		
SECOBARBITAL	ETHANOL	1	2
	Concurrent use of SECOBARBITAL and ETHANOL may result in excessive CNS depression.		
SERTRALINE	ETHANOL	1	2
	Concurrent use of SERTRALINE and ETHANOL may increase the risk of mental and motor-skill impairment.		
SULFAMETHOXAZOLE	ETHANOL	1	1
	Concurrent use of SULFAMETHOXAZOLE and ETHANOL may result in disulfiram-like reactions (flushing, sweating, palpitations, drowsiness).		
TACROLIMUS	ETHANOL	1	3
	Concurrent use of TACROLIMUS and ETHANOL may result in alcohol-related flushing and rash.		
TADALAFIL	ETHANOL	1	2
	Concurrent use of TADALAFIL and ETHANOL may result in an increased risk of hypotension and orthosiatic signs and symptoms.		
TEMAZEPAM	ETHANOL	1	2
	Concurrent use of TEMAZEPAM and ETHANOL may result in impaired psychomotor functions.		
THIETHYLPERAZINE	ETHANOL	1	2
	Concurrent use of THIETHYLPERAZINE and ETHANOL may result in increased CNS depression and an increased risk of extrapyramidal reactions.		
THIEOPENTAL	ETHANOL	1	2
	Concurrent use of THIEOPENTAL and ETHANOL may result in excessive CNS depression.		
THIORIDAZINE	ETHANOL	1	2
	Concurrent use of THIORIDAZINE and ETHANOL may result in increased CNS depression and an increased risk of extrapyramidal reactions.		
TIZANIDINE	ETHANOL	1	2
	Concurrent use of TIZANIDINE and ETHANOL may increase the risk of tizanidine adverse effects (excessive CNS depression).		
TOLAZAMIDE	ETHANOL	1	1
	Concurrent use of TOLAZAMIDE and ETHANOL may result in prolonged hypoglycemia and disulfiram-like reactions.		

(Continued on next page)

Product	Interaction	Onset	Severity
TOLAZOLINE	ETHANOL	2	1
	Concurrent use of TOLAZOLINE and ETHANOL may result in disulfiram-like reactions.		
TOLBUTAMIDE	ETHANOL	1	1
	Concurrent use of TOLBUTAMIDE and ETHANOL may result in prolonged hypoglycemia and disulfiram-like reactions.		
TRAMADOL	ETHANOL	1	2
	Concurrent use of TRAMADOL and ETHANOL may increase the risk of excessive CNS depression.		
TRANYLCYPROMINE	ETHANOL	1	2
	Concurrent use of TRANYLCYPROMINE and ETHANOL may result in hypertensive urgency or emergency.		
TRIAZOLAM	ETHANOL	1	2
	Concurrent use of TRIAZOLAM and ETHANOL may result in increased sedation.		
TRIFLUPERAZINE	ETHANOL	1	2
	Concurrent use of TRIFLUPERAZINE and ETHANOL may result in increased CNS depression and an increased risk of extrapyramidal reactions.		
TRIFLUPROMAZINE	ETHANOL	1	2
	Concurrent use of TRIFLUPROMAZINE and ETHANOL may result in increased CNS depression and an increased risk of extrapyramidal reactions.		
TRIMETHOPRIM	ETHANOL	1	1
	Concurrent use of ETHANOL and COTRIMOXAZOLE may result in disulfiram-like reactions.		
TRIMIPRAMINE	ETHANOL	1	2
	Concurrent use of TRIMIPRAMINE and ETHANOL may result in enhanced drowsiness and impairment of motor skills.		
VALERIAN	ETHANOL	1	2
	Concurrent use of VALERIAN and ETHANOL may result in increased sedation.		
VENLAFAXINE	ETHANOL	1	3
	Concurrent use of VENLAFAXINE and ETHANOL may result in an increased risk of CNS effects.		
VERAPAMIL	ETHANOL	1	2
	Concurrent use of VERAPAMIL and ETHANOL may result in enhanced ethanol intoxication (impaired psychomotor functioning).		
WARFARIN	ETHANOL	2	2
	Concurrent use of WARFARIN and ETHANOL may result in increased or decreased international normalized ratio (INR) or prothrombin time.		
YOHIMBINE	ETHANOL	1	2
	Concurrent use of YOHIMBINE and ETHANOL may result in increased ethanol intoxication and increased anxiety and blood pressure.		
ZALEPLON	ETHANOL	1	2
	Concurrent use of ZALEPLON and ETHANOL may result in impaired psychomotor functions.		
ZOLPIDEM	ETHANOL	1	2
	Concurrent use of ZOLPIDEM and ETHANOL may result in increased sedation.		

ONSET: 0 = Unspecified
    1 = Rapid (within 24 hours)
    2 = Delayed (after 24 hours)
SEVERITY: 1 = Major (possibly life threatening or potential permanent damage)
    2 = Moderate (may exacerbate patient's condition)
    3 = Minor (little if any clinical effect)
Note: Disulfiram-like reactions include nausea, vomiting, diarrhea, flushing, tachycardia, and hypotension. Reprinted with permission from *The Drug Topics Red Book*. Montvale, NJ: Thomson Medical Economics, 2007.

DRUG/TOBACCO INTERACTIONS

Product	Interaction	Onset	Severity
ALPRAZOLAM	TOBACCO	0	2
	Concurrent use of ALPRAZOLAM and TOBACCO may result in decreased alprazolam plasma concentrations and efficacy.		
CONTRACEPTIVES, COMBINATION	TOBACCO	2	3
	Concurrent use of CONTRACEPTIVES, COMBINATION and TOBACCO may result in an increased risk of cardiovascular disease.		
ERLOTINIB	TOBACCO	0	2
	Concurrent use of ERLOTINIB and TOBACCO may result in increased erlotinib clearance and reduced serum concentrations.		
FLUVOXAMINE	TOBACCO	2	3
	Concurrent use of FLUVOXAMINE and TOBACCO may result in increased fluvoxamine metabolism.		
IMIPRAMINE	TOBACCO	2	2
	Concurrent use of IMIPRAMINE and TOBACCO may result in decreased imipramine concentrations.		
PENTAZOCINE	TOBACCO	2	2
	Concurrent use of PENTAZOCINE and TOBACCO may result in decreased pentazocine concentrations.		
PROPOXYPHENE	TOBACCO	2	2
	Concurrent use of PROPOXYPHENE and TOBACCO may result in decreased propoxyphene concentrations.		
ROPINIROLE	TOBACCO	0	2
	Concurrent use of ROPINIROLE and TOBACCO may result in decreased ropinirole plasma concentrations and efficacy.		
THEOPHYLLINE	TOBACCO	2	2
	Concurrent use of THEOPHYLLINE and TOBACCO may result in decreased theophylline concentrations.		
TOLBUTAMIDE	TOBACCO	2	2
	Concurrent use of TOLBUTAMIDE and TOBACCO may result in decreased tolbutamide concentrations.		
WARFARIN	TOBACCO	2	2
	Concurrent use of WARFARIN and TOBACCO may result in increased or decreased international normalized ratio (INR) or prothrombin time.		

ONSET: 0 = Unspecified
1 = Rapid (within 24 hours)
2 = Delayed (after 24 hours)
SEVERITY: 1 = Major (possibly life threatening or potential permanent damage)
2 = Moderate (may exacerbate patient's condition)
3 = Minor (little if any clinical effect)
Note: Disulfiram-like reactions include nausea, vomiting, diarrhea, flushing, tachycardia, and hypotension. Reprinted with permission from *The Drug Topics Red Book*. Montvale, NJ: Thomson Medical Economics, 2007.

USE-IN-PREGNANCY RATINGS

The U.S. Food and Drug Administration's Use-in-Pregnancy rating system weighs the degree to which available information has ruled out risk to the fetus against the drug's potential benefit to the patient. Below is a listing of drugs (by generic name) for which ratings are available.

X

CONTRAINDICATED IN PREGNANCY

Studies in animals or humans, or investigational or post-marketing reports, have demonstrated fatal risk which clearly outweighs any possible benefit to the patient.

Acetohydroxamic Acid
Acitretin
Amlodipine Besylate/Atorvastatin Calcium
Amprenavir
Anisindione
Atorvastatin Calcium
Bexarotene
Bicalutamide
Bosentan
Cetrorelix Acetate
Choriogonadotropin Alfa
Chorionic Gonadotropin
Clomiphene Citrate
Desogestrel/Ethinyl Estradiol
Diclofenac Sodium/Misoprostol
Dihydroergotamine Mesylate
Dutasteride
Estazolam
Estradiol
Estradiol Acetate
Estradiol Cypionate/ Medroxyprogesterone Acetate
Estradiol Valerate
Estradiol/Levonorgestrel
Estradiol/Norethindrone Acetate
Estrogens, Conjugated
Estrogens, Conjugated, Synthetic A
Estrogens, Conjugated/ Medroxyprogesterone Acetate
Estrogens, Esterified
Estrogens, Esterified/ Methyltestosterone
Estropipate
Ethinyl Estradiol/Drospirenone
Ethinyl Estradiol/Ethynodiol Diacetate

Ethinyl Estradiol/Etonogestrel
Ethinyl Estradiol/Ferrous Fumarate/ Norethindrone Acetate
Ethinyl Estradiol/Levonorgestrel
Ethinyl Estradiol/Norelgestromin
Ethinyl Estradiol/Norethindrone
Ethinyl Estradiol/Norethindrone Acetate
Ethinyl Estradiol/Norgestimate
Ethinyl Estradiol/Norgestrel
Ezelimibe/Simvastatin
Finasteride
Fluorouracil
Fluoxymesterone
Flurazepam Hydrochloride
Fluvastatin Sodium
Follitropin Alfa
Follitropin Beta
Ganirelix Acetate
Goserelin Acetate
Histrelin Acetate
Hydromorphone Hydrochloride
Interferon Alfa-2B, Recombinant/ Ribavirin
Iodine 1 131 Tositumomab/ Tositumomab
Isotretinoin
Leflunomide
Leuprolide Acetate
Levonorgestrel
Lovastatin
Lovastatin/Niacin
Medroxyprogesterone Acetate
Megestrol Acetate
Menotropins
Mequinol/Tretinoin
Mestranol/Norethindrone
Methotrexate Sodium
Methyltestosterone
Miglustat
Misoprostol
Nafarelin Acetate
Norethindrone
Norethindrone Acetate
Norgestrel
Oxandrolone
Oxymetholone

Pilcamycin
Pravastatin Sodium
Pravastatin Sodium/Aspirin Buffered
Raloxifene Hydrochloride
Ribavirin
Rosuvastatin Calcium
Simvastatin
Tazarotene
Testosterone
Testosterone Enanthate
Thalidomide
Tositumomab
Triptorelin Pamoate
Urofollitropin
Warfarin Sodium

D

POSITIVE EVIDENCE OF RISK

Investigational or postmarketing data show risk to the fetus. Nevertheless, potential benefits may outweigh the potential risk.

Alitretinoin
Alprazolam
Altretamine
Amiodarone Hydrochloride
Amiodipine Besylate/Benazepril Hydrochloride
Anastrozole
Arsenic Trioxide
Aspirin Buffered/Pravastatin Sodium
Aspirin/Dipyridamole
Atenolol
Azathioprine
Azathioprine Sodium
Benazepril Hydrochloride*
Benazepril Hydrochloride/ Hydrochlorothiazide*
Bortezomib
Busulfan
Candesartan Cilexetil*
Candesartan Cilexetil/ Hydrochlorothiazide*

*Category C or D depending on the trimester the drug is given.

Capecitabine
Captopril*
Carbamazepine
Carboplatin
Carmustine (Bcnu)
Chlorambucil
Cladribine
Clofarabine
Clonazepam
Cytarabine Liposome
Dactinomycin
Daunorubicin Citrate Liposome
Daunorubicin Hydrochloride
Demeclocycline Hydrochloride
Diazepam
Divalproex Sodium
Docetaxel
Doxorubicin Hydrochloride
Doxorubicin Hydrochloride
    Liposome
Doxycycline Calcium
Doxycycline Hyclate
Doxycycline Monohydrate
Efavirenz
Enalapril Maleate*
Enalapril Maleate/
    Hydrochlorothiazide*
Epirubicin Hydrochloride
Eprosartan Mesylate
Eriotinib
Exemestane
Felodipine/Enalapril Maleate
Floxuridine
Fludarabine Phosphate
Flutamide
Fosinopril Sodium*
Fosinopril Sodium/
    Hydrochlorothiazide*
Fosphenytoin Sodium
Fulvestrant
Gefitinib
Gemcitabine Hydrochloride
Gemtuzumab Ozogamicin
Goserelin Acetate
Ibritumomab Tiuxetan
Idarubicin Hydrochloride
Ifosfamide
Imatinib Mesylate
Irbesartan*
Irbesartan/Hydrochlorothiazide*
Irinotecan Hydrochloride
Letrozole

Lisinopril*
Lisinopril/Hydrochlorothiazide*
Lithium Carbonate
Losartan Potassium*
Losartan Potassium/
    Hydrochlorothiazide*
Mechlorethamine Hydrochloride
Melphalan
Melphalan Hydrochloride
Mephobarbital
Mercaptopurine
Methimazole
Midazolam Hydrochloride
Minocycline Hydrochloride
Mitoxantrone Hydrochloride
Moexipril Hydrochloride*
Moexipril Hydrochloride/
    Hydrochlorothiazide*
Nelarabine
Neomycin Sulfate/Polymyxin
    B Sulfate
Nicotine
Olmesartan Medoxomil
Oxaliplatin
Pamidronate Disodium
Pemetrexed
Penicillamine
Pentobarbital Sodium
Pentostatin
Perindropil Erbumine*
Phenytoin
Procarbazine Hydrochloride
Quinapril Hydrochloride*
Quinapril Hydrochloride/
    Hydrochlorothiazide*
Ramipril*
Sorafenib
Streptomycin Sulfate
Sunitinib
Tamoxifen Citrate
Telmisartan
Telmisartan/Hydrochlorothiazide
Temozolomide
Thioguanine
Tigecycline
Tobramycin
Topotecan Hydrochloride
Toremifene Citrate
Trandolapril*
Trandolapril/Verapamil
    Hydrochloride*
Tretinoin

Valproate Sodium
Valproic Acid
Valsartan*
Valsarlan/Hydrochlorothiazide*
Vinorelbine Tartrate
Voriconazole
Zoledronic Acid

C

RISK CANNOT BE RULED OUT

Human studies are lacking, and animal studies are either positive for risk or are lacking as well. However, potential benefits may outweigh the potential risk.

Abacavir Sulfate
Abacavir Sulfate/Lamivudine
Abacavir Sulfate/Lamivudine/
    Zidovudine
Abciximab
Acamprosate Calcium
Acetaminophen
Acetaminophen/Butalbital/Caffeine
Acetaminophen/Caffeine/
    Chlorpheniramine Maleate/
    Hydrocodone Bitartrate/
    Phenylephrine Hydrochloride
Acetazolamide
Acetazolamide Sodium
Acyclovir
Adapalene
Adefovir Dipivoxil
Adenosine
Alatroflaxacin Mesylate
Albendazole
Albumin (Human)
Albuterol
Albuterol Sulfate
Albuterol Sulfate/Ipratropium
    Bromide
Alclometasone Dipropionate
Aldesleukin
Alemtuzumab
Alendronate Sodium
Alendronate Sodium/Cholecalciferol
Altopurinol Sodium
Almotriptan Malate
Alpha1-Proteinase Inhibitor (Human)
Alprostadil

(Continued on next page)

---

*Category C or D depending on the trimester the drug is given.

Alteplase
Amantadine Hydrochloride
Amifostine
Aminocaproic Acid
Aminohippurate Sodium
Aminolevulinic Acid Hydrochloride
Aminosalicylic Acid
Amlodipine Besylate
Amlodipine Besylate/Benazepril
    Hydrochloride
Amoxicillin/Clarithromycin/
    Lansoprazole
Amphetamine Aspartate/
    Amphetamine Sulfate/
    Dextroamphetamine Saccharate/
    Dextroamphetamine Sulfate
Amprenavir
Anagrelide Hydrochloride
Anthralin
Antihemophilic Factor (Human)
Antihemophilic Factor (Recombinant)
Anti-Inhibitor Coagulant Complex
Anti-Thymocyte Globulin
Apomorphine Hydrochloride
Aripiprazole
Arnica Montana/Herbals, Multiple/
    Sulfur
Asparaginase
Atomoxetine Hydrochloride
Atovaquone
Atovaquone/Proguanil Hydrochloride
Atropine Sulfate/Benzoic
    Acid/Hyoscyamine Sulfate/
    Mathenamine/Methylene Blue/
    Phenyl Salicylate
Atropine Sulfate/Hyoscyamine
    Sulfate/Scopolamine
    Hydrobromide
Azelastine Hydrochloride
Bacitracin Zinc/Neomycin Sulfate/
    Polymyxin B Sulfate
Baclofen
Bcg. Live (Intravesical)
Becaplermin
Beclomethasone Dipropionate
Beclomethasone Dipropionate
    Monohydrate
Benzepril Hydrochloride*
BenzeprilHydrochloride/
    Hydrochlorothlazide*
Bendroflumethiazide
Benzocaine
Benzonatate

Benzoyl Peroxide
Benzoyl Peroxide/Clindamycin
Benzoyl Peroxide/Erythromycin
Betamethasone Dipropionate
Betamethasone Dipropionate/
    Chlotrimazole
Betamethasone Valerate
Betaxolol Hydrochloride
Bethanechol Chloride
Bevacizumab
Bimatoprost
Bisacodyl/Polyethylene Glycol/
    Potassium Chloride/ Sodium
    Bicarbonate/ Sodium Chloride
Bisoprolol Fumarate
Bisoprolol Fumarate/
    Hydrochlorothiazide
Bitolterol Mesylate
Black Widow Spider Antivenin
    (Equine)
Botulinum Toxin Type A
Botulinum Toxin Type B
Brinzolamide
Brompheniramine Maleate/
    Dextromethorphan
    Hydrobromide/Phenylephrine
    Hydrochloride
Budesonide
Bupivacaine Hydrochloride
Bupivacaine Hydrochloride/
    Epinephrine Bitartrate
Buprenorphine Hydrochloride
Buprenorphine Hydrochloride/
    Naloxone Hydrochloride
Butabarbital/Hyoscyamine
    Hydrobromide/Phenazopyridine
    Hydrochloride
Butalbital/Acetaminophen
Butenafine Hydrochloride
Butoconazole Nitrate
Butorphanol Tartrate
Caffeine Citrate
Calcipotriene
Calcitonin-Salmon
Calcitriol
Calcium Acetate
Candesartan Cilexetil*
Candesartan Cilexetil/
    Hydrochlorothiazide*
Capreomycin Sulfate
Captropil*
Carbetapentane Tannate/
    Chlorpheniramine Tannate

Carbetapentane Tannate/
    Chlorpheniramine Tannate/
    Ephedrine Tannate/Phenylephrine
    Tannate
Carbidopa/Entacapone/Levodopa
Carbidopa/Levodopa
Carbinoxamine Maleate/
    Daxtromathorphan
    Hydrobromide/Pseudoephedrine
    Hydrochloride
Carteolol Hydrochloride
Carvedilol
Caspofungin Acetate
Celecoxib
Cetirizine Hydrochloride
Cetuximab
Cevimeline Hydrochloride
Chloramphenicol
Chloroprocaine Hydrochloride
Chlorothiazide
Chlorothiazide Sodium
Chlorpheniramine Maleate/
    Methscopolamine Nitrate/
    Phenylephrine Hydrochloride
Chlorpheniramine Maleate/
    Pseudoephedrine Hydrochloride
Chlorpheniramine Polistirex/
    Hydrocodone Polistirex
Chlorpheniramine Tannate/
    Phenylephrine Tannate
Chlorpropamide
Chlorhalidone/Clonidine
    Hydrochloride
Choline Magnesium Trisalicylate
Cidofovir
Cilostazol
Cinacalcet Hydrochloride
Ciprofloxacin Hydrochloride
Ciprofloxacin Hydrochloride/
    Hydrocortisone
Ciprofloxacin/Dexamethasone
Citalopram Hydrobromide
Clarithromycin
Clobetasol Propionate
Clonidine
Clonidine Hydrochloride
Codeine Phosphate/Acetaminophen
Colistimethate Sodium
Colistin Sulfate/Hydrocortisone
    Acetate/Neomycin Sulfate/
    Thonzonium Bromide
Corticorelin Ovine Triflutate
Cycloserine

---

*Category C or D depending on the trimester the drug is given.

Cyclosporine
Cytomegalovirus Immune Globulin
Dacarbazine
Daclizumab
Dantrolene Sodium
Dapsone
Darbepoetin Alfa
Darifenacin
Deferoxamine Mesylate
Delavirdine Masylate
Denileukin Diftitox
Desloratadine Desloratadine/
    Pseudoephedrine Sulfate
Desoximetasone
Dexamethasone
Dexamethasone Sodium Phosphate
Dexmethylphenidate Hydrochloride
Dexrazoxane
Dextroamphetamine Sulfate
Diazoxide
Dichlorophenamide
Diclofenac Potassium
Diclofenac Sodium
Diflorasone Diacetate
Diflunisal
Digoxin
Digoxin Immune Fab (Ovine)
Diltiazem Hydrochloride
Dimethyl Sulfoxide
Dinoprostone
Diphtheria & Tetanus Toxoids
    and Acellular Pertussis Vaccine
    Adsorbed
Diphtheria & Tetanus Toxoids
    and Acellular Pertussis Vaccine
    Adsorbed/Hepatitis B Vaccine,
    Recombinant/Poliovirus Vaccine
    Inactivated
Dirithromycin
Dofetilide
Donepezil Hydrochloride
Dorzolamide Hydrochloride
Dorzolamide Hydrochloride/Timolol
    Maleate
Doxazosin Mesylate
Dronabinol
Drotrecogin Alfa (Activated)
Duloxetine Hydrochloride
Echothiophate Iodide
Econazole Nirate
Efalizumab
Elfornithine Hydrochloride

Eletriptan Hydrobromide
Enalapril Maleate*
Enalapril Maleate/Felodipine*
Enalapril Maleate/Hydrochlorothiazide*
Entacapone
Entecavir
Epinastine Hydrochloride
Epinephrine
Epoetin Alfa
Eprosartan Mesylate
Erythromycin Ethylsuccinate/
    Sulfisoxazole Acetyl
Escitalopram Oxalate
Esmolol Hydrochloride
Eszopiclone
Ethionamide
Ethotoin
Etidronate Disodium
Exenatide
Ezetimibe
Factor Ix Complex
Felodipine
Fenofibrate
Fentanyl
Fentanyl Citrate
Ferrous Fumarate/Folic Acid/
    Intrinsic Factor Concentrate/
    Liver Preparations/Vitamin B12/
    Vitamin C/Vitamins with Iron
Fexofenadine Hydrochloride
Fexofenadine Hydrochloride/
    Pseudoephedrine Hydrochloride
Filgrastim
Flecainide Acetate
Fluconazole
Flucytosine
Fludrocortisone Acetate
Flumazenil
Flunisolide
Fluocinolone Acetonide
Fluocinolone Acetonide/
    Hydroquinone/Tretinoin
Fluocinonide
Fluoromethalone
Fluorometholone/Sulfacetamide
    Sodium
Fluoxetine Hydrochloride
Fluoxetine Hydrochloride/Olanzapine
Flurandrenolide
Flurbiprofen Sodium
Fluticasone Propionate
Fluticasone Propionate Hfa

Fluticasone Propionate/Salmeterol
    Xinafoate
Fomivirsen Sodium
Formoterol Fumarate
Fosamprenavir Calcium
Foscarnet Sodium*
Fosinopril Sodium*
Fosinopril Sodium/
    Hydrochlorothiazide*
Frovatriptan Succinate
Furosamide
Gabapentin
Gallium Nitrate
Ganciclovir
Ganciclovir Sodium
Gatifloxacin
Gemfibrozil
Gemifloxacin Mesylate
Gentamicin Sulfate
Gentamicin Sulfate/Prednisolone
    Acetate
Glimepiride
Glipzide
Glipizide/Metformin Hydrochloride
Globulin, Immune (Human)
Globulin, Immune (Human)/Rho (D)
    Immune Globulin (Human)
Glyburid
Gramicidin/Neomycin Sulfate/
    Polymyxin B Sulfate
Guaifenesin/Hydrocodone Bitartrate
Haemophilus B Conjugate Vaccine
Haemophilus B Conjugate Vaccine/
    Hepatitis B Vaccine, Recombinant
Halobetasol Propionate
Haloperidol Decanoate
Hemin
Heparin Sodium
Hepatitis A Vaccine, Inactivated
Hepatitis A Vaccine, Inactivated/
    Hepatitis B Vaccine, Recombinant
Hepatitis B Immune Globulin (Human)
Hepatitis B Vaccine, Recombinant
Homatropine Methylbromide/
    Hydrocodone Bitartrate
Homeopathic Formulations
Hydralazine Hydrochloride/
    Isosorbide Dinitrate
Hydrochlorothiazide
Hydrocodone Bitartrate
Hydrocodone Bitartrate/
    Acetaminophen

(Continued on next page)

*Category C or D depending on the trimester the drug is given.

Hydrocodone Bitartrate/Ibuprofen
Hydrocortisone
Hydrocortisone Acetate
Hydrocortisone Acetate/
    Neomycin Sulfate/Polymyxin B
    Sulfate
Hydrocortisone Acetate/Pramoxine
    Hydrochloride
Hydrocortisone Butyrate
Hydrocortisone Probutate
Hydrocortisone/Neomycin Sulfate/
    Polymyxin B Sulfate
Hydromorphone Hydrochloride
Hydroquinone
Hyoscyamine Sulfate
Ibandronate Sodium
Ibutilide Fumarate
Iloprost
Imiglucerase
Imipenem/Cilastatin
Imiquimod
Immune Globulin Intravenous
    (Human)
Indinavir Sulfate
Indocyanine Green
Influenza Virus Vaccine
Insulin Aspart
Insulin Aspart Protamine, Human/
    Insulin Aspart, Human
Insulin Glargine
Insulin Glulisine
Interferon Alfa-2A, Recombinant
Interferon Alfa-2B, Recombinant
Interferon Alfacon-1
Interferon Alfa-N3 (Human
    Leukocyte Derived)
Interferon Beta-1A
Interferon Beta-1B
Interferon Gamma-1B
Iodoquinol/Hydrocortisone
Irbesartan*
Irbesarran/Hydrochlorothiazide*
Iron Dextran
Isoniazid/Pyrazinamide/Rifampin
Isosorbide Mononitrate
Isradipine
Itraconazole
Ivermectin
Ketoconazole
Ketorolac Tromethamine
Ketotifen Fumarate
Labetalol Hydrochloride
Lamivudine

Lamivudin/Zidovudine
Lamotrigine
Lanthanum Carbonate
Latanoprost
Levalbuterol Hydrochloride
Levalbuterol Tartrate
Levamisole Hydrochloride
Levetiracetam
Levobunolol Hydrochloride
Levofloxacin
Linezolid
Lisinopril*
Lisinopril/Hydrochlorothiazide*
Lopinavir Ritonavir
Losartan Potassium*
Losartan Potassium/
    Hydrochlorothiazide*
Loteprednol Etabonate
Mafenide Acetate
Magnesium Salicylate Tetrahydrate
Measles Virus Vaccine, Live
Measles, Mumps & Rubella Virus
    Vaccine, Live
Mebendazole
Mecamylamine Hydrochloride
Mecasermin |Rdna Origin|
Medrysone
Mefenamic Acid
Mefloquine Hydrochloride
Meloxicam
Meningoccal Polysaccharide
    Diphtheria Toxoid Conjugate
    Vaccine
Meningoccal Polysaccharide Vaccine
Meperidine Hydrochloride
Mepivacaine Hydrochloride
Metaproterenol Sulfate
Mitaraminol Bitartate
Metformin Hydrochloride/
    Pioglitazone Hydrochloride
Metformin Hydrochloride/
    Rosiglitazone Maleate
Methamphetamine Hydrochloride
Methazolamide
Methenamine Mandelate/Sodium
    Acid Phosphate
Methocarbamol
Methoxsafen
Methscopolamine Nitrate/
    Pseudoephedrine Hydrochloride
Methyldopa/Chlorothiazide
Methyldopa/Hydrochlorothiazide
Methylphenidate Hydrochloride

Metipranolol
Metoprolol Succinate
Metoprolol Tartrate
Metoprolol Tartrate/
    Hydrochlorolhiazide
Metyrosine
Mexiletine Hydrochloride
Micafungin Sodium
Midodrine Hydrochloride
Mivacurium Chloride
Modafinil
Moexipril Hydrochloride*
Moexipril Hydrochloride/
    Hydrochlorothiazide*
Mometasone Furoate
Mometasone Furoate Monohydrate
Morphine Sulfate
Morphine Sulfate, Liposomal
Moxifloxacin Hydrochloride
Mumps Virus Vaccine, Live
Muromonab-Cd3
Mycophenolate Mofetil
Mycophenolate Mofetil Hydrochloride
Mycophenolic Acid
Nabumetone
Nadolol
Nadolol/Bendroflumethiazide
Naloxone Hydrochloride/Pentazocine
    Hydrochloride
Naltrexone Hydrochloride
Naphazoline Hydrochloride
Naproxen
Naproxen Sodium
Naratriptan Hydrochloride
Natamycin
Nateglinide
Nefazodone Hydrochloride
Neomycin Sulfate/Dexamethasone
    Sodium Phosphate
Neomycin Sulfate/Polymyxin B
    Sulfate/Prednisolone Acetate
Nesiritide
Nevirapine
Niacin
Nicardipine Hydrochloride
Nifedipine
Nilutamide
Nimodipine
Nisoldipine
Nitroglycerin
Norfloxacin
Ofloxacin
Olanzapine

*Category C or D depending on the trimester the drug is given.

Olmesartan Medoxomil/
    Hydrochlorothiazide
Olopatadine Hydrochloride
Olsalazine Sodium
Omega-3-Acid Ethyl Esters
Omeprazole
Oprelvekin
Orphenadrine Citrate
Oseltamivir Phosphate
Oxcarbazepine
Oxycodone Hydrochloride/
    Acetaminophen
Oxycodone Hydrochloride/Ibuprofen
Oxymorphone Hydrochloride
Palifermin
Palivizumab
Pancrelipase
Paricalcitol
Paroxetine Hydrochloride
Paroxetine Mesylate
Peg-3350/Potassium Chloride/
    Sodium Bicarbonate/Sodium
    Chloride
Pegademase Bovine
Pegaspargase
Pegfilgrastim
Peginterferon Alfa-2A
Peginterferon Alfa-2B
Pemirolast Potassium
Pentazocine Hydrochloride/
    Acetaminophen
Pentoxifylline
Perindopril Erbumine*
Phenoxybenzamine Hydrochloride
Phentermine Hydrochloride
Pilocarpine Hydrochloride
Pimercrolimus
Pimozide
Pioglitazone Hydrochloride
Pirbuterol Acetate
Piroxicam
Plasma Fractions, Human/Rabies
    Immune Globulin (Human)
Plasma Protein Fraction (Human)
Pneumococcal Vaccine, Diphtheria
    Conjugate
Pneumococcal Vaccine, Polyvalent
Podofilox
Polyethylene Glycol
Polyethylene Glycol/Potassium
    Chloride/Sodium Bicarbonate/
    Sodium Chloride

Polyethylene Glycol/Potassium
    Chloride/Sodium Bicarbonate/
    Sodium Chloride/Sodium Sulfate
Polymyxin B Sulfate/Trimethoprim
    Sulfate
Polythiazide/Prazosin Hydrochloride
Porfimer Sodium
Potassium Acid Phosphate
Potassium Chloride
Potassium Citrate
Potassium Phosphate/Sodium
    Phosphate
Pralidoxime Chloride
Pramipexole Dihydrochloride
Pramlintide Acetate
Pramoxine Hydrochloride/Hydrocor-
    tisone Acetate
Prazosin Hydrochloride
Prednisolone Acetate
Prednisolone Acetate/Sulfaceramide
    Sodium
Prednisolone Sodium Phosphate
Pregabalin
Proclainamide Hydrochloride
Promethazine Hydrochloride
Propafenone Hydrochloride
Proparacaine Hydrochloride
Propranolol Hydrochloride
Pseudoephedrine Hydrochloride
Pyrimethamine
Quetiapine Fumarate
Quinapril Hydrochloride*
Quinidine Sulfate
Rabies Vaccine
Ramelteon
Ramipril*
Rasburicase
Remifentanil Hydrochloride
Repaglinide
Reteplase
Rho (D) Immune Globulin (Human)
Rifampin
Rifapentine
Rifamixin
Riluzole
Rimantadine Hydrochloride
Risedronate Sodium
Risedronate Sodium/Calcium
    Carbonate
Risperidone
Rituximab
Rizatriptan Benzoate

Rocuronium Bromide
Rofecoxib
Ropinirole Hydrochloride
Rosiglitazone Maleate
Rubella Virus Vaccine, Live
Salmeterol Xinafoate
Sargamostim
Scopolamine
Selegiline Hydrochloride
Sertaconazole Nitrate
Sertraline Hydrochloride
Sevelamer Hydrochloride
Sibutramine Hydrochloride
    Monohydrate
Sirolimus
Sodium Benzoate/Sodium
    Phenylacelate
Sodium Phenylbutyrate
Sodium Sulfacetamide/Sulfur
Solifenacin Succinate
Somatropin
Somatropin (rDNA Origin)
Stavudine
Streptokinase
Succimer
Sulfacetamide Sodium
Sulfamethoxazole/Trimethoprim
Sulfanilamide
Sumatriptan
Sumatriptan Succinate
Tacrine Hydrochloride
Tacrolimus
Telithromycin
Telmisartan*
Telmisartan/Hydrochlorothiazide*
Tenecteplase
Terazosin Hydrochloride
Teriparatide
Tetanus & Diphtheria Toxoids
    Adsorbed
Tetanus Immune Globulin (Human)
Theophylline
Theophylline Anhydrous
Thiabendazole
Thrombin
Thyrotropin Alfa
Tiagabine Hydrochloride
Tiludronate Disodium
Timolol Hemihydrate
Timolol Maleate
Timolol Maleate/
    Hydrochlorothiazide

(Continued on next page)

---

*Category C or D depending on the trimester the drug is given.

Tinidazole
Tiotropium Bromide
Tipranavir
Tizanidine Hydrochloride
Tobramycin/Dexamethasone
Tobramycin/Loteprednol Etabonate
Tolcapone
Tolterodine Tartrate
Topiramate
Tramadol Hydrochloride
Tramadol Hydrochloride/
    Acetaminophen
Trandolapril*
Trandolapril/Verapamil
    Hydrochloride*
Travoprost
Tretinoin
Triamcinolone Acetonide
Triamterene
Triamterene/Hydrochlorothiazide
Trientine Hydrochloride
Triethanolamine Polypeptide
    Oleate-Condensate
Trifluridine
Trimethoprim Hydrochloride
Trimipramine Maleate
Tropicamide/Hydroxyamphetamine
    Hydrobromide
Trospium Chloride
Trovafloxacin Mesylate
Tuberculin Purified Protein
    Derivative, Diluted
Typhoid Vaccine Live Oral Ty21A
Unoprostone Isopropyl
Urea
Valdecoxib
Valganciclovir Hydrochloride
Valsartan*
Valsartan/Hydrochlorothiazide*
Varicella Virus Vaccine, Live
Venlafaxine Hydrochloride
Verapamil Hydrochloride
Verteporfin
Vitamin K$_1$
Yellow Fever Vaccine
Zalcitabine
Zaleplon
Zanamivir
Zidovudine
Zileuton
Ziprasidone Mesylate
Zolmitriptan
Zonisamide

B

NO EVIDENCE OF RISK IN HUMANS

Either animal findings show risk while human findings do not, or, if no adequate human studies have been done, animal findings are negative.

Acarbose
Acrivastine
Acyclovir
Acyclovir Sodium
Adalimumab
Agalsidase Beta
Alefacept
Alfuzosin Hydrochloride
Alosetron Hydrochloride
Amiloride Hydrochloride
Amiloride Hydrochloride/
    Hydrochlorothiazide
Amoxicillin
Amoxicillin/Clavulanate Potassium
Amphotericin B
Amphotericin B Lipid Complex
Amphotericin B Liposomal
Amphotericin B/Cholesteryl Sulfate
    Complex
Ampicillin Sodium/Sulbactam
    Sodium
Anakinra
Antithrombin III
Aprepitant
Aprotinin
Argatroban
Arginine Hydrochloride
Atazanavir Sulfate
Azalaic Acid
Azithromycin
Azithromycin Dihydrate
Aztreonam
Balsalazide Disodium
Basiliximab
Bivalirudin
Brimonidine Tartrate
Budesonide
Bupropion Hydrochloride
Cabergoline
Carbenicillin Indanyl Sodium
Cefaclor
Cefazolin Sodium
Cefdinir
Cefditoren Pivoxil

Cefepime Hydrochloride
Cefixime
Cefoperazone Sodium
Cefotaxime Sodium
Cefotetan Disodium
Cefoxitin Sodium
Cefpodoxime Proxetil
Cefprozil
Ceftazidime Sodium
Ceftibuten Dihydrate
Ceftizoxime Sodium
Ceftriaxone Sodium
Cefuroxime
Cefuroxime Axetil
Cephalexin
Cetirizine Hydrochloride
Ciclopirox
Ciclopirox Olamine
Cimetidine
Cimetidine Hydrochloride
Cisatracurium Besylate
Clindamycin Hydrochloride/
    Clindamycin Phosphate
Clindamycin Palmitate Hydrochloride
Clindamycin Phosphate
Clopidogrel Bisulfate
Clotrimazole
Clozapine
Colesevelam Hydrochloride
Cromolyn Sodium
Cyclobenzaprine Hydrochloride
Cyproheptadine Hydrochloride
Dalfopristin/Quinupristin
Dalteparin Sodium
Dapiprazole Hydrochloride
Daptomycin
Desflurane
Desmopressin Acetate
Dicyclomine Hydrochloride
Didanosine
Diphenhydramine Hydrochloride
Dipivefrin Hydrochloride
Dipyridamole
Dolasetron Mesylate
Dornase Alfa
Doxapram Hydrochloride
Doxepin Hydrochloride
Doxercalciferol
Edetate Calcium Disodium
Emtricitabine
Emtricitabine/Tenofovir Disoproxil
    Fumarate
Enfuvirtide

---

*Category C or D depending on the trimester the drug is given.

Enoxaparin Sodium
Eplerenone
Epoprostenol Sodium
Ertapenem
Erythromycin
Erythromycin Ethylsuccinate
Erythromycin Stearate
Esomeprazole Magnesium
Esomeprazole Sodium
Etanercept
Ethacrynate Sodium
Ethacrynic Acid
Famciclovir
Famotidine
Fanoldopam Mesylate
Fondaparinux Sodium
Galantamine Hydrobromide
Glatiramer Acetate
Glucagon
Glyburide/Metformin Hydrochloride
Granisetron Hydrochloride
Hydrochlorothiazide
Ibuprofen
Indapamide
Infliximab
Insulin Lispro Protamine, Human/
    Insulin Lispro, Human
Insulin Lispro, Human
Ipratropium Bromide
Iron Sucrose
Isosorbide Mononitrate
Lactulose
Lansoprazole
Lansoprazole/Naproxen
Laronidase
Lepirudin
Levocarnitine
Lidocaine
Lidocaine Hydrochloride
Lidocaine/Prilocaine
Lindane
Loperamide Hydrochloride
Loracarbef
Loratadine
Malathion
Meclizine Hydrochloride
Memantine Hydrochloride
Meropenem
Mesalamine
Metformin Hydrochloride

Methohexital Sodium
Methyldopa
Metolazone
Metronidazole
Miglitol
Montelukast Sodium
Mupirocin
Mupirocin Calcium
Naftifine Hydrochloride
Nalbuphine Hydrochloride
Nalmefene Hydrochloride
Naloxone Hydrochloride
Naproxen Sodium
Nedocromil Sodium
Nelfinavir Mesylate
Nitazoxanide
Nitrofurantoin Macrocrystals
Nitrofurantoin Macrocrystals/
    Nitrofurantoin Monohydrate
Nizatidine
Ocreotide Acelate
Omalizumab
Ondansetron
Ondansetron Hydrochloride
Orlistat
Oxiconazole Nitrate
Oxybutynin
Oxybutynin Chloride
Oxycodone Hydrochloride
Palonosetron Hydrochloride
Pancrelipase
Pantoprazole Sodium
Pegvisomant
Pemoline
Penciclovir
Penicillin G Benzathine
Penicillin G Benzathine/Penicillin G
    Procaine
Penicillin G Potassium
Pentosan Polysulfate Sodium
Pergolide Mesylate
Permethrin
Piperacillin Sodium
Piperacillin Sodium/Tazobactam
    Sodium
Praziquantel
Progesterone
Propofol
Pseudoephedrine Hydrochloride
Pseudoephadrine Sulfate

Psyllium Preparations
Rabeprazole Sodium
Ranitidine Hydrochloride
Rifabutin
Ritonavir
Rivastigmine Tartrate
Ropivacaine Hydrochloride
Saquinavir
Saquinavir Mesylate
Sevoflurane
Sildenafil Citrate
Silver Sulfadiazine
Sodium Ferric Gluconate
Somatropin
Sotalol Hydrochloride
Sucralfate
Sulfasalazine
Tadalafil
Tamsulosin Hydrochloride
Tegaserod Maleate
Tenofovir Disoproxil Fumarate
Terbinafine Hydrochloride
Ticarcillin Disodium/Clavulanate
    Potassium
Ticlopidine Hydrochloride
Tirofiban Hydrochloride
Torsemide
Trastuzumab
Treprostinil Sodium
Urokinase
Ursodiol
Valacyclovir Hydrochloride
Vancomycin Hydrochloride
Vardenafil Hydrochloride
Zafirlukast
Zolpidem Tartrate

A

CONTROLLED STUDIES SHOW NO RISK

Adequate, well-controlled studies in pregnant women have failed to demonstrate risk to the fetus.

Levothyroxine Sodium
Liothyronine Sodium
Liotrix
Nystatin

DRUGS EXCRETED IN BREAST MILK

The following list is not comprehensive; generic forms and alternate brands of some products may be available. When recommending drugs to pregnant or nursing patients, always check product labeling for specific precautions.

Accolate
Accuretic
Aciphex
Actiq
Activella
Actonel with Calcium
ActoPlus Met
Actos
Adalat
Adderall
Advicor
Aggrenox
Aldactazide
Aldactone
Aldomet
Aldoril
Alesse
Allegra-D
Alfenta
Aloprim
Altace
Ambien
Anaprox
Ancef
Androderm
Antara
Apresoline
Aralen
Arthrotec
Asacol
Ativan
Augmentin
Avalide
Avandia
Avetox
Axid
Axocet
Azactam
Azasari
Azathloprine
Azulfidine
Bactrim
Baraclude
Benadryl
Bentyl
Betapace
Bextra
Bexxar
Bicllin
Biocadren
Boniva
Brethine

Brevicone
Brontex
Byetta
Caduet
Cafergot
Calan
Campral
Capoten
Capozide
Captopril
Carbatrol
Cardizem
Cataflam
Catapres
Ceclor
Cefizox
Cefobid
Cefotan
Ceftin
Celebrex
Celexa
Ceptaz
Cerebyx
Ceredase
Cipro
Ciprodex
Claforan
Clarinex
Claritin
Claritin-D
Cleocin
Climara
Clozaril
Codeine
CombiPatch
Combipres
Combivir
Combunox
Compazine
Cordarone
Corgard
Cortisporin
Corzide
Cosopt
Coumadin
Covera-HS
Cozaar
Crestor
Crinone
Cyclessa
Cymbalta
Cystospaz

Cytomel
Cytotec
Cytoxan
Dapsone
Daraprim
Darvon
Darvon-N
Decadron
Deconsal II
Demerol
Demulen
Depacon
Depakene
Depakote
DepoDur
Depo-Provera
Desogen
Desoxyn
Desyrel
Dexedrine
DextroStat
D.H.E.45
Diabinese
Diastat
Diflucan
Digitek
Dilacor
Dilantin
Dilaudid
Diovan
Diprivan
Diuril
Dolobid
Dolophine
Doral
Doryx
Droxia
Duracion
Duragesic
Duramorph
Duratuss
Duricef
Dyazide
Dyrenium
E.E.S.
EC-Naprosyn
Ecotrin
Effexor
Elestat
EMLA
Enduron
Epzicom

Equetro
ERYC
EryPed
Ery-Tab
Erythrocin
Erythromycin
Esgic-plus
Eskalith
Estrogel
Estrostep
Ethmozine
Evista
FazaClo
Felbatol
Feldene
Femhrt
Florinal
Flagyl
Florinef
Floxin
Foradil
Fortamet
Fortaz
Fosamax Plus D
Furosemide
Gabitril
Galzin
Garamycin
Glucophage
Glyset
Guaifed
Halcion
Haldol
Helidac
Hydrocet
Hydrocortone
HydroDIURIL
Iberet-Folic
Ifex
Imitrex
Imuran
Inderal
Ideride
Indocin
INFed
Inspra
Invanz
Inversine
Isoptin
Kadlan
Keflex
Keppra
Kerlone
Ketek
Klonopin
Kronofed-A
Kutrase

Lamictal
Lamisil
Lamprene
Lanoxicaps
Lanoxin
Lariam
Lescol
Levbid
Levitra
Levlen
Levlite
Levora
Levothroid
Levoxyl
Levsin
Levsinex
Lexapro
Lexiva
Lexxel
Lindane
Lioresal
Lipitor
Lithium
Lithobid
Lo/Ovral
Loestrin
Lomotil
Loniten
Lopressor
Lortab
Lostensin
Lotrel
Luminal
Luvox
Lyrica
Macrobid
Macrodantin
Marinol
Maxipime
Maxzide
Mefoxin
Menostar
Methergine
Methotrexate
MetroCream/
Gel/Lotion
Mexitil
Micronor
Microzide
Midamor
Migranal
Miltown
Minizide
Minocin
Mirapex
Mircette
M-M-R II

Mobic
Modicon
Moduretic
Monodox
Monopril
Morphine
MS Contin
MSIR
Myambutol
Mycamine
Mysoline
Namenda
Naprelan
Naprosyn
Nascobal
Necon
NegGram
Nembutal
Neoral
Niaspan
Nicotrol
Niravam
Nizoral
Norco
Nor-QD
Nordette
Norinyl
Noritate
Normodyne
Norpace
Norplant
Novantrone
Nubain
Nucofed
Nydrazid
Oramorph
Oretic
Ortho-Cept
Ortho-Cyclen
Ortho-Novum
Ortho Tri-Cyclen
Orudis
Ovcon
Oxistat
OxyContin
OxyFast
OxyIR
Pacerone
Pamelor
Pancrease
Paxil
PCE
Pediapred
Pediazole
Pediotic
Pentasa
Pepcid

(Continued on next page)

Periostat
Persantine
Pfizerpen
Phenergan
Phenobarbital
Phrenilin
Pipracil
Plan B
Ponstel
Pravachol
Premphase
Prempro
Prevacid
Prevacid NapraPAC
PREVPAC
Prinzide
Procanbid
Prograf
Proloprim
Prometrium
Pronestyl
Propofol
Prosed/DS
Protonix
Provera
Prozac
Pseudoephedrine
Pulmicort
Pyrazinamide
Quinidex
Quinine
Raptiva
Reglan
Relpax
Renese
Requip
Reserpine
Restoril
Retrovir
Rifadin
Rifamate
Rifater
Rimactane
Risperdal
Rocaltrol
Rocephin
Roferon A
Roxanol
Rozerem
Sanctura
Sandimmune
Sarafem
Seconal
Sectral
Semprex-D

Septra
Seroquel
Sinequan
Slo-bid
Soma
Sonata
Spiriva
Sporanox
Stadol
Streptomycin
Stromectol
Symbyax
Symmetrel
Synthroid
Tagamet
Tambocor
Tapazole
Tarka
Tavist
Tazicef
Tazidime
Tegretol
Tenoretic
Tenormin
Tenuate
Tequin
Testoderm
Thalitone
Theo-24
The-Dur
Thorazine
Tiazac
Timolide
Timoptic
Tindamax
Tobi
Tofranil
Tolectin
Toprol-XL
Toradol
Trandate
Tranxene
Trental
Tricor
Triglide
Trilafon
Trileptal
Tri-Levlen
Trilisate
Tri-Norinyl
Triostat
Triphasil
Trivora
Trizivir
Trovan

Truvada
Tygacil
Tylenol
Tylenol with Codeine
Ultane
Ultram
Unasyn
Uniphyl
Uniretic
Unithroid
Urimax
Valium
Valtrex
Vanceril
Vancocin
Vantin
Vascor
Vaseretic
Vasotec
Ventavis
Verelan
Vermox
Versed
Vibramycin
Vibra-Tabs
Vicodin
Vigamox
Viramune
Voltaren
Vytorin
Wellbutrin
Xanax
Xolair
Zantac
Zarontin
Zaroxolyn
Zegerid
Zemplar
Zestoretic
Zetia
Ziac
Zinacef
Zithromax
Zocor
Zomig
Zonalon
Zonegran
Zosyn
Zovia
Zovirax
Zyban
Zydone
Zyloprim
Zyprexa
Zyrtec

LOW POTASSIUM DIET
Lexi-Drugs Online

Potassium is a mineral found in most all foods except sugar and lard. It plays a role in maintaining normal muscle activity and helps to keep body fluids in balance. Too much potassium in the blood can lead to changes in heartbeat and can lead to muscle weakness. The kidneys normally help to keep blood potassium controlled, but in kidney disease or when certain drugs are taken, dietary potassium must be limited to maintain a normal level of potassium in the blood. The following guideline includes 2–3 g of potassium per day.

Milk Group: Limit to one cup serving of milk or milk product (yogurt, cottage cheese, ice cream, pudding).

Fruit Group: Limit to two servings daily from the low potassium choices. Watch serving sizes. Avoid the high potassium choices.

Low Potassium

Apple, 1 small
Apple juice, applesauce ½ cup
Apricot, 1 medium or ½ cup canned in syrup
Blueberries, ½ cup
Cherries, canned in syrup ⅓ cup
Cranberries, cranberry juice ½ cup
Fruit cocktail, canned in syrup ½ cup
Grapes, 10 fresh
Lemon, lime 1 fresh
Mandarin orange, canned in syrup ½ cup

Nectar: apricot, pear, peach ½ cup
Peach, 1 small or ½ cup canned with syrup
Pear, 1 small or ½ cup canned with syrup
Pineapple, ½ cup raw or canned with syrup
Plums, 1 small or ½ cup canned with syrup
Tangerine, 1 small
Watermelon, ½ cup

High Potassium

Avocado
Banana
Cantaloupe
Cherries, fresh
Dried fruits
Grapefruit, fresh and juice
Honeydew melon
Kiwi
Mango
Nectarine
Orange, fresh and juice
Papaya
Prunes, prune juice
Raisins

Avoid use of the following salt substitutes due to their high potassium contents: Adolph's, Lawry's Season Salt Substitute, No Salt, Morton Season Salt Free, Nu Salt, Papa Dash, and Morton Lite Salt.

TYRAMINE CONTENT OF FOODS

Food[1]	Allowed	Minimize Intake	Not Allowed
Beverages	Decaffeinated beverages (eg, coffee, tea, soda); milk, soy milk, chocolate beverage	Caffeine-containing drinks, clear spirits, wine, bottled/canned beers	**Tap** beer
Breads/cereals	All except those containing cheese	None	Cheese bread and crackers
Dairy products	Cottage cheese, farmers or pot cheese, cream cheese, ricotta cheese, all milk, eggs, ice cream, pudding, yogurt, sour cream, processed cheese, mozzarella	None	All other cheeses (**aged** cheese, American, Camembert, cheddar, Gouda, gruyere, parmesan, provolone, romano, Roquefort, stilton)
Meat, fish, and poultry	All fresh packaged or processed (eg, hot dogs, bologna), or frozen	Pepperoni	**Aged** chicken and beef liver, dried and pickled fish, shrimp paste, summer or dry sausage, dried meats (eg, salami, cacciatore), meat extracts, liverwurst
Starches— potatoes/rice	All	None	Soybean (including paste), tofu

(Continued on next page)

Food[1]	Allowed	Minimize Intake	Not Allowed
Vegetables	All fresh, frozen, canned, or dried vegetable juices except those not allowed	Chili peppers, Chinese pea pods	Sauerkraut, broad or fava bean pods (not beans)
Fruit	Fresh, frozen, or canned fruits and fruit juices	Avocado, figs	Banana peel, avocado (over-ripened)
Soups	All soups not listed to limit or avoid	None	Soups which contain **aged** cheese, **tap** beer, any made with flavor cubes or meat extract, miso soup, broad or fava bean pods (not beans)
Fats	All except fermented	None	None
Sweets	Sugar, hard candy, honey, molasses, syrups, chocolate candy	None	None
Desserts	Cakes, cookies, gelatin, pastries, sherbets, sorbets, chocolate desserts	None	None
Miscellaneous	Salt, nuts, spices, herbs, flavorings, Worcestershire sauce, Brewer's or Baker's yeast, monosodium glutamate, vitamins with Brewer's yeast	Peanuts	Soy sauce, all aged and fermented products, marmite and other concentrated yeast extracts

[1]Freshness is of primary importance. Food that is spoiled or improperly stored should be avoided. *Copyright © 1978-2008 Lexi-Comp Inc. All Rights Reserved.*

REFERENCES

Shulman KI and Walker SE, "A Reevaluation of Dietary Restrictions for Irreversible Monoamine Oxidase Inhibitors" *Psychiatr Ann*, 2001, 31(6):378–84.

Shulman KI and Walker SE, "Refining the MAOI Diet: Tyramine Content of Pizza and Soy Products," *J Clin Psychiatry*, 1999, 60(3):191–3.

Walker SE, Shulman KI, Tailor SAN, et al., "Tyramine Content of Previously Restricted Foods in Monoamine Oxidase Inhibitor Diets," *J Clin Psychopharmacol*, 1996, 16(5):383–8.

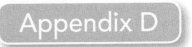

National and State Boards of Pharmacy Contact Information

This appendix contains the most recent contact information for the national and state boards of pharmacy. A current listing of contact information for state boards of pharmacy is maintained at the National Association of Boards of Pharmacy Web site, http://www.nabp.com. In addition, contact information for all the pharmacy schools in the United States can be found at the American Association of Colleges of Pharmacy Web site, http://www.aacp.org.

National Association of Boards of Pharmacy
Carmen A. Catizone
Executive Director
1600 Feehanville Drive
Mount Prospect, IL 60056
Phone: 847/391-4406
Fax: 847/391-4502
Web site: http://www.nabp.net

State Boards of Pharmacy Alabama State Board of Pharmacy
Louise Foster Jones
Executive Secretary
10 Inverness Center, Suite 110
Birmingham, AL 35242
Phone: 205/981-2280
Fax: 205/981-2330
Web site: http://www.albop.com
E-mail: ljones@albop.com

Alaska Board of Pharmacy
Sher Zinn
Licensing Examiner
PO Box 110806
Juneau, AK 99811-0806
Phone: 907/465-2589
Fax: 907/465-2974
Web site: http://www.commerce.state.ak.us/occ/ppha.htm
E-mail: sher_zinn@commerce.state.ak.us
(through the Division of Occupational Licensing)

Arizona State Board of Pharmacy
Harlan Wand
Executive Director
4425 West Olive Avenue, Suite 140
Glendale, AZ 85302-3844
Phone: 623/463-2727
Fax: 623/934-0583
Web site: http://www.pharmacy.state.az.us
E-mail: hwand@azsbp.com

Arkansas State Board of Pharmacy
Charles S. Campbell
Executive Director
101 East Capitol, Suite 218
Little Rock, AR 72201
Phone: 501/682-0190
Fax: 501/682-0195
Web site: http://www.arkansas.gov/asbp
E-mail: charlie.campbell@arkansas.gov

California State Board of Pharmacy
Patricia F. Harris
Executive Officer
1625 North Market Boulevard, N219
Sacramento, CA 95834
Phone: 916/574-7900
Fax: 916/574-8618
Web site: http://www.pharmacy.ca.gov
E-mail: patricia_harris@dca.ca.gov

Colorado State Board of Pharmacy
Susan L. Warren
Program Director
1560 Broadway, Suite 1310
Denver, CO 80202-5143
Phone: 303/894-7800
Fax: 303/894-7764
Web site: http://www.dora.state.co.us/pharmacy
E-mail: susan.warren@dora.state.co.us

Connecticut Commission of Pharmacy
Michelle Sylvestre
Drug Control Agent and Board Administrator
State Office Building, 165 Capitol Avenue, Room 147
Hartford, CT 06106
Phone: 860/713-6070
Fax: 860/713-7242
Web site: http://www.ct.gov/dcp/site/default.asp
E-mail: michelle.sylvestre@ct.gov

Delaware State Board of Pharmacy
David W. Dryden
Executive Secretary
Division of Professional Regulation
Cannon Building
861 Silver Lake Boulevard, Suite 203
Dover, DE 19904
Phone: 302/744-4526
Fax: 302/739-2711
Web site: http://www.dpr.delaware.gov
E-mail: debop@state.de.us

District of Columbia Board of Pharmacy
Bonnie Rampersaud
Executive Director
717 Fourteenth Street NW, Suite 600
Washington, DC 20005
Phone: 202/724-4900
Fax: 202/727-8471
Web site: http://www.dchealth.dc.gov
E-mail: graphelia.ramseur@dc.gov

Florida Board of Pharmacy
Rebecca Poston
Executive Director
4052 Bald Cypress Way, Bin #C04
Tallahassee, FL 32399-3254
Phone: 850/245-4292
Fax: 850/413-6982
Web site: http://www.doh.state.fl.us/mga
E-mail: rebecca_poston@doh.state.fl.us

Georgia State Board of Pharmacy
Sylvia L. "Sandy" Bond
Executive Director
Professional Licensing Boards
237 Coliseum Drive
Macon, GA 31217-3858
Phone: 478/207-1640
Fax: 478/207-1660
Web site: http://www.sos.state.ga.us/plb/pharmacy
E-mail: sibond@sos.state.ga.us

Guam Board of Examiners for Pharmacy
Jane M. Diego
Secretary for the Board
PO Box 2816
Hagatna, GU 96932
Phone: 671/735-7406 ext 11
Fax: 671/735-7413
E-mail: jmdiego@dphss.govguam.net

Hawaii State Board of Pharmacy
Lee Ann Teshima
Executive Officer
PO Box 3469
Honolulu, HI 96801
Phone: 808/586-2694
Fax: 808/586-2874
Web site: http://www.hawaii.gov/dcca/areas/pvl/boards/
    pharmacy
E-mail: pharmacy@dcca.hawaii.gov

Idaho Board of Pharmacy
Richard Markuson
Executive Director
3380 Americana Terrace, Suite 320
Boise, ID 83706
Phone: 208/334-2356
Fax: 208/334-3536
Web site: http://www.accessidaho.org/bop
Email: rmarkuson@bop.state.id.us

Illinois Department of Financial and Professional
    Regulation, Division of Professional Regulation-State
    Board of Pharmacy
Kim Scott
Pharmacy Board Liaison
320 West Washington, 3rd Floor
Springfield, IL 62786
Phone: 217/782-8556
Fax: 217/782-7645
Web site: http://www.idfpr.com
E-mail: PRFGROUP10@idfpr.com (through Department of
    Professional Regulation)

Indiana Board of Pharmacy
Marty Allain
Director
402 West Washington Street, Room W072
Indianapolis, IN 46204-2739
Phone: 317/234-2067
Fax: 317/233-4236
Web site: http://www.in.gov/pla/bandc/isbp
E-mail: pla4@pla.IN.gov

Iowa Board of Pharmacy Examiners
Lloyd K. Jessen
Executive Director/Secretary
400 Southwest Eighth Street, Suite E
Des Moines, IA 50309-4688
Phone: 515/281-5944
Fax: 515/281-4609
Web site: http://www.state.ia.us/ibpe
E-mail: Lloyd.jessen@ibpe.state.ia.us

Kansas State Board of Pharmacy
Debra L. Billingsley
Executive Secretary/Director
Landon State Office Building, 900 Jackson, Room 560
Topeka, KS 66612-1231
Phone: 785/296-4056
Fax: 785/296-8420
Web site: http://www.kansas.gov/pharmacy
E-mail: pharmacy@pharmacy.state.ks.us

Kentucky Board of Pharmacy
Michael A. Burleson
Executive Director
Spindletop Administration Building, Suite 302
2624 Research Park Drive,
Lexington, KY 40511
Phone: 859/246-2820
Fax: 859/246-2823
Web site: http://pharmacy.ky.gov
E-mail: mike.burleson@ky.gov

Louisiana Board of Pharmacy
Malcolm J. Broussard
Executive Director
5615 Corporate Boulevard, Suite 8E
Baton Rouge, LA 70808-2537
Phone: 225/925-6496
Fax: 225/925-6499
Web site: http://www.labp.com
E-mail: mbroussard@labp.com

Maine Board of Pharmacy
Geraldine Betts
Board Administrator
Department of Professional/Financial Regulation
35 State House Station
Augusta, ME 04333
Phone: 207/624-8689
Fax: 207/624-8637
Hearing Impaired: 207/624-8563
PFR/OLR Web site: http://www.maineprofessionalreg.org
E-mail: for all Licensing and Board Meeting Information/
    Inquires and for Application packets:
    kelly.l.mclaughlin@maine.gov
Enforcement inquiries: gregory.w.cameron@maine.gov
Administration and all other Inquiries:
    geraldine.l.betts@maine.gov

Maryland Board of Pharmacy
La Verne George Naesea
Executive Director
4201 Patterson Avenue
Baltimore, MD 21215-2299
Phone: 410/764-4755
Fax: 410/358-6207
Web site: http://www.dhmh.state.md.us/pharmacyboard
E-mail: lnaesea@dhmh.state.md.us

Massachusetts Board of Registration in Pharmacy
Charles R. Young
Executive Director
239 Causeway Street, 2nd Floor
Boston, MA 02114
Phone: 617/973-0800
Fax: 617/973-0983
Web site: http://www.mass.gov/dpl/boards/ph/index.htm
E-mail: charles.young@state.ma.us

Michigan Board of Pharmacy
Rae Ramsdell
Director, Licensing Division
611 West Ottawa, 1st Floor
PO Box 30670
Lansing, MI 48909-8170
Phone: 517/335-0918
Fax: 517/373-2179
Web site: http://www.michigan.gov/healthlicense
Email: rhramsd@michigan.gov

Minnesota Board of Pharmacy
Cody C. Wiberg
Executive Director
2829 University Avenue SE, Suite 530
Minneapolis, MN 55414-3251
Phone: 612/617-2201
Fax: 612/617-2212
Web site: http://www.phcybrd.state.mn.us
E-mail: Cody.Wiberg@state.mn.us

Mississippi State Board of Pharmacy
Leland McDivitt
Executive Director
204 Key Drive, Suite C
Madison, MS 39110
Phone: 601/605-5388
Fax: 601/605-9546
Web site: http://www.mbp.state.ms.us
E-mail: lmcdivitt@mbp.state.ms.us

Missouri Board of Pharmacy
Kevin E. Kinkade
Executive Director
PO Box 625
Jefferson City, MO 65102
Phone: 573/751-0091
Fax: 573/526-3464
Web site: http://www.pr.mo.gov/pharmacists.asp
E-mail: kevin.kinkade@pr.mo.gov

Montana Board of Pharmacy
Ronald J. Klein
Executive Director
PO Box 200513
301 South Park Avenue, 4th Floor
Helena, MT 59620-0513
Phone: 406/841-2355
Fax: 406/841-2305
Web site: http://mt.gov/dli/bsd/license/bsd_boards/
    pha_board/board_page.asp
E-mail: dlibsdpha@state.mt.us

Nebraska Board of Pharmacy
Becky Wisell
Executive Secretary
PO Box 94986
Lincoln, NE 68509-4986
Phone: 402/471-2118
Fax: 402/471-3577
Web site: http://www.hhs.state.ne.us
E-mail: becky.wisell@hhss.ne.gov

Nevada State Board of Pharmacy
Larry L. Pinson
Executive Secretary
555 Double Eagle Circuit, Suite 1100
Reno, NV 89521
Phone: 775/850-1440
Fax: 775/850-1444
Web site: http://state.nv.us/pharmacy
E-mail: pharmacy@govmail.state.nv.us

New Hampshire Board of Pharmacy
Paul G. Boisseau
Executive Secretary
57 Regional Drive
Concord, NH 03301-8518
Phone: 603/271-2350
Fax: 603/271-2856
Web site: http://www.nh.gov/pharmacy
E-mail: pharmacy.board@nh.gov

New Jersey Board of Pharmacy
Joanne Boyer
Executive Director
124 Halsey Street
Newark, NJ 07101
Phone: 973/504-6450
Fax: 973/648-3355
Web site: http://www.state.nj.us/lps/ca/boards.htm
E-mail: boyerj@dca.lps.state.nj.us

New Mexico Board of Pharmacy
William Harvey
Executive Director/Chief Drug Inspector
5200 Oakland NE, Suite A
Albuquerque, NM 87113
Phone: 505/222-9830
Fax: 505/222-9845
Web site: http://www.state.nm.us/pharmacy
E-mail: William.Harvey@state.nm.us

New York Board of Pharmacy
Lawrence H. Mokhiber
Executive Secretary
89 Washington Avenue, 2nd Floor W
Albany, NY 12234-1000
Phone: 518/474-3817 ext. 130
Fax: 518/473-6995
Web site: http://www.op.nysed.gov
E-mail: pharmbd@mail.nysed.gov

North Carolina Board of Pharmacy
Jack W. Campbell IV
Executive Director
PO Box 4560
Chapel Hill, NC 27515-4560
Phone: 919/942-4454
Fax: 919/967-5757
Web site: http://www.ncbop.org
E-mail: jcampbell@ncbop.org

North Dakota State Board of Pharmacy
Howard C. Anderson Jr
Executive Director
PO Box 1354
Bismarck, ND 58502-1354
Phone: 701/328-9535
Fax: 701/328-9536
Web site: http://www.nodakpharmacy.com
E-mail: ndboph@btinet.net

Ohio State Board of Pharmacy
William T. Winsley
Executive Director
77 South High Street Room 1702
Columbus, OH 43215-6126
Phone: 614/466-4143
Fax: 614/752-4836
Web site: http://www.pharmacy.ohio.gov
E-mail: exec@bop.state.oh.us

Oklahoma State Board of Pharmacy
Bryan H. Potter
Executive Director
4545 Lincoln Boulevard, Suite 112
Oklahoma City, OK 73105-3488
Phone: 405/521-3815
Fax: 405/521-3758
Web site: http://www.pharmacy.ok.gov
E-mail: pharmacy@pharmacy.ok.gov

Oregon State Board of Pharmacy
Gary A. Schnabel
Executive Director
800 Northeast Oregon Street, Suite 150
Portland, OR 97232
Phone: 971/673-0001
Fax: 971/673-0002
Web site: http://www.pharmacy.state.or.us
E-mail: pharmacy.board@state.or.us

Pennsylvania State Board of Pharmacy
Melanie Zimmerman
Executive Secretary
PO Box 2649
Harrisburg, PA 17105-2649
Phone: 717/783-7156
Fax: 717/787-7769
Web site: http://www.dos.state.pa.us/pharm
E-mail: st-pharmacy@state.pa.us

Puerto Rico Board of Pharmacy
Madga Bouet
Executive Director, Department of Health, Board of Pharmacy
Call Box 10200
Santurce, PR 00908
Phone: 787/724-7282
Fax: 787/725-7903
E-mail: mbouet@salud.gov.pr

Rhode Island Board of Pharmacy
Catherine A. Cordy
Executive Director
3 Capitol Hill, Room 205
Providence, RI 02908-5097
Phone: 401/222-2837
Fax: 401/222-2158
Web site: http://www.health.ri.gov/hsr/professions/pharmacy.php
E-mail: cathyc@doh.state.ri.us

South Carolina Department of Labor, Licensing, and Regulation-Board of Pharmacy
LeeAnn Bundrick
Administrator
Kingstree Building
110 Centerview Drive, Suite 306
Columbia, SC 29210
Phone: 803/896-4700
Fax: 803/896-4596
Web site: http://www.llronline.com/POL/pharmacy
E-mail: bundrici@llr.sc.gov

South Dakota State Board of Pharmacy
Dennis M. Jones
Executive Secretary
4305 South Louise Avenue, Suite 104
Sioux Falls, SD 57106
Phone: 605/362-2737
Fax: 605/362-2738
Web site: http://www.state.sd.us/doh/pharmacy
E-mail: dennis.jones@state.sd.us

Tennessee Board of Pharmacy
Terry Webb Grinder
Interim Executive Director
Tennessee Department of Commerce and Insurance,
Board of Pharmacy
Davy Crockett Tower, 2nd Floor
500 James Robertson Pkwy
Nashville, TN 37243-1149
Phone: 615/741-2718
Fax: 615/741-2722
Web site: http://www.state.tn.us/commerce/boards/pharmacy
E-mail: terry.grinder@state.tn.us

Texas State Board of Pharmacy
Gay Dodson
Executive Director
333 Guadalupe, Tower 3, Suite 600
Austin, TX 78701-3942
Phone: 512/305-8000
Fax: 512/305-8082
Web site: http://www.tsbp.state.tx.us
E-mail: gay.dodson@tsbp.state.tx.us

Utah Board of Pharmacy
Diana L. Baker
Bureau Manager
PO Box 146741
Salt Lake City, UT 84114-6741
Phone: 801/530-6179
Fax: 801/530-6511
Web site: http://www.dopl.utah.gov
E-mail: dbaker@utah.gov (through Division of Occupational
 and Professional Licensing)

Vermont Board of Pharmacy
Peggy Atkins
Board Administrator
Office of Professional Regulation
26 Terrace Street
Montpelier, VT 05609-1106
Phone: 802/828-2373
Fax: 802/828-2465
Web site: http://www.vtprofessionals.org
E-mail: patkins@sec.state.vt.us

Virgin Islands Board of Pharmacy
Lydia T. Scott
Executive Assistant
Department of Health
Schneider Regional Center
48 Sugar Estate
St. Thomas, VI 00802
Phone: 340/774-0117
Fax: 340/777-4001
E-mail: lydia.scott@usvi-doh.org

Virginia Board of Pharmacy
Elizabeth Scott Russell
Executive Director
6603 West Broad Street, 5th Floor
Richmond, VA 23230-1712
Phone: 804/662-9911
Fax: 804/662-9313
Web site: http://www.dhp.state.va.us/pharmacy/deafault.htm
(or through Department of Health Professions at
 http://www.dhp.state.va.us)
E-mail: scotti.russell@dhp.virginia.gov

Washington State Board of Pharmacy
Steven M. Saxe
Executive Director
PO Box 47863
Olympia, WA 98504-7863
Phone: 360/236-4825
Fax: 360/586-4359
Web site: https://fortress.wa.gov/doh/hpqa1/hps4/
pharmacy/default.htm
E-mail: Steven.Saxe@doh.wa.gov

West Virginia Board of Pharmacy
William T. Douglass Jr
Executive Director and General Counsel
232 Capitol Street
Charleston, WV 25301
Phone: 304/558-0558
Fax: 304/558-0572
Web site: http://www.wvbop.com
E-mail: wdouglass@wvbop.com

Wisconsin Pharmacy Examining Board
Tom Ryan
Bureau Director
1400 East Washington
PO Box 8935
Madison, WI 53708-8935
Phone: 608/266-2112
Fax: 608/267-0644
Web site: http://www.drl.state.wi.us
E-mail: thomas.ryan@drl.state.wi.us

Wyoming State Board of Pharmacy
James T. Carder
Executive Director
632 South David Street
Casper, WY 82601
Phone: 307/234-0294
Fax: 307/234-7226
Web site: http://pharmacyboard.state.wy.us
E-mail: wybop@state.wy.us

Reprinted with permission from National Association of Boards of Pharmacy, Mount Prospect, IL.

Budgeting for Drug Information Resources

Basic Library

References	Cost[a]
American Hospital Formulary Service (AHFS) Drug Information	$ 239.00
Drug Facts and Comparisons	$ 226.95
Handbook on Injectable Drugs	$ 234.00
Handbook of Non-Prescription Drugs: An Interactive Approach to Self-Care	$ 149.95
Martindale: The Complete Drug Reference	$ 550.00
Nonprescription Product Therapeutics	$ 94.95
Physicians' Desk Reference	$ 94.95
Remington's Pharmaceutical Sciences	$ 137.00
USP DI (three-volume set)	$ 412.00

Additional Resources

References	Cost[a]
Drug–drug interaction	
Drug Interactions Analysis and Management	$ 210.00
Drug Interaction Facts	$ 235.00
Evaluations of Drug Interactions	$ 240.00
Herbal	
PDR for Herbal Medicines	$ 59.95
The Review of Natural Products	$ 169.00
Natural Medicine Comprehensive Database	$ 92.00
Natural Standard Herb and Supplement Reference	$ 133.00
Internal medicine	
Cecil Medicine	$ 219.00
Harrison's Principles of Internal Medicine	$ 137.75
Pediatrics	
Pediatric Dosage Handbook	$ 49.95
The Harriet Lane Handbook	$ 54.95
Pharmacokinetics	
Applied Biopharmaceutics and Pharmacokinetics	$ 62.95
Clinical Pharmacokinetics	$ 46.00
Concepts in Clinical Pharmacokinetics	$ 66.00
Applied Pharmacokinetics and Pharmacodynamics: Principles of Therapeutic Drug Monitoring	$ 79.95
Pharmacology	
Goodman and Gilman's The Pharmacological Basis of Therapeutics	$ 140.00
Pregnancy/breast-feeding	
Drugs in Pregnancy and Lactation	$ 99.00

(Continued on next page)

(Continued)

References	Cost[a]
Therapeutics	
Applied Therapeutics: The Clinical Use of Drugs	$ 213.00
Pharmacotherapy: A Pathophysiologic Approach	$ 206.00
Textbook of Therapeutics: Drug and Disease Management	$ 213.00
CD ROM computer systems/programs	
Clinical Pharmacology	$ 5,800.00
Lexi–Comp Online	$ 3,000.00
DataKinetics	$ 1,225.00
Facts and Comparisons 4.0 (online)	$ 2,000.00
Iowa Drug Information System	$ 9,000+
IPA	$ 3,000+
Medline	$ 20,000+
MedTeach Patient Education Program	$ 611.00
UPTODATE (stand alone)	$ 1,611.93
Micromedex	
Diseasedex	Must contact representative for price
Drugdex	Must contact representative for price
Poisindex	Must contact representative for price
Other Micromedex databases	
CareNotes	Must contact representative for price
Drug–Reax	Must contact representative for price
Kinetidex	Must contact representative for price
Martindale: The Complete Drug Reference	Must contact representative for price
PDR	Must contact representative for price
P&T Quik	Must contact representative for price
Reprorisk	Must contact representative for price

Major Online Vendors

American Chemical Society
Dialog
EBSCO
Elsevier
Gale Group
National Library of Medicine
Ovid
OCLC First Search
ProQuest
ScienceDirect
Thomson
Wolters Kluwer

[a]Costs are approximate and are based on 2007 figures. Costs vary depending upon selection of format site versus individual license fees, concurrent users, number of beds in facility, or number of students enrolled. Institutional subscriptions are more expensive than individual subscriptions. It is important to have the appropriate site license.

Common Systems of Measurement and Intersystem Conversion

The International System of Units (SI) is the official system for weights and measures as stated in the *United States Pharmacopeia—National Formulary*.[1] However, other so-called *common systems of measurement* are encountered in pharmacy and must be recognized and understood. The *apothecaries' system of measurement* is the traditional system of pharmacy, and although it is now largely of historic significance, components of this system are occasionally found on prescriptions. The *avoirdupois system* is the common system of commerce, employed along with the SI in the United States. It is through this system that items are purchased and sold by the ounce and pound. This appendix defines these common systems, expresses their quantitative relationship to one another and to the SI, and provides the means for intersystem conversion. Conversion of temperature between the Fahrenheit and Celsius (or centigrade) scales, and alcohol conversion of proof strength are also included in this appendix.

APOTHECARIES' FLUID MEASURE

60 minims (m)	= 1 fluidrachm or fluidram (f$\mathfrak{z}$ or $\mathfrak{z}$)[a]
8 fluidrachms (480 minims)	= 1 fluid ounce (f$\breve{\mathfrak{z}}$ or $\breve{\mathfrak{z}}$)[a]
16 fluid ounces	= 1 pint (pt)
2 pints (32 fluid ounces)	= 1 quart (qt)
4 quarts (8 pints)	= 1 gallon (gal)

This table may also be written:

gal	pt	Pt	f$\breve{\mathfrak{z}}$	f$\mathfrak{z}$	m
1	4	8	128	1,024	61,440
	1	2	32	256	15,360
		1	16	128	7,680
			1	8	480
				1	60

---

[a]When it is clear that a liquid is to be measured, the *f* may be omitted in this symbol.

APOTHECARIES' MEASURE OF WEIGHT

20 grains (gr)	= 1 scruple ($\ni$)
3 scruples (60 grains)	= 1 drachm or dram ($\mathfrak{z}$)
8 drachms (480 grains)	= 1 ounce ($\breve{\mathfrak{z}}$)
12 ounces (5760 grains)	= 1 pound (℔)

This table may also be written:

℔	$\breve{\mathfrak{z}}$	$\mathfrak{z}$	$\ni$	gr
1	12	96	288	5760
	1	8	24	480
		1	3	60
			1	20

A typical set of Apothecaries' weights consists of the following units:

$\breve{\mathfrak{z}}$ii	$\breve{\mathfrak{z}}$I $\breve{\mathfrak{z}}$ss	$\mathfrak{z}$ii $\mathfrak{z}$i	$\mathfrak{z}$ss $\ni$ii	$\ni$i	$\ni$ss
5 grain,	4 grain,	3 grain,	2 grain,	1 grain,	½ grain

AVOIRDUPOIS MEASURE OF WEIGHT

437½ or 437.5 grain (gr)	= 1 ounce (oz)
16 ounces (7000 grains)	= 1 pound (lb)

This table may also be written:

lb	oz	gr
1	16	7000
	1	437.5

FUNDAMENTAL OPERATIONS AND CALCULATIONS

Only one denomination has a value common to the apothecaries' and avoirdupois systems of measuring weight: the grain. The other denominations bearing the same name have different values.

Bulk or stock packages of powdered drugs and chemicals (and occasionally some liquids when they are sold by weight) are customarily provided to the pharmacist in avoirdupois units of weight by manufacturers and wholesalers. The pharmacist likewise sells bulk packages of non-prescription drug and chemical items by the avoirdupois system.

In contrast with the invariable use of *simple* quantities in the metric system, measurements in the common systems are recorded whenever possible in *compound quantities* (i.e., quantities expressed in two or more denominations). So, 20 f℥ maybe used during the process of calculating but, as a final result, it should be recorded as 1 pt 4 f℥. The process of reducing a quantity to a compound quantity beginning with the highest possible denomination is called *simplification*. Decimal fractions may be used in calculation, but the subdivision of a minim or a grain in a final result is recorded as a *common fraction*.

In days gone by, when prescriptions were written in the apothecaries' system, the following format was used, with Roman numerals placed after the abbreviations or symbols for the denominations.

Codeine sulfate	gr iv
Ammonium chloride	℥ iss
Cherry syrup ad	f℥
Sig. ℥i as directed.	

Example Calculations in the Apothecaries' System

Usually, before a compound quantity can be used in a calculation, it must be expressed in terms of a single denomination. To do so, each denomination in the compound quantity must be reduced to the required denomination and the results added.

Reduce ℥ss ℥ii Ɔi to grains.

$$℥ss = ½ × 480 \text{ gr} = \quad 240 \quad gr$$
$$℥ii = 2 \ × \ 60 \text{ gr} = \quad 120 \quad gr$$
$$Ɔi = 1 \ × \ 20 \text{ gr} = \quad \underline{20} \quad gr$$
$$380 \text{ gr, } answer.$$

Reduce f℥iv f℥iiss to fluidrachms.

$$f℥iv = 4 × 8 \text{ f℥} \quad = \quad 32 \quad f℥$$
$$f℥iiss \quad\quad = \quad \underline{2½} \ f℥$$
$$34½ \text{ f℥, } answer.$$

Before being weighed, a given quantity should be expressed in denominations equal to the actual weights on hand. Before a volume is measured, a given quantity should be expressed in denominations represented by the calibrations on the graduate.

Change 165 gr to weighable apothecaries' units.

By selecting larger weight units to account for as many of the required grains as possible, beginning with the largest, we find that we may use following weights:

℥ii, ℥ss, Ɔss, 5 gr, *answer.*

$$Check: \quad\quad ℥ii = \quad 120 \quad gr$$
$$℥ss = \quad 30 \quad gr$$
$$Ɔss = \quad 10 \quad gr$$
$$5 \text{ gr} = \quad \underline{5} \quad gr$$
$$165 \text{ gr, } total.$$

In enlarging a formula, we are to measure 90 f℥ of a liquid. Using two graduates, if necessary, in what denominations may we measure this quantity?

11 f℥ and 2 f℥, *answer.*

$$Check: \quad\quad 11 \text{ f℥} = \quad 88 \quad f℥$$
$$2 \text{ f℥} = \quad \underline{2} \ f℥$$
$$90 \text{ f℥, } total.$$

Addition or Subtraction

To add or subtract quantities in the common systems, reduce to a common denomination, add or subtract, and reduce the result (unless it is to be used in further calculations) to a compound quantity.

A formula contains Ɔii of ingredient A, ℥i of ingredient B, ℥iv of ingredient C, and gr viss of ingredient D. Calculate the total weight of the ingredients.

$$Ɔii = 2 × 20 \text{ gr} = \quad 40 \quad gr$$
$$℥i = 1 × 60 \text{ gr} = \quad 60 \quad gr$$
$$℥iv = 4 × 60 \text{ gr} = \quad 240 \quad gr$$
$$\text{gr viss} \quad\quad = \quad \underline{7½} \quad gr$$
$$347½ \text{ gr} = 5 \ ℥ \ 2 \ Ɔ \ 7½ \text{ gr, } answer.$$

A pharmacist had 1 gal of alcohol. At different times, he dispensed f℥iv, 2 pt, f℥viii, and f℥iv. What volume of alcohol was left?

$$f℥iv = \quad 4 \quad f℥$$
$$2 \text{ pt} = 2 × 16 \text{ f℥} = \quad 32 \quad f℥$$
$$f℥viii = \quad 8 \quad f℥$$
$$f℥iv = \quad \underline{½} \quad f℥$$
$$44½ \text{ f℥, } total \ dispensed.$$

$$1 \text{ gal} = \quad 128 \quad f℥$$
$$- \quad \underline{44½} \text{ f℥}$$
$$83½ \text{ f℥} = \text{pt 3 f℥ 4 f℥, } answer.$$

Multiplication and Division

A *simple* quantity may be multiplied or divided by any pure number, such as *12 × 10 oz = 120 oz* or *7 lb 8 oz.*

If, however, *both* terms in division are derived from denominate numbers (as when we express one quantity as a fraction of another), they must be reduced to a *common* denomination before division.

A *compound* quantity is most easily multiplied or divided, and with least chance of careless error, if it is first reduced to a *simple* quantity: $2 \times 8\,f\text{℥}\,6\,f\text{Ʒ} = 2 \times 70\,f\text{Ʒ} = 140\,f\text{Ʒ}$ or $17\,f\text{℥}\,4\,f\text{Ʒ}.$

The *result* of multiplication should be (1) left as it is, if it is to be used in further calculations, (2) simplified, or (3) reduced to weighable or measurable denominations.

A prescription for 24 powders calls for ¼ gr of ingredient A, Ʒss of ingredient B, and gr v of ingredient C in each powder. How much of each ingredient should be used in compounding the prescription?

$$24 \times \tfrac{1}{4}\ \text{gr} = 6\ \text{gr of ingredient A}$$

$$24 \times \tfrac{1}{2}\ \text{Ʒ} = 12\ \text{Ʒ, or } 4\ \text{Ʒ of ingredient B}$$

$$24 \times \text{gr v} = 120\ \text{gr, or } 2\ \text{Ʒ of ingredient C, } answer.$$

How many 15-minim does can be obtained from a mixture containing f℥iii of one ingredient and fƷ of another?

$$\text{f℥iii} = 3 \times 480\ \text{♏} = 1440\ \text{♏}$$

$$\text{fƷii} = 2 \times\ 60\ \text{♏} = \underline{120\ \text{♏}}$$

$$1560\ \text{♏, total.}$$

$$\frac{1560}{15}\ \text{doses} = 104\ \text{doses, } answer.$$

RELATIONSHIP BETWEEN AVOIRDUPOIS AND APOTHECARIES' WEIGHTS

As noted previously, the *grain* is the same in both the avoirdupois and apothecaries' systems of weight, but other denominations with the same names are not equal.

To convert from either system to the other, first reduce the given quantity to grains in the one system, and then reduce to any desired denomination in the other system.

The custom of buying chemicals by avoirdupois weight and compounding prescriptions by apothecaries' weight leads to problems, many of which can be most conveniently solved by proportion.

Example Calculations Involving the Avoirdupois System

Convert ℥ii Ʒii to avoirdupois weight.

$$\text{℥ii} = 2 \times 480\ \text{gr} = 960\ \text{gr}$$

$$\text{Ʒii} = 2 \times\ 60\ \text{gr} = \underline{120\ \text{gr}}$$

$$\text{Total:} \qquad\qquad 1080\ \text{gr}$$

$$1\ \text{oz} = 437.5\ \text{gr}$$

$$\frac{1080}{437.5}\ \text{oz} = 2\ \text{oz, 205 gr, } answer.$$

How many grains of a chemical are left in a 1-oz (avoir) bottle after Ʒvii are dispensed from it?

$$1\ \text{oz} = 1 \times 437.5\ \text{gr} = 437.5\ \text{gr}$$

$$\text{Ʒvii} = 7 \times 60\ \text{gr}\quad = \underline{420.0\ \text{gr}}$$

$$\text{Difference:} \qquad\qquad 17.5\ \text{gr, } answer.$$

If a drug costs $8.75 per oz (avoir), what is the cost of 2 Ʒ?

$$1\ \text{oz} = 437.5\ \text{gr, and } 2\ \text{Ʒ} = 120\ \text{gr}$$

$$\frac{4375.5\ (\text{gr})}{120\ (\text{gr})} = \frac{8.75\ (\$)}{\text{x}\ (\$)}$$

$$\text{x} = \$2.40, answer.$$

INTERSYSTEM CONVERSION

In pharmacy and medicine, the SI currently predominates in use over the common systems. Most prescriptions and medication orders are written in the SI, and labeling on prefabricated pharmaceutical products has drug strengths and dosages described in SI units. Manufacturing formulas are similarly expressed almost exclusively in SI units, replacing use of the common systems of measurement.

On occasion, however, it may be necessary to translate a weight or measurement from units of one system to units of another system. This translation is called *conversion*. The translation of a denomination of one system to that of another system requires a *conversion factor* or *conversion equivalent*.

Table F-1 presents both practical and precise conversion equivalents. In most pharmacy practice applications, the practical equivalents may be used. The precise equivalents show their derivation. *The practical equivalents should be memorized.*

Note that such equivalents may be used in two ways. For example, to convert a number of fluid ounces to milliliters, *multiply* by 29.57; to convert a number of milliliters to fluid ounces, divide by 29.57.

Some individuals prefer to set up a ratio of a known equivalent and solve conversion problems by proportion. For example, in determining the number of milliliters in 8 f℥, an equivalent relating *milliliters to fluid ounces is selected* (1 f℥ = 29.57 mL) and the problem is solved by proportion as follows:

$$\frac{1(\$\$\$)}{8(\$\$\$)} = \frac{29.57\ (\text{mL})}{\text{x}\ (\text{mL})}$$

$$\text{x} = 236.56\ \text{mL, } answer.$$

In using the ratio and proportion method, the equivalent that contains both the units named in the problem is the best one to use. Sometimes, more than one equiva-

TABLE F-1 PRACTICAL AND PRECISE CONVERSION EQUIVALENTS

Unit	Practical Pharmacy Equivalent	Precise Equivalent[a]
Conversion Equivalents of Length		
1 m	39.37 in	39.37008 in
1 in	2.54 cm (exact)	
Conversion Equivalents of Volume		
1 mL	16.23 ℳ	16.23073 ℳ
1 ℳ	0.06 mL	0.06161152 mL
1 f℥	3.69 mL	3.696691 mL
1 f℥	29.57 mL	29.57353 mL
1 pt	473 mL	473.1765 mL
1 gal (U.S.)[b]	3785 mL	3785.412 mL
Conversion Equivalents of Weight		
1 g	15.432 gr	15.43236 gr
1 kg	2.20 lb (avoir)	2.204623 lb (avoir)
1 gr	0.065 g (65 mg)	0.06479891 g
1 oz (avoir)	28.35 g	28.349523125 g
1 ℥	31.1 g	31.1034768 g
1 lb (avoir)	454 g	453.59237 g
1 lb (apoth)	373 g	373.2417216 g
Other Useful Equivalents		
1 oz (avoir)	437.5 gr (exact)	
1 ℥	480 gr (exact)	
1 gal (U.S.)	128 f℥ (exact)	

[a]Precise equivalents from the National Institute of Standards and Technology. http://ts.nist.gov/htdocs/200/2002/mpohome.htm. Accessed September 25, 2008.
[b]The U.S. gallon is specified because the British imperial gallon and other counterpart measures differ substantially, as follows: British imperial gallon, 4545 mL; pint, 568.25 mL; f℥, 28.412 mL; f℥, 3.55 mL; and ℳ, 0.059 mL. Note, however, that the SI is used in both the *United States Pharmacopeia* and *British Pharmacopeia*.

lent may be appropriate. For instance, in converting grams to grains, or vice versa, the gram-to-grain relationship is found in the following basic equivalents, 1 g = 15.432 gr and 1 gr = 0.065 g, as well as in *derived equivalents*, such as 31.1 g = 480 grand 28.35 g = 437.5 gr. It is best to use the basic equivalents when converting from one system to another and to select the equivalent that provides the answer most readily.

In response to the question, *must we round off results so as to contain no more significant figures than are contained in the conversion factor?*, the answer is yes. If we desire greater accuracy, we should use a more accurate conversion factor. But to the question, *If a formula includes the one-figure quantity 5 g, and we convert it to grains, must we round off the result to one significant figure?*, the answer is decidedly no. We should interpret the quantity given in a formula as expressing the precision we are expected to achieve in compounding—usually not less than three-figure accuracy. Hence, 5 g in a formula or prescription should be interpreted as meaning 5.00 g or greater precision.

For prescriptions and all other problems stated in the apothecaries' or avoirdupois systems of measurement, it is recommended that all such quantities be converted to equivalent metric quantities before solving in the usual manner described in this text.

CONVERSION OF LINEAR QUANTITIES

Example Calculations of Linear Conversion

The fiber length of a sample of purified cotton is 6.35 mm. Express the length in inches.

$$6.35 \text{ mm} = 0.635 \text{ cm}$$
$$1 \text{ in} = 2.54 \text{ cm}$$

Solving by proportion:

$$\frac{1 \text{ (in)}}{x \text{ (in)}} = \frac{2.54 \text{ (cm)}}{0.635 \text{ (cm)}}$$

$$x = 0.250 \text{ in, or } \tfrac{1}{4} \text{ in, } answer.$$

Or, solving by dimensional analysis:

$$6.35 \text{ mm} \times \frac{1 \text{ cm}}{10 \text{ mm}} \times \frac{1 \text{ in}}{2.54 \text{ cm}} = 0.250 \text{ in, } answer.$$

A medicinal plaster measures 4½ in. by 6½ in. What are its dimensions in centimeters?

Assuming three-figure precision in the measurement,

4½ or 4.50 × 2.54 cm = 11.4 cm wide,

6½ or 6.50 × 2.54 cm = 16.5 cm long, *answers.*

Rulers are often calibrated in dual scale.

CONVERSION OF LIQUID QUANTITIES

Example Calculations of Fluid Volume Conversions

Convert 0.4 mL to minims.
To achieve two-figure precision,

$$0.40 \times 16.23 \, \text{m} = 6.492 \text{ or } 6.5 \, \text{m, } \textit{answer.}$$

Or, solving by dimensional analysis:

$$0.4 \text{ mL} \times \frac{16.23 <\$\$\$>}{1 \text{ mL}} = 6.492 \text{ or } 6.5 <\$\$\$>, \textit{answer.}$$

Convert 2.5 L to fluid ounces.

$$2.5 \text{ L} = 2500 \text{ mL}$$

Solving by proportion:

$$\frac{1 \, (\text{f} <\$\$\$>)}{\text{x} \, (\text{f} <\$\$\$>)} = \frac{29.57 \, (\text{mL})}{2500 \, (\text{mL})}$$

$$\text{x} = 84.5 \text{ f} <\$\$\$>, \textit{answer.}$$

Or, solving by dimensional analysis:

$$2.5 \text{ L} \times \frac{1000 \text{ mL}}{1 \text{ L}} \times \frac{1 \text{ f} <\$\$\$>}{29.57 \text{ mL}} = 84.5 \text{ f} <\$\$\$>, \textit{answer.}$$

Convert 2½ pt to milliliters.

$$2½ \text{ pt} = 2½ \times 16 \text{ f} \tilde{3} = 40 \text{ f} \tilde{3}$$

$$40 \times 29.57 \text{ mL} = 1182.8 \text{ or } 1180 \text{ mL, } \textit{answer.}$$

Or, solving by dimensional analysis:

$$2½ \text{ pt} \times \frac{16 \text{ f} <\$\$\$>}{1 \text{ pt}} \times \frac{29.57 \text{ mL}}{1 \text{ f} <\$\$\$>} = 11.82.8 \text{ or}$$

$$1180 \text{ mL, } \textit{answer.}$$

CONVERSION OF WEIGHTS

Example Calculations of Weight Conversion

Convert 12.5 g to grains.

$$12.5 \times 15.432 \text{ gr} = 192.9 \text{ or } 193 \text{ gr, } \textit{answer.}$$

Alternate solution (about 0.5% less accurate):

$$\frac{12.5}{0.065} \text{ gr} = 192.3 \text{ or } 192 \text{ gr, } \textit{answer.}$$

Convert 5 mg to grains.
Solving by proportion:

$$\frac{1 \, (\text{gr})}{\text{x} \, (\text{gr})} = \frac{65 \, (\text{mg})}{5 \, (\text{mg})}$$

$$\text{x} = \frac{5}{65} \text{ gr} = \frac{1}{13} \text{ gr, } \textit{answer.}$$

Convert 15 kg to avoirdupois pounds.
Solving by proportion:

$$\frac{1 \, (\text{kg})}{15 \, (\text{kg})} = \frac{2.2 \, (\text{lb})}{\text{x} \, (\text{lb})}$$

$$\text{x} = 33.0 \text{ lb, } \textit{answer.}$$

Convert 6.2 gr to milligrams.

$$6.2 \times 65 \text{ mg} = 403 \text{ or } 400 \text{ mg, } \textit{answer.}$$

Or, solving by dimensional analysis:

$$6.2 \text{ gr} \times \frac{1 \text{ g}}{15.432 \text{ gr}} \times \frac{1000 \text{ mg}}{1 \text{ g}} = 401.8 \text{ or } 400 \text{ mg, } \textit{answer.}$$

Convert 176 avoirdupois pounds to kilograms.

$$\frac{176}{2.2} \text{ kg} = 80.0 \text{ kg, } \textit{answer.}$$

CONVERSION OF TEMPERATURES

In 1709, the German scientist Gabriel Fahrenheit discovered that according to the scale he had marked on a thermometer, ice melted at 32° and water boiled at 212°, a difference of 180 degrees. In 1742, Anders Celsius, a Swedish astronomer, suggested the convenience of a thermometer with a scale having a difference of 100° between two fixed points, with 0° for the freezing point and 100° for the boiling point of water. Thus, the *Fahrenheit* and the *Celsius*, or *centigrade*, thermometers were established.

Because 100 degrees centigrade (°C) measures the same difference in temperature that is measured by 180 degrees Fahrenheit (°F), each degree centigrade is the equivalent of 1.8 or 9/5 the size of each degree Fahrenheit.

There are a number of different arithmetic methods for the conversion of temperatures from the centigrade scale to the Fahrenheit scale and vice versa, as described in an earlier edition of this text.[2] One of these methods, as used in the *United States Pharmacopeia* (*USP*), is described by the following equations. It should be noted that temperatures in the *USP* are expressed in degrees centigrade.[3]

$$°F = \frac{9}{5} °C + 32, \text{ and}$$

$$°C = \frac{5}{9} \times (°F - 32)$$

Example Calculations of Temperature Conversions

Convert 26°C to corresponding degrees Fahrenheit.

$$°F = \frac{9}{5} (26°C) + 32 = 78.8°F, \textit{answer.}$$

Convert 98.6°F to corresponding degrees centigrade.

$$°C = \frac{5}{9} \times (98.6°F - 32) = \times 37°C, \textit{answer.}$$

CLINICAL ASPECTS OF THERMOMETRY

The instrument used to measure body temperature is termed a *clinical* or *fever thermometer*. Traditional clinical thermometers include (1) the *oral thermometer*, slender in the design of stem and bulb reservoir; (2) the *rectal thermometer*, having a blunt, pear-shaped, thick-bulb reservoir for both safety and to ensure retention in the rectum; and (3) a *universal or security thermometer*, which is stubby in design, for both oral and rectal use. In addition, *oral electronic digital fever thermometers* and *infrared emission detection (IRED) ear thermometers* are widely used. The oral electronic digital fever thermometer works by the absorption of heat from the point of body contact. Heat causes the expansion and rise of mercury in the thermometer and the response of the thermocouple. The IRED ear thermometer measures heat radiated from the tympanic membrane without actually touching the membrane.

A recent innovation is a thermometry system of *single-use disposable* clinical thermometers that reduce the risk of passing harmful microorganisms between patients.[4] These disposable thermometers are commercially available in both nonsterile and sterile units. The thermometers use a dot sensor matrix consisting of temperature-sensitive indicating dots. Each dot changes color at a specific temperature relative to the melting point of the specific chemical mixture in the dot. Each dot changes color at a temperature of 0.2°F or 0.1°C higher than the preceding dot. Body temperature is read from a numerical temperature scale. Clinically accurate oral body temperatures are obtained in 60 seconds and axillary temperatures in 3 minutes.

Specialized thermometers include *basal thermometers* and *low-reading thermometers*. The *basal temperature* is the body's normal resting temperature, generally taken immediately on awakening in the morning. In women, body temperature normally rises slightly because of hormonal changes associated with ovulation. Basal thermometers, calibrated in tenths of a degree, are designed to measure these slight changes in temperature. When charted over the course of a month, these changes are useful in assessing optimal times for conception.

Low-reading thermometers are required in diagnosing hypothermia. The standard clinical thermometer reads from 34.4°C (94°F) to 42.2°C (108°F), which is not fully satisfactory for measuring hypothermia, which may involve body temperatures of 35°C (95°F) or lower. A low-reading thermometer registers temperatures between 28.9°C (84°F) and 42.2°C (108°F). Examples of various thermometers are shown in *Figure F-1*.

In the past, the *normal* body temperature for healthy adults was accepted to be 37°C (98.6°F) based on studies

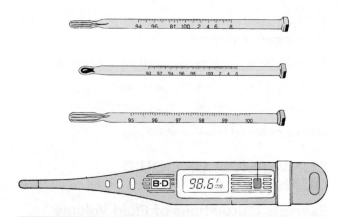

Figure F-1. Examples of various clinical thermometers. From top to bottom: oral fever thermometer, rectal thermometer, basal thermometer, oral digital fever thermometer. (Courtesy of Becton Dickinson and Company.)

performed over a century ago.[5] The use of advanced electronic digital thermometers, however, has shown that normal adult temperature may vary widely between individuals (from 96.3°F to 99.9°F in one study).[6] Lowest body temperatures generally occur in the early morning and peak high temperatures in the late afternoon, with an average diurnal variation of approximately 0.9°F.

Pharmaceutical Aspects of Temperature

Temperature control is an important consideration in the manufacture, shipping, and storage of pharmaceutical products. Excessive temperature can result in chemical or physical instability of a therapeutic agent or its dosage form. For this reason, the labeling of pharmaceutical products contains information on the appropriate temperature range under which the product should be maintained. The *United States Pharmacopeia* provides the following definitions for the storage of pharmaceuticals.[7]

> *Freezer* – between −25°C and −10°C (−13°F and 14°F)
>
> *Cold* – not exceeding 8°C (46°F)
>
> *Refrigerator* – between 2°C and 8°C (36°F and 46°F)
>
> *Cool* – between 8°C and 15°C (46°F and 59°F)
>
> *Warm* – between 30°C and 40°C (86°F and 104°F)
>
> *Excessive Heat* – above 40°C (104°F)
>
> *Controlled Room Temperature* – between 20°C and 25°C (68°F and 77°F)

ALCOHOL PROOF STRENGTH CONVERSIONS

Alcohol is commonly employed in the small- and large-scale manufacturing of pharmaceuticals. There are special terms associated with alcohol that require understanding for correct interpretation and conversion.

Proof spirit is an aqueous solution containing 50% v/v of *absolute alcohol* (100% v/v ethyl alcohol). Alcohols of other percentage strengths are said to be *above proof* or *below proof*, depending on whether they contain more or less than 50% v/v of absolute alcohol.

Proof strength is twice the percentage strength of alcohol and thus 50% v/v alcohol is 100 proof. In reverse then, alcohol that is 90 proof is equivalent to 45% v/v alcohol.

Alcohol for manufacturing use may be purchased by the *proof gallon*. A proof gallon is a gallon by measure of proof spirit; that is, a gallon of 100 proof or 50% v/v absolute alcohol.

Example Calculations Involving Proof Strength and Proof Gallons

To calculate the number of proof gallons contained in a given quantity of alcohol of specified strength, observe the following. Because a proof gallon has a percentage strength of 50% (v/v), the equivalent number of proof gallons may be calculated by the formula:

$$\text{Proof gallons} = \frac{\text{gallons} \times \text{Percentage strength of solution}}{50\ (\%)}$$

Because proof strength is twice percentage strength, the formula may be revised as follows:

$$\text{Proof gallons} = \frac{\text{gallons} \times \text{Proof strength of solution}}{100\ (\text{proof})}$$

How many proof gallons are contained in 5 gal of 75% v/v alcohol?

First method:
1 proof gallon = 1 gallon of 50% v/v strength

$$\frac{5\ (\text{gallons}) \times 75\ (\%)}{50\ (\%)} = 7.5 \text{ proof gallons, } answer.$$

Second method:
75% v/v = 150 proof

$$\frac{5\ (\text{gallons}) \times 150\ (\text{proof})}{100\ (\text{proof})} = 7.5 \text{ proof gallons, } answer.$$

To calculate the number of gallons of alcohol of specified strength equivalent to a given number of proof gallons, observe the following:

$$\text{gallons} = \frac{\text{Proof gallons} \times 50\ (\%)}{\text{Percentage strength of solution}}$$

or,

$$\text{gallons} = \frac{\text{Proof gallons} \times 100\ (\text{proof})}{\text{Proof strength of solution}}$$

How many gallons of 20% v/v alcohol would be the equivalent of 20 proof gallons?

First method:
1 proof gallon = 1 wine gallon of 50% v/v strength

$$\frac{20\ (\text{proof gallons}) \times 50\ (\%)}{20\ (\%)} = 50 \text{ gal, } answer.$$

Second method:
20% v/v = 40 proof

$$\frac{20\ (\text{proof gallons}) \times 100\ (\text{proof})}{40\ (\text{proof})} = 50 \text{ gal, } answer.$$

To calculate the tax on a given quantity of alcohol of a specified strength, observe the following:

If the tax on alcohol is quoted at $13.50 per proof gallon, how much tax would be collected on 10 gal of alcohol marked 190 proof?

$$\frac{10\ (\text{gallons}) \times 190\ (\text{proof})}{100\ (\text{proof})} = 19 \text{ proof gallons}$$

$13.50 \times 19\ (\text{proof gallons}) = \$256.50, answer.$

Note: When specific equations, as those described above, are difficult to recall, it is always an option to perform calculations in a stepwise and logical fashion. Although a greater number of steps may be required, the outcome is worth the time.

For example, in the above-stated problem, "How many proof gallons are contained in 5 gal of 75% v/v alcohol?" If one worked logically on the basis of the amount of absolute alcohol in 5 gal of 75% v/v alcohol, the answer to the problem may be deduced as follows:

$$5 \text{ gal} \times 75\% \text{ v/v} = 3.75 \text{ gal of absolute alcohol}$$
$$(100\% \text{ v/v})$$

then, it follows that

$$3.75 \text{ gal of absolute alcohol} \times 2 =$$
$$7.5 \text{ proof gallons, } answer.$$

The student may wish to work the same problem in terms of milliliters (3785 mL/gallon) to arrive at the same answer.

Practice Problems

Calculations of the Avoirdupois and Apothecaries' Systems

1. Reduce each of the following quantities to grains:

    (A) ℨii ℈iss.
    (B) ℥ii ℨiss.
    (C) ℥i ℨss ℈i.
    (D) ℨi ℈i gr x.

2. Reduce 1 pt, f℥ii to fluidrachms.

3. Reduce each of the following quantities to weighable apothecaries' denominations:

    (A) 158 gr
    (B) 175 gr
    (C) 210 gr
    (D) 75 gr
    (E) 96 gr

4. How many f℥ii bottles of cough syrup can be obtained from 5 gal of the cough syrup?

5. Low-dose aspirin tablets contain 1¼ gr of aspirin in each tablet. How many tablets can be prepared from 1 avoirdupois pound of aspirin?

6. How many 1/400-gr tablets of nitroglycerin can a manufacturer prepare from a quantity of a trituration of nitroglycerin that contains ⅛ oz of the drug?

Intersystem Conversion Calculations

7. A brand of nitroglycerin transdermal patch measures 2.5 in. in diameter. Express this dimension in centimeters.

8. Urethral suppositories are traditionally prepared to the following lengths: 50 mm for women and 125 mm for men. Convert these dimensions to inches.

9. A pharmacist received a prescription calling for 30 capsules, each to contain 1/200 gr of nitroglycerin. How many 0.4-mg nitroglycerin tablets would supply the amount required?

10. If a physician prescribed 4 g of aspirin to be taken by a patient daily, about how many 5-gr tablets should the patient take each day?

11. <$$$> Codeine Sulfate 30 mg
    Acetaminophen 325 mg
    M. ft. cap. D.T.D. no. 24
    Sig. One capsule tid for pain.

    How many grains each of codeine sulfate and acetaminophen would be contained in the prescription?

12. If a child accidentally swallowed 2 f℥ of Feosol Elixir, containing ⅔ gr of ferrous sulfate per 5 mL, how many milligrams of ferrous sulfate did the child ingest?

13. Sustained-release tablets of nitroglycerin contain the following amounts of drug: 1/25 gr, 1/10 gr, and 1/50 gr. Express these quantities as milligrams.

14. A physician advises an adult patient to take a children's tablet (81 mg of aspirin per tablet) daily as a precaution against a heart attack. Instead, the patient decides to cut 5-gr aspirin tablets into dosage units. How many doses could be obtained from each 5-gr tablet?

15. A hematinic tablet contains 525 mg of ferrous sulfate, which is equivalent to 105 mg of elemental iron. How many grains each of ferrous sulfate and elemental iron would a patient receive from one tablet?

16. The usual dose of colchicine for an acute gout attack is 1/120 gr every hour for 8 doses. How many milligrams of colchicine are represented in the usual dose?

17. If f℥i of a cough syrup contains 10 gr of sodium citrate, how many milligrams are contained in 5 mL?

18. A formula for a cough syrup contains ⅛ gr of codeine phosphate per teaspoonful (5 mL). How many grams of codeine phosphate should be used in preparing 1 pt of the cough syrup?

19. A drug substance has been shown to be embryotoxic in rats at doses of 50 mg/kg/day. Express the dose on the basis of micrograms per pound per day.

20. Tetracycline has been shown to form a calcium complex in bone-forming tissue in infants given oral tetracycline in doses of 0.011 g/lb of body weight every 6 hours. Express the dose in terms of milligrams per kilogram of body weight.

Temperature Conversions

21. Convert the following from centigrade to Fahrenheit:

  (A) 10°C
  (B) −30°C
  (C) 4°C
  (D) −173°C

22. Convert the following from Fahrenheit to centigrade:

  (A) 77°F
  (B) 240°F
  (C) 98.9°F
  (D) 227.1°F

23. A patient's rectal temperature reading is frequently 1°F higher than the oral temperature reading. Express this difference in degrees centigrade.

24. A woman charting her basal temperature finds that her body temperature on day 14 is 97.7°F and on day 18 is 98.6°F. Express this temperature range and the difference in degrees centigrade.

Proof Strength Conversions

25. If the tax on alcohol is $13.50 per proof gallon, how much tax must be paid on 5 gal of alcohol, *USP*, which contains 94.9% v/v of pure alcohol?

26. On the first of the month, a hospital pharmacist had on hand a drum containing 54 gal of 95% alcohol. During the month, the following amounts were used:

  • 10 gal in the manufacture of bathing lotion
  • 20 gal in the manufacture of medicated alcohol
  • 5 gal in the manufacture of soap solution

How many proof gallons of alcohol were on hand at the end of the month?

Answer to Practice Problems

1. (A) 150 gr
   (B) 1050 gr
   (C) 530 gr
   (D) 90 gr

2. 144 f ʒ

3. (A) 2 ʒ ½ ʒ 8 gr, or 2 ʒ 1 ϶ ½ ϶ 8 gr

   (B) 2 ʒ 2 ϶ ½ ϶ 5 gr, or 2 ʒ ½ ʒ 1 ϶ 5 gr

   (C) 2 ʒ 1 ʒ 1 ϶ ½ ϶, or 3 ʒ 1 ϶ ½ ϶

   (D) 1 ʒ ½ ϶ 5 gr

   (E) 1 ʒ ½ ʒ 6 gr, or 1 ʒ 1 ϶ ½ ϶ 6 gr.

4. 320 tablets

5. 5600 tablets

6. 21,875 tablets

7. 6.35 cm

8. 1.97 in, 4.92 in

9. 24.4 or 25 tablets

10. 12 tablets

11. 11 7/100 or 11.08 gr of codeine sulfate 120 gr of acetaminophen

12. 512.55 mg

13. 2.6 mg (1/25 gr)
   6.5 mg (1/10 gr)
   1.3 mg (1/50 gr)

14. 4 doses

15. 8 7/100 or 8.08 gr of ferrous sulfate
   1 62/100 or 1 3/5 or 1.62 gr of elemental iron

16. 0.54 mg

17. 109.9 mg

18. 0.769 g

19. 22,727 μg/lb/day

20. 24.2 mg/kg

21. (A) 50°F
    (B) −22°F
    (C) 39.2°F
    (D) −279.4°F

22. (A) 25°C
    (B) 115.6°C
    (C) 37.2°C
    (D) 108.4°C

23. 0.56°C

24. 36.5° to 37°C
    0.5°C

25. $128.12

26. 361.1 proof gallons

REFERENCES

1. *United States Pharmacopeia,* 31st Rev. National Formulary 26. Rockville, MD: United States Pharmacopeial Convention; 2008;1:13.

2. Ansel HC, Stoklosa MJ. *Pharmaceutical Calculations.* 11th ed. Baltimore, MD: Lippincott Williams & Wilkins; 2001:299–304.

3. *United States Pharmacopeia,* 31st Rev. National Formulary 26. Rockville, MD: United States Pharmacopeial Convention; 2008;1:8, 905–906.

4. 3M. Tempa-DOT Thermometer. http://www.3m.com/Product/information/Tempa-DOT-Thermometer.html. Accessed January 11, 2008.

5. Wunderlich CR, Sequin E. *Medical Thermometry and Human Temperature.* New York, NY: William Wood; 1871.

6. Mackowiak PA, Wasserman SS, Levine MM. A critical appraisal of 98.6°F, the upper limit of the normal body temperature and other legacies of Carl Reinhold Wunderlich. *JAMA.* 1992;268:1578.

7. *The United States Pharmacopeia,* 31st Rev. National Formulary 26. Rockville, MD: The United States Pharmacopeial Convention; 2008;1:10.

Glossary of Pharmaceutical Dosage Forms and Drug Delivery Systems*

AEROSOLS

Pharmaceutical aerosols are products packaged under pressure that contain therapeutically active ingredients that are released as a fine mist, spray, or foam on actuation of the valve assembly. Some aerosol emissions are intended to be inhaled deep into the lungs (*inhalation aerosol*), whereas others are intended for topical application to the skin or to mucous membranes. Aerosols with metered valve assemblies permit a specific quantity of emission for dosage regulation.

AROMATIC WATERS

Aromatic waters are clear, saturated solutions of volatile oils or other aromatic substances in water. They are used orally, topically, or pharmaceutically for the characteristics of the aromatic material they contain.

BOLUSES

Boluses are large elongated tablets intended for administration to animals.

CAPSULES

Capsules are solid dosage forms in which one or more medicinal and/or inert substances are enclosed within small shells of gelatin. Capsule shells are produced in varying sizes, shapes, color, and hardness. *Hard-shell* capsules, which have two telescoping parts, are used in the manufacture of most commercial capsule products and in the extemporaneous filling of prescriptions. They are filled with powder mixtures or granules.

Soft-shell gelatin capsules are formed, filled, and sealed in a continuous process by specialized large-scale equipment. They may be filled with powders, semisolids, or liquids.

Capsules contain a specific quantity of fill, with the capsule size selected to accommodate that quantity. In addition to their medication content, capsules usually contain inert substances, such as fillers. When swallowed, the gelatin capsule shell is dissolved by gastrointestinal fluids, releasing the contents.

Delayed-release capsules are prepared in such a manner as to resist the release of the contents until the capsules have passed through the stomach and into the intestines.

Extended-release capsules are prepared in such a manner as to release the medication from the capsules over an extended period following ingestion.

CREAMS

Creams are semisolid preparations containing one or more drug substances dissolved or dispersed in a suitable base. Many creams are either oil-in-water emulsions or aqueous microcrystalline dispersions in a water-washable base. Compared to ointments, creams are easier to spread and remove. Creams are used for administering drugs to the skin and, to a lesser extent, to mucous membranes.

DRUG DELIVERY SYSTEMS

Drug delivery systems are physical carriers used to deliver medications to site-specific areas. They include transdermal, ocular, and intrauterine systems.

Transdermal drug delivery systems support the passage of drug substances from the surface of the skin, through its various layers, and into the systemic circulation. These systems are sophisticated skin patches containing a drug formulation within a reservoir for the controlled delivery of drug.

Ocular drug delivery systems consist of drug-impregnated membranes that, when placed in the lower conjunctival sac, release medication over an extended period.

Intrauterine drug delivery systems consist of a drug-containing intrauterine device that releases medication over an extended period after insertion into the uterus.

ELIXIRS

Elixirs are sweetened, flavored, hydroalcoholic solutions intended for oral administration. They may be medicated or nonmedicated. Compared to syrups, elixirs are usually less

---

*Some portions of this Glossary have been abstracted from the *United States Pharmacopeia 31—National Formulary 26*. Copyright 2008, United States Pharmacopeial Convention, Inc. Permission granted.

sweet and less viscous because they contain a lesser amount of sugar. Because of their hydroalcoholic character, elixirs are better able than are syrups to maintain both water-soluble and alcohol-soluble components in solution.

EMULSIONS

An emulsion is a type of dispersal system in which one liquid is dispersed throughout another liquid in the form of fine droplets. The two liquids, generally an oil and water, are immiscible and constitute two phases that would separate into layers without the presence of a third agent, an *emulsifier* or *emulsifying agent*. The latter facilitates the emulsification process and provides physical stability to the system.

If oil is the internal phase, then the emulsion is termed an oil-in-water, or o/w, emulsion. If water is the internal phase, then the emulsion is termed a water-in-oil, or w/o, emulsion. The type of emulsion produced is largely determined by the emulsifying agent, with hydrophilic agents generally producing oil-in-water emulsions and lipophilic agents generally producing water-in-oil emulsions. Emulsifying agents may have both hydrophilic and lipophilic characteristics, hence the term hydrophilic-lipophilic balance (HLB).

Depending on their formulation, emulsions may be administered orally, topically, or by intravenous injection.

EXTRACTS

Extracts are concentrated preparations of vegetable or animal drugs prepared by extracting the constituents from the natural source and drying the extractive to the desired pilular or powdered form.

FLUID EXTRACTS

Fluid extracts are liquid extractives of vegetable drugs generally prepared such that 1 mL represents the active constituents from 1 g of the vegetable drug.

GELS

Gels are semisolid systems consisting of either suspensions of small inorganic particles or large organic molecules interpenetrated by a liquid.

IMPLANTS OR PELLETS

Implants or pellets are small, sterile, solid dosage forms containing a concentrated drug for subcutaneous implantation in the body where they continuously release their medication over prolonged periods.

INHALATIONS

Inhalations are finely powdered drug substances, solutions, or suspensions of drug substances administered by the nasal or oral respiratory route for local or systemic effects. Special devices are used to facilitate their administration.

INJECTIONS

Injections are sterile preparations intended for parenteral administration by needle or pressure syringe. Drugs may be injected into most any vessel or tissue of the body, but the most common routes are intravenous (IV), intramuscular (IM), and subcutaneous (SC). Injections may be solutions or suspensions of a drug substance in an aqueous or nonaqueous vehicle. They may be small-volume injections, packaged in ampules for single-dose administration, or vials for multiple-dose injections. Large-volume parenterals, containing 100 mL to 1 L of fluid, are intended for the slow intravenous administration (or infusion) of medications and/or nutrients in the institutional or home care setting.

IRRIGATIONS

Irrigations are sterile solutions intended to bathe or flush open wounds or body cavities. They are not intended for injection.

LINIMENTS

Liniments are alcoholic or oleaginous solutions, suspensions, or emulsions of medicinal agents intended for external application to the skin, generally by rubbing.

LOTIONS

Lotions are liquid preparations intended for external application to the skin. They are generally suspensions or emulsions of dispersed solid or liquid materials in an aqueous vehicle. Their fluidity allows rapid and uniform application over a wide skin surface. Lotions are intended to soften the skin and leave a thin coat of their components on the skin's surface as they dry.

LOZENGES

Lozenges are solid preparations containing one or more medicinal agents in a flavored, sweetened base intended to dissolve or disintegrate slowly in the mouth, releasing medication generally for localized effects.

MAGMAS

Magmas are pharmaceutical suspensions of fine particles that, because of a high degree of physical attraction to the aqueous vehicle, form a gelatinous mixture. This characteristic maintains the uniformity and stability of the suspension. Magmas are administered orally.

OINTMENTS

Ointments are semisolid preparations intended for topical application to the skin, eye, ear, or various mucous membranes. With some exceptions, ointments are applied for their local effects on the tissue membrane rather than for systemic effects. *Ophthalmic ointments* are sterile preparations intended for application to the eye.

Nonmedicated ointments serve as vehicles, or as *ointment bases*, in the preparation of medicated ointments. Because ointments are semisolid preparations, they are prepared and dispensed on a weight basis.

PASTES

Pastes are semisolid dosage forms that contain one or more drug substances intended for topical application to the skin. Generally, pastes contain a higher proportion of solid materials than do ointments and thus are more stiff, less greasy, and more absorptive of serous secretions.

PLASTERS

Plasters are solid or semisolid adhesive masses spread across a suitable backing material and intended for external application to a part of the body for protection or for the medicinal benefit of added agents.

POWDERS

Powders are dry mixtures of finely divided medicinal and nonmedicinal agents intended for internal or external use. Powders may be dispensed in bulk form, or they may be divided into single-dosage units and packaged in folded papers or unit-of-use envelopes.

PREMIXES

Premixes are mixtures of one or more drug substances with suitable vehicles intended for admixture to animal feedstuffs before administration. They are generally in powdered, pelletized, or granulated form.

SOLUTIONS

Solutions are liquid preparations that contain one or more chemical substances (*solutes*) dissolved in a solvent or mixture of solvents. The most common solvent used in pharmaceuticals is water; however, alcohol, glycerin, and propylene glycol also are widely used as solvents or cosolvents.

Depending on their purpose, solutions are formulated and labeled for use by various routes, including oral, topical, ophthalmic, otic, nasal, rectal, urethral, and parenteral. The concentration of active ingredients in solutions varies widely depending on the nature of the therapeutic agent and its intended use. The concentration of a given solution may be expressed in molar strength, milliequivalent strength, percentage strength, ratio strength, milligrams per milliliter, or another expression describing the amount of active ingredient per unit of volume.

SPIRITS

Spirits are alcoholic or hydroalcoholic solutions of volatile substances. Depending on their contents, some spirits are used orally for medicinal purposes and others as flavoring agents.

SUPPOSITORIES

Suppositories are solid dosage forms intended for insertion into body orifices. They are used rectally, vaginally, and, occasionally, urethrally. Suppositories are of various weights, sizes, and shapes, depending on their intended use. Various types of *suppository bases* are used as vehicles for the medication, including cocoa butter (theobroma oil), glycerinated gelatin, polyethylene glycols, hydrogenated vegetable oils, and fatty acid esters of polyethylene glycol. Depending on the base used, the suppository either softens, melts, or dissolves after insertion, releasing its medication for the intended local action or for absorption and systemic effects.

SUSPENSIONS

Suspensions are preparations containing finely divided, undissolved drug particles dispersed throughout a liquid vehicle. Because the drug particles are not dissolved, suspensions assume a degree of opacity depending on the concentration and size of the suspended particles. Because particles tend to settle when left standing, suspensions should be shaken to redistribute any settled particles before use to ensure uniform dosing. Depending on their formulation, suspensions are administered orally, by intramuscular injection, and topically to the eye.

SYRUPS

Syrups are concentrated aqueous solutions of a sugar or sugar substitute. Syrups may be medicated or nonmedicated. *Nonmedicated syrups* are used as vehicles for medicinal substances to be added later, either in the extemporaneous compounding of prescriptions or in the preparation of a formula for a medicated syrup. In addition to the sugar or sweetener, syrups also contain flavoring agents, colorants, cosolvents, and antimicrobial preservatives to prevent microbial growth. Syrups are administered orally for the therapeutic value of the medicinal agent(s).

TABLETS

Tablets are solid dosage forms containing one or more medicinal substances. Most tablets also contain added pharmaceutical ingredients, as diluents, disintegrants, colorants, binders, solubilizers, and coatings. Tablets may be coated for appearance, for stability, to mask the taste of the medication, or to provide controlled drug release. Most tablets are manufactured on an industrial scale by compression, using highly sophisticated machinery. Punches and dies of various shapes and sizes enable the preparation of a wide variety of tablets of distinctive shapes, sizes, and surface markings.

Most tablets are intended to be swallowed whole. However, some are prepared to be chewable, others to be dissolved in the mouth (*buccal tablets*) or under the tongue (*sublingual tablets*), and still others to be dissolved in water before taking (*effervescent tablets*). Tablets are formulated to contain a specific quantity of medication. To enable flexibility in dosing, manufacturers commonly make available various tablet strengths of a given medication. Some tablets are scored, or grooved, to permit breaking into portions that the patient can take.

TINCTURES

Tinctures are alcoholic or hydroalcoholic solutions of either pure chemical substances or of plant extractives. Most chemical tinctures are applied topically (e.g., iodine tincture). Plant extractives are used for their content of active pharmacologic agents.

TABLE G.1 ROUTES OF DRUG ADMINISTRATION AND PRIMARY DOSAGE FORMS AND DRUG DELIVERY SYSTEMS

Route	Site	Dosage Forms/Drug Delivery Systems
Oral	Mouth	Tablets, capsules, oral solutions, drops, syrups, elixirs, suspensions, magmas, gels, powders, troches, and lozenges (oral cavity)
Sublingual	Under the tongue	Tablets
Parenteral		Solutions, suspensions
Intravenous	Vein	
Intra-arterial	Artery	
Intracardiac	Heart	
Intraspinal/Intrathecal	Spine	
Intraosseous	Bone	
Intra-articular	Joint	
Intrasynovial	Joint fluid	
Intracutaneous/ Intradermal/ Subcutaneous	Skin	
Intramuscular	Muscle	
Epicutaneous	Skin surface	Ointments, creams, pastes, plasters, powders, aerosols, lotions, transdermal patches, solutions (topical)
Conjunctival	Eye conjunctiva	Ointments
Intraocular	Eye	Solutions, suspensions
Intranasal	Nose	Solutions, ointments
Aural	Ear	Solutions and suspensions (drops)
Intrarespiratory	Lung	Solutions (aerosols)
Recta	Rectum	Solutions, ointments, suppositories
Vaginal	Vagina	Solutions, ointments, emulsion foams, gels, tablets/inserts
Urethral	Urethra	Solutions and suppositories